the
kind
mama

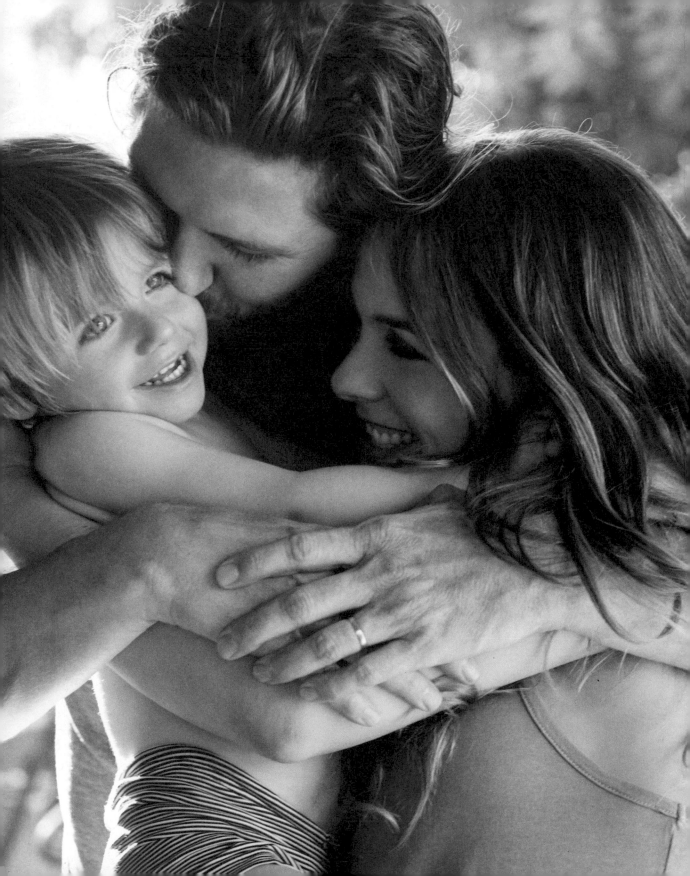

the
kind
mama

A Simple Guide to Supercharged Fertility,
a Radiant Pregnancy, a Sweeter Birth,
and a Healthier, More Beautiful Beginning

alicia silverstone

Photography by Amy Neunsinger

RODALE

Rodale books may be purchased for business or promotional use or for special sales.
For information, please write to:
Special Markets Department, Rodale Inc., 733 Third Avenue, New York, NY 10017.

Printed in the United States of America

Rodale Inc. makes every effort to use acid-free ♾, recycled paper ♻.

Book design by Kara Plikaitis

Photographs by Amy Neunsinger

Additional photographs by Anamaria Brandt (pages 169, 172, 198),
Claire Weiss (pages 86, 136, 153, 155), and Stephanie Todaro (page 289)

Library of Congress Cataloging-in-Publication Data is on file with the publisher.

ISBN-13: 978–1–62336–040–5 paperback

Distributed to the trade by Macmillan

2   4   6   8   10   9   7   5   3   1   paperback

We inspire and enable people to improve their lives and the world around them.
rodalebooks.com

For Bear Blu
and all the babies yet to come into this world

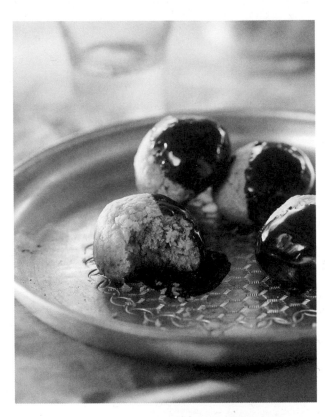
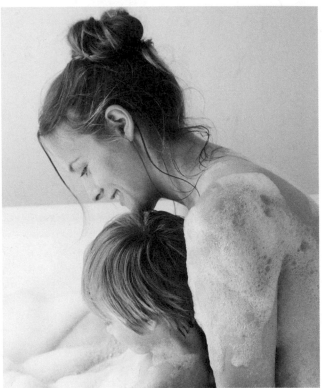
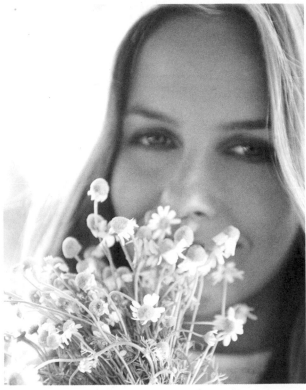
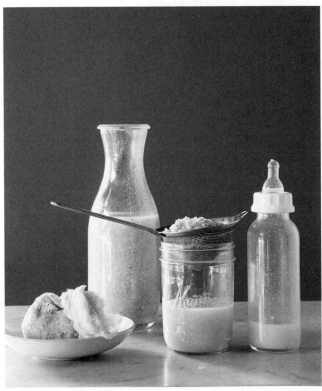

Contents

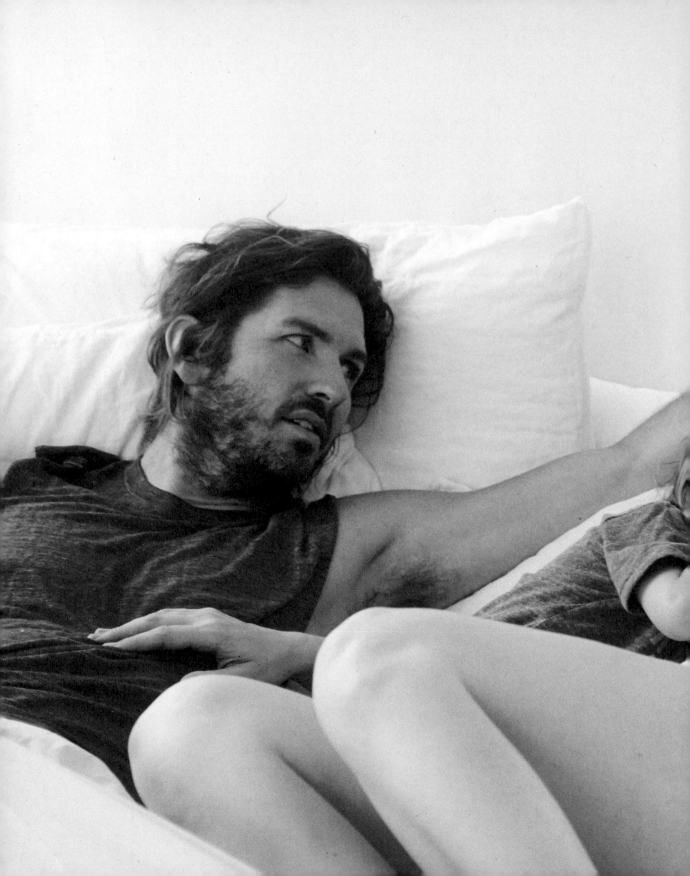

Hello, babies. Welcome to Earth. It's hot in the summer and cold in the winter. It's wet and round and crowded. At the outside, babies, you've got about a hundred years here. There's only one rule that I know of, babies—"God damn it, you've got to be kind."

–Kurt Vonnegut

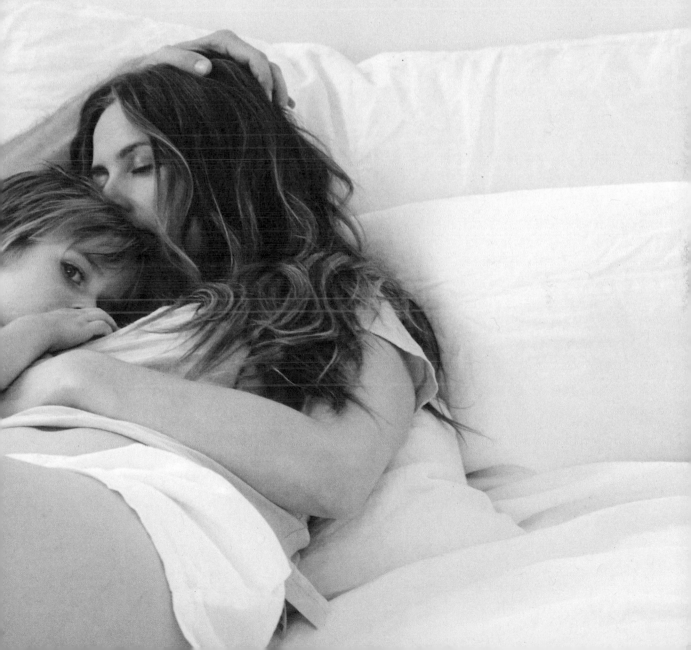

Foreword

Over the last couple of years, I've had conversations with Alicia Silverstone about pregnancy, birth, breastfeeding, and nutrition and I love her point of view on these topics—so I happily accepted her request to write this foreword. Frankly, I thought I would skim the manuscript to meet my deadline—it being my office's busy season, though there aren't a lot of *un*busy seasons in pediatrics—and then I started reading . . . and couldn't stop. And found I had no urge to skim or to skip chapters.

Not only do you need this book but *I* needed this book.

The Kind Mama is a unique positive statement about how wonderfully well prebirth, pregnancy, birth, and child raising can be experienced.

The American Academy of Pediatrics has accepted my dues for 30 years and I have remained a member in good standing for all that time. By that, I don't mean to suggest that I have won awards from them, or that I'd win a pediatricians' popularity contest for my opinions on breastfeeding, the family bed, childhood nutrition, or other matters. They do a pretty good job advocating for the members of the Academy—us pediatricians—but I have found that they are often lacking in strong advocacy for breastfeeding and other crucial children's health issues.

I have also worked for 30 years with doctors of the American College of Obstetrics and Gynecology. These docs have delivered most of the babies I've cared for throughout my career, although I have seen hundreds of babies born at home, too. Obstetricians may someday return to an evidence-based and research-based model for the practice of obstetrics and childbirth, but right now the C-section rate in America hovers around 33 percent. This is a huge increase from the less than 5 percent cesarean deliveries 50 years ago. Just consider that the World Health Organization (WHO) has suggested that for the best health of mothers, the Caesarean section rate should be about 10 to 15 percent.

By the way, this large number of surgical deliveries does not promote safer pregnancy outcomes: In 2010 the WHO's official report on cesarean sections was published in the world's most highly respected journal, *The Lancet*, and one of the study's authors, Dr. A. Metin Gülmezoglu, said, "The relative safety of the operation leads people to think it's as safe as vaginal birth. That's unlikely to be the case." The WHO Study also pointed to increased ICU admissions, transfusion, and later complications for women who underwent operative delivery that was not medically indicated. Other medical research has shown that babies delivered via C-section have more respiratory issues immediately following birth.

According to the Centers for Disease Control, the United States ranked 50th in the world in rates of maternal death and 32nd in infant mortality. We earn this distinction in a nation that operated on one-third of pregnant women in 2013 and puts more babies in newborn intensive care units than any other country on the planet.

Mothers and fathers need to inform themselves before birth about hospital procedures and how to keep your newborn safe, unmedicated, and close to you. *The Kind Mama* offers the newest and best information I've ever seen. It covers everything from the natural approach to treating postpartum depression to babies' varying poop schedules.

Carry this book with you when you interview pediatricians, who should be honored to care for your conscious, healthy, new family. And later, take *The Kind Mama* to each doctor's visit. Vegan and vegetarian doctors are hard to find, so *The Kind Mama's* nutritional guidance is a godsend to those of us who skip burgers, fries, and chocolate cereal in favor of fruits, vegetables, and beans and want to feed our babies and children that way, too. (To give you a feeling for the American Academy of Pediatrics' approach to feeding moms and babies, please know that for years the chairwoman of the AAP's Committee on Nutrition was also a paid consultant for the American Cattlemen's Beef Association. You can imagine her opinion and her influence on the agency.)

The Kind Mama can help you create a nontoxic life for yourself before, during, and after delivery. Your best friends won't be offended by your shower invitation or birth announcement telling them you respectfully request no plastic toys as gifts. In fact, they'll be grateful for the insight—and the guidance.

Thank you, Alicia, for saving my babies and their parents.

Jay Gordon, MD, FAAP
January 20, 2014

Introduction

I Promise There's a Better Way

When did making babies become so *hard*?

First there are the drugs and injections just to get pregnant; then what seems like the inevitable 9 months of being a bloated, hormonal bitch; topped off by a hectic delivery under bright lights while strapped to beeping machines. Not to mention the impending doom of having to deal with a screaming baby while feeling sick, tired, and helpless. Whatever happened to starting with sweet baby-making love, enjoying 9 months of glowing fertility-goddess joy, then giving birth with confidence and raising a baby with clarity? Well, listen up, ladies: It *can* be that way. Did you hear what I said?! Having a super-healthy, super-vibrant, soul-satisfying pregnancy, birth, and mamahood is a complete and total reality.

Whether you believe in God, the Divine Spirit, or Mother Nature, this fact remains the same: We have been blessed with everything we need to carry, birth, and care for a child. Full stop. What you and I are going to do is unlock this amazing potential. If you're having trouble conceiving, I'll do my best to get you knocked up. If you're just starting to think about getting pregnant, we'll talk about how to just let it flow—no crazy planning or calendar tracking required. If you're already expecting—and have maybe hit a couple of bumps in the road—then I'll show you the way to have a luminous, present, ailment-free pregnancy. And just when you think it can't get any more gooey and delicious than having that little one in your belly, we'll talk about how to get that scrumptious light of a baby into this world in the most gentle, beautiful way.

Oh, and while we're at it, we're going to help prevent or even cure your PMS, irregular periods, high blood pressure, insomnia, allergies, breakouts, weight struggles, thyroid condition, lupus, and multiple sclerosis—while significantly lowering your risk of heart disease, diabetes, and cancer. We'll boost your immune system and unclutter your mind. You'll have more energy, sleep better at night, maintain an ideal weight, and exude a glow that's more than just hormonal frenzy. You'll be able to listen to what your body really needs and then relax into the yumminess of it all.

This is not a book about the day-to-day affairs of your uterus. This book is a recipe for how to have a pregnancy, birth, and ever after free of fear, anxiety, and all the not-fun things that everyone says are unavoidable. I was inspired to follow this path because I watched some of my friends being pregnant, then birthing and raising their kids beautifully and easily and naturally. The choices I made regarding raising my own son, Bear Blu, came from witnessing the difference between their way and the "normal" way that didn't feel so right to me.

I'll share with you my choices and the choices that many women around the world are making so that you can find the path that feels best for you. This book will be a guiding hand to offer another way. I recommend you read this book all the way through first—then you can refer to each section as need be. Believe me, it's a lot easier to set your intentions for a beautiful mama-hood *before* the baby is born. In these pages, we'll talk about all the things you might have been told—whether from friends, doctors, or family members—and why there may be better alterna-tives. We'll help you create the best protective shield for fragile new life while tapping into your most grounded self. You'll connect more deeply with your own needs, which means you'll be more receptive to your baby's. You'll have a lot of questions along the way, and I'm here to help. But nature's already provided the answers. All you have to do is get kind, tap in, and receive the gifts of the incredible road ahead.

Now, let's go make a baby!

With love,

Alicia

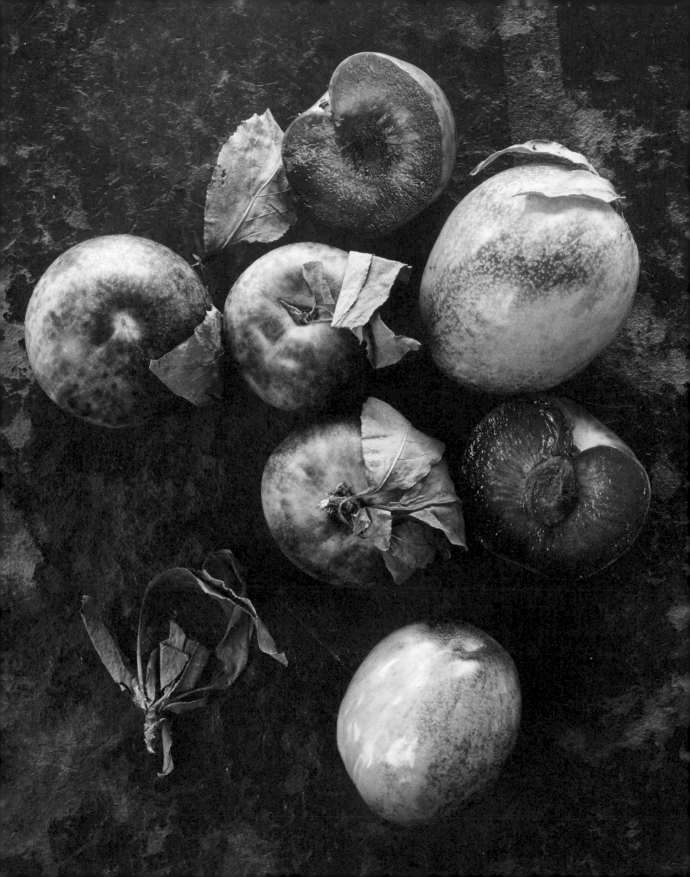

PART I

preparing your baby house:

Getting Your Body Ready for a
Beautiful Pregnancy and Birth

I

Becoming a Kind Mama

Before we dive in, I'd first like to talk to all those ladies out there having trouble in the baby department. If it's been a struggle getting pregnant, let's focus on how we can turn what might feel like a curse into a blessing. I know that might be the last thing you want to hear after what may have been months or years of stressing about things like ovulation and endometrial lining, but if you're still fertility challenged, then something has to change, right? Think of all the people who go through their entire lives never knowing what's keeping them from reaching their full, glorious potential. Now you have the opportunity to feel your best, get happy, become centered, and try to do this nature's way. It's a gentler, easier, and certainly more fun path to becoming the mama you were meant to be.

Now, to all the pregos out there: Listen up. Believe me when I say that I hear you when you lament the aches and pains and tribulations of being pregnant. I know what almost everyone is telling you—that this time in your life will be a constant battle between you and your seemingly out-of-control body. But a radiant, buoyant, nourished, stress-free pregnancy is within your grasp. And we are going to get you there.

And guess what, everyone? The secret to a blissed-out pregnancy and mamahood is the same for all of you. It doesn't matter whether you are trying to get pregnant or have already conceived, are expecting your first baby or your fourth, or are giving birth in 9 months or 9 days—you are all on same journey, and it's what I call becoming a Kind Mama.

We usually think of kindness in terms of how we treat others, and while that is always important, the kindness I'm calling for is—first and foremost—toward yourself. It's not about being selfish; it's about realizing that honoring your own wants and needs is the sweetest thing you can do. Because when you're happy and healthy, it's easier to be the best version of you. And most important, it's how we're going to bring your baby into the world in a healthier, happier way.

Being a Kind Mama is not only the key to building the ideal place for your baby to thrive and grow but also the secret to having a soulful, sexy pregnancy that's liberated from digestive issues, bloating, swollen feet, insomnia, and all the other yucky things we think come automatically with carrying a small person inside of us. You'll be protecting both you and your baby from a wide range of diseases as well as from pollutants and toxic influences that can cause nasty long-term effects. If your journey has been difficult up until now, then you'll finally be able to shed all that manic energy surrounding baby making. You'll be on your way toward having a pregnancy that's magical and delightful—the kind that makes you envy other pregnant women after you've given birth because you can't wait to do it all over again.

The good habits that you start here will make your journey through parenthood that much smoother. They'll set you up to channel your inner-warrior strength for labor; heal more quickly after birth; make the most ambrosial breast milk elixir; bond more deeply with your baby; and set a healthy, wise example for your child. Sure, you'll face challenging moments, but you'll be able to glide right through them. Have I gotten less sleep in the past 2 years than I'd like? *Definitely*. Do I sometimes leave the house in yesterday's pajamas? Often. But has being a Kind Mama been the most delicious, world-rocking undertaking in my time on this planet so far? Without a doubt.

Regardless of where you are in this adventure, know that from this moment forward, you have a choice—you can *choose* whether to feel amazing or to just be getting by. Take this opportunity to set the bar for how you want to live the rest of your life. I promise you'll come out the other side feeling more incredible than you ever thought possible.

What you'll find in the pages of this book is the wisdom I've taken to heart on my own path to Kind Mamahood. It's a precious and potent stew of advice that comes from some of the smartest obstetricians, gurus, midwives, pediatricians, experts, healers, and friends I've been lucky enough to know. I've sifted through pages and pages of research, read stacks of books, looped in readers of my blog, and asked experts question after question to confirm what I know in the depth of my soul to be right. Clearly, it was too much to ask for one easy-to-follow resource that was as inspiring as it was informative! Believe me, if it were out there, I wouldn't be writing it now—I'd be handing out a copy to everyone I know. So instead, I started thinking about all the amazing information and insight I was lucky enough to have at my fingertips. I thought about it during checkups, while out for walks, when figuring out how to stick it to ridiculous naysayers—I was even thinking about this book during labor! Now I get to pass it all on to you. So let's get started!

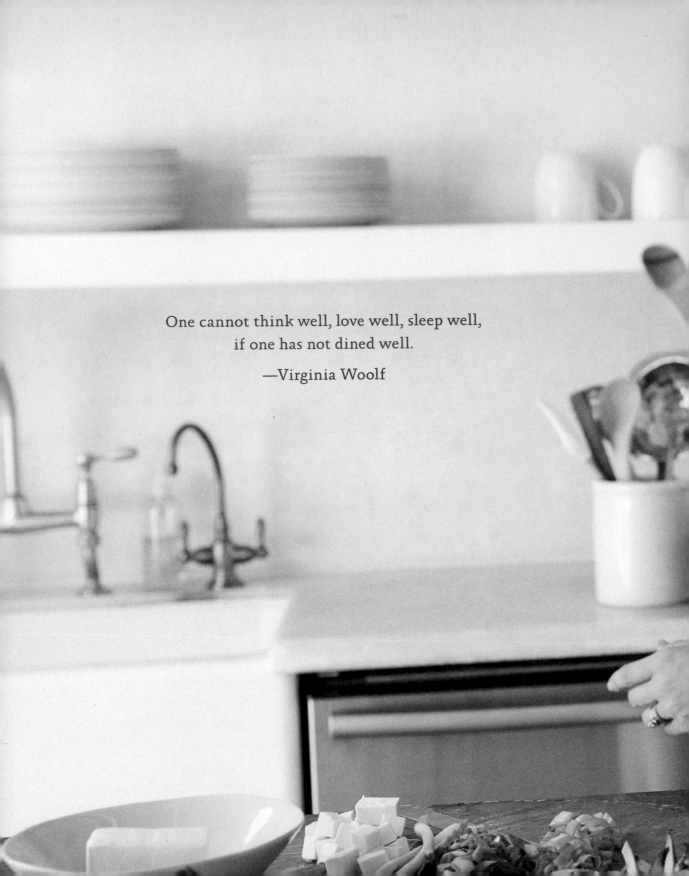

One cannot think well, love well, sleep well,
if one has not dined well.

—Virginia Woolf

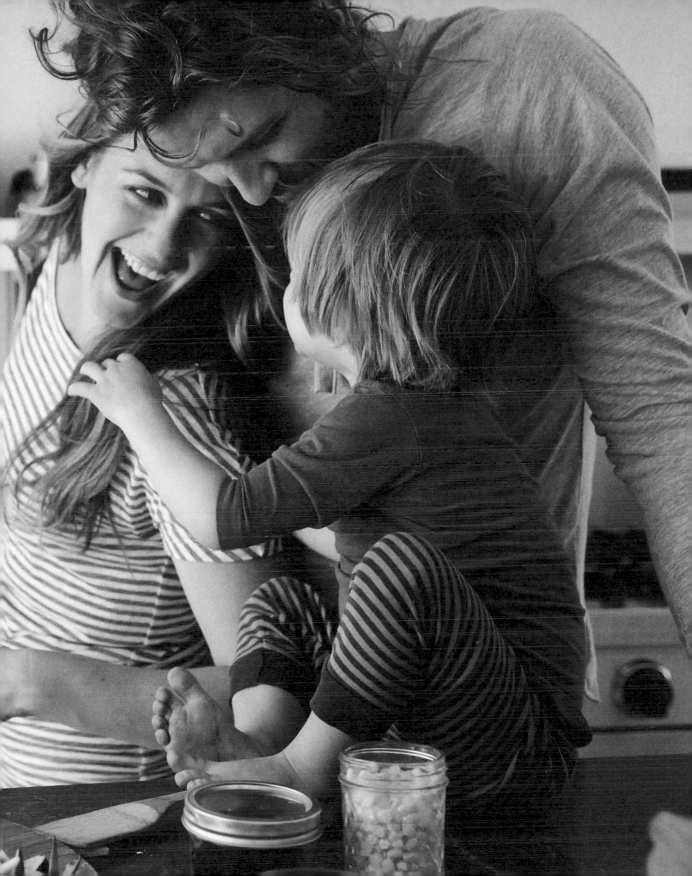

2

Let's Get You Pregnant

Your baby house is the special part of you that will shelter and nourish your baby for the first 9 months of his or her life. You can think of it as your uterus, sure, but it's more than that. It includes your organs, intestines, veins, heart, blood, bones, and tissues, too. Because your body is like a little machine. All the parts work *together* to get you pregnant. They work *together* to keep you healthy. And the most genius thing of all is that this machine knows how to fix itself when something's broken. That's what's so brilliant—your body *wants* to be healthy! When you're sleeping at night and your parts are resting, that little machine is working to make new blood cells, repair your organs and tissues, and otherwise hit "refresh" on the whole operation.

The one catch, though, is that it can use only the materials you give it to make those repairs. So if you're indulging in not-so-healthy habits, then your body is working overtime to keep that outside nastiness from doing harm to the rest of you. And that means basic upkeep starts to fall by the wayside. Soon your skin isn't clearing up the way it used to, your poop is all backed up, your menstrual cycle is all over the place, your allergy flare-ups are worse, your aches and pains are more persistent, and so goes the list. If you're having trouble conceiving, then your body most likely isn't getting what it needs—or is getting too much of what it doesn't—and it's taking it out on your baby house. But if you give your body the nourishing, restorative resources it needs to repair and rebuild, then it can do what it does best: heal!

Your baby house needs maintenance, too. When you're pregnant, it's like your body becomes a walking, talking baby condo. You wouldn't want to bring your baby into a junk-filled house with a leaky roof and backed-up plumbing, right? Chances are your baby is on the same page. As obstetrician-gynecologist Tracy Gaudet, MD, said in an interview with *US News and World Report*, "Sometimes the body's refusal to get pregnant can be a sign of its wisdom." She explained that if you're overweight, for example, you're at an increased risk for pregnancy complications like high blood pressure, diabetes, and an abnormally large baby. So it might not be a coincidence that all the estrogen that's made by excess body fat messes with ovulation.[1] And as Randine Lewis, PhD, who is a healer and fertility expert and the author of *The Way of the Fertile Soul,* sums it up, "Nature knows when you are in harmony with yourself and your environment. When animals in the wild are stressed and deprived, they don't go into heat. Nature knows this is incompatible with life. When humans go through the same, we frantically go to a doctor to see if they can 'fix it.' They can't; only you can."

Just because you don't take medication every day doesn't mean you're well. I hate to burst your bubble, but needing coffee and soda for a pick-me-up, aspirin for that nagging headache, antacids to wash down lunch, and another pill to fall asleep isn't the picture of health. When I was backstage at a daytime TV show to talk about my first book, *The Kind Diet,* I got to watch while the segment before mine finished taping. It featured a woman who couldn't get pregnant and was clearly at the end of her rope. For 20 minutes, the panel of experts rattled off a long list of all the tests she could undergo to get to the bottom of her infertility. But consider this: She was overweight and a smoker. This woman was clearly sick! Her baby house couldn't have been in any shape to support a growing baby. There she was, facing what some might consider the oracles of medicine—an obstetrics specialist, a pediatrician, a surgeon, and a physician—and yet it took *20 minutes* for someone to tell her to stop smoking and clean up her diet.

Now, don't get me wrong—I'm fully aware that there are plenty of women out there who are popping out babies and basically live on cigarettes, Coca-Cola, and potato chips. Does that mean those babies are healthy and that the mamas are happy and able to embrace the joy and simplicity of total goddess mamahood? I'm not so sure. Plus, the fact remains: If you're having trouble getting pregnant, something's got to give. So let's not keep this magical secret under wraps any longer! It's time to shout from the rooftops what is really the culprit behind your broken-down baby house. It's time to get back in balance. It's time to clean out your baby house.

WHY YOUR BABY HOUSE MIGHT NOT BE REACHING ITS POTENTIAL

According to the Centers for Disease Control and Prevention, the most commonly cited causes of infertility—defined as not getting pregnant after 12 months or more of regular unprotected sex—are being overweight, problems with ovulation and irregular or absent periods, polycystic ovary syndrome (PCOS), endometriosis, uterine fibroids, and pelvic inflammatory disease.[2] In almost every case, the problem is linked to inflammation and/or hormonal imbalance,[3] which can be caused by diet. A number of mucky culprits are at work: animal fats, dairy, sugar, and toxic chemicals. These foods may increase your estrogen levels,[4] which then can throw off your menstrual cycle.[5] They cause inflammation *and,* especially in the case of animal fats, carry nasty toxic chemicals that increase your risk for endometriosis and hormonal imbalance issues.[6] (Don't worry, we'll explore all of this in *much* more detail in just a bit!)

We aren't talking about consuming these foods in excess either. Harvard Medical School's Nurses' Health Study, one of the largest and longest-running investigations of factors that influence women's health, showed that adding just one serving a day of red meat, chicken, or turkey to your diet could increase your risk of infertility by a *third.* In women with the highest intake of animal protein, ovulatory infertility was 39 percent more likely. Animal fats and trans fats— which are often hidden in fast food and most manufactured foods—can even get in the way of ovulation, cause endometriosis, and affect early development of your baby.[7] As for dairy, another study done at Harvard Medical School found a positive correlation between drinking milk and infertility, which only gets worse as you age. But before you think that "old" is a long ways away, consider that the study saw a decline in fertility in subjects as young as 20 to 24.[8]

Plus, our bodies aren't made to have babies forever. It's simply nature at work, the cosmic design made us most fertile in our late teens and twenties. The longer in life we wait to have babies, the less vibrant our machinery becomes, and the more worn down our bodies can get from bad habits. And yet, more and more American women now wait to have their first child until after age 35. But *a third* of the couples in which the woman is older than 35 have fertility problems.[9] While I'm certainly not advocating that you go out and have a baby ASAP, I am advocating that you do everything in your power to get yourself as healthy as possible. I know firsthand how important that is because I had Bear when I was 34 and I definitely plan to have another baby one day.

Here comes the really, really good news: We can change all this! And what's more, it's never too late to get healthy. I've seen so many people transform their lives. So now are you dying to know what the remedy is? The cure-all solution that prepares your body for having a baby, wards off totally unnecessary (and potentially dangerous) pregnancy side effects, costs dramatically less than expensive fertility treatments, and is the key to a balanced, vibrant life for you and your baby? It's as simple as what you *eat.*

What you put in your mouth is one of the biggest factors affecting how your body works and feels. The cleaner, more cell-loving, oxygen-pumping, nutrient-rocking food you put in your body, the better your body can do what you ask of it. Getting pregnant and having a blissful 9 months are no exceptions. But don't just take it from me—or Harvard. Listen to these experts:

WHAT THE DOCS SAY: Katherine Thurer, MD, an integrative gynecologist at the Raby Institute for Integrative Medicine at Northwestern University

> Diet is huge! It has an enormous role in every aspect of our health across the board, and fertility is part of that. Switching to an anti-inflammatory diet is the number one thing I recommend. It can help ovulation-related difficulties and conditions that are inflammatory or estrogen dominant like PCOS, endometriosis, and thyroid problems. Plus, infertility is often something that feels so out of control for a couple, and one element that a woman can control is what she puts in her mouth.

Suzanne Gilberg-Lenz, MD, OB-GYN and clinical Ayurvedic specialist at Women's Care of Beverly Hills

> While there's not much scientific evidence on diet and conception, that may be because there's not a lot of money in it. And that's where I end up having my own personal and professional dilemma, because we live in a world that requires empirical scientific support for everything. . . . But my common sense—and my Ayurvedic guidance—tells me that we are literally what we eat. The truth is that we're constantly changing, which is amazing, but what those cells are being created from is what we consume. So it stands to reason that what we eat has a major influence on how we function.

WHAT THE HEALER SAYS: Diane Avoli, macrobiotic counselor and instructor at the Kushi Institute

> The clogging up of the reproductive system seems to be one of the main causes of infertility, and that comes from diet. But we can absolutely turn things around, at any age.

So let's go make room for that tiny special guest and, while we're at it, get you feeling better than you ever have in your life.

The Octomomification of America: The Scary Truth about Fertility Drugs

We've found ourselves in a baby crisis. Married women in the prime of their childbearing years are having fewer babies than ever, and infertility affects 10 percent or 6.1 *million* women ages 15 to 44 in the United States.[10] That's like the entire state of Missouri not being able to have a baby![11] What's worse, women are being convinced to navigate a scary and expensive maze of no-sure-thing promises—because the truth is there's no money in the recommendation to clean up your diet. Can you imagine a world where doctors got kickbacks from the kale lobby?! There's also not a lot of education about food as medicine. A majority of medical schools still fail to meet the bare-minimum recommendation of 25 hours for nutrition-related instruction.[12] So the best prescription for total wellness just isn't being talked about enough.

The current reality for infertile couples looking to get pregnant goes something like this: Your doctor will most likely first prescribe low-potency fertility pills, which, while good at boosting ovulation, are also great for boosting the chances you'll conceive multiples (more on that in a bit). If that treatment doesn't take, you might move on to intrauterine insemination (IUI), which has a low success rate (only 5 to 20 percent per treatment),[13] though when it does work, it frequently leads to multiples, too.

That leaves in vitro fertilization (IVF).[14] What would ideally happen is your doctor would implant a *single* embryo in your uterus and let your body finish the job of creating a single child. But even though the industry's guidelines encourage the single-embryo approach,[15] many doctors routinely ignore the advice. Instead, many believe that more embryos equals a higher chance of conception, which is great for their success rate and therefore excellent for their bottom line.[16] The only problem is, carrying multiples—of which you now have a 20 to 40 percent chance if you've been implanted with two or more embryos[17]—can lead to a host of risks that affect both your life and the babies'. And that risk gets greater with methods like IUI. Sixty percent of twins are born prematurely, a rate that increases with each additional baby. Premature birth is a risk factor for death in the first few days of life and for problems like bleeding in the brain, eye and ear impairments, developmental delays, and learning disabilities. You run a higher risk for preeclampsia and gestational diabetes with multiples.[18]

Is it impressive that we've achieved the technology to create babies in women who maybe can't get pregnant? Sure. But just how far should we take it? And what if we spent all the time and money it took to create that technology and actually taught people how to get well?

3

Transforming Your Body into a Clean, Mean, Baby-Making Machine

Embracing foods that heal is the ultimate solution for maximizing your baby-making prowess. (It helps, too, that a naturally balanced diet will make you feel sexier than ever!) And once pregnant, you won't need to worry about having the bloated, moody, and otherwise miserable experience that has become the norm. You'll feel more comfortable in your own dewy, delicious skin and be more confident. You'll have more energy, your immune system will work more efficiently, and your body will be better at mending itself after you give birth.

Plus, once you clear away the gunk that's clogging up your body, you unclog your mind as well. You'll be able to tap into your most grounded, truest self, which is so crucial for being a mama. Because when you can tune in to your own needs, you get better at hearing your baby's, too. And a healthy baby is a happy baby.

All of this starts with lovely, wonderful plants—or what I like to call kind food.

These incredible, life-changing, life-*creating* foods are the ultimate baby house–scrubbing task force. Eating a plant-based diet is one of the biggest boosts to your chances of getting pregnant.[19] Plants help balance our hormones, maintain stable blood sugar and pressure, and generally fuel all of our machinery in a cleaner, more efficient way. Eating them means not only boosting the odds of conceiving but also setting the stage for a transcendent pregnancy, a smoother birth, a healthier baby, and long-term protection from almost every disease there is.

Plant-based foods—or kind foods—are nature's way of giving us sun-powered health at its most delicious. There are virtually no nutrients in animal-based foods—including protein and iron—that aren't better provided by plants.[20] Kind foods can supercharge fertility; reduce the likelihood of miscarriage;[21] infuse breast milk with all kinds of nutrient goodness that make your kid smart and healthy; and help stave off diseases like cancer, heart disease, diabetes, osteoporosis, and high blood pressure. Groundbreaking authorities like Drs. T. Colin Campbell, Caldwell B. Esselstyn Jr., and John McDougall have demonstrated that changing your diet to include more kind food and less nasty food (more on this in Chapter 4) can help you live longer, feel younger, lose weight, have more energy, preserve your eyesight, keep your mind sharp, and have a more vibrant sex life. They also assert that it can demolish your need for pharmaceutical drugs, especially for the treatment of things like depression, type 2 diabetes, and hypertension. And because the Food and Drug Administration estimates that 10 percent or more of birth defects result from medications taken during pregnancy—things like prescription painkillers, antidepressants, and thyroid medications[22]—that's a pretty big deal. These doctors agree that eating a diet rich in Mama Earth's little miracles can turn you into a super-healthy clean machine, and isn't that the kind of house you want to build for your baby?

So how exactly are plants going to get you pregnant, keep you healthy, make you feel beautiful, and protect both you and your baby from a huge number of ailments? Check this out:

KIND CAN FIX THE BABY HOUSE

As integrative gynecologist Katherine Thurer, MD, illuminated in the previous chapter, inflammation is at the root of a number of baby house ills. And where inflammation isn't the culprit, hormonal imbalance often is. Well, guess what? Plants have an incredible alkalizing effect on the body, which combats inflammation. And a diet that is high in whole plant foods can help rebalance the body's estrogen levels,[23] since all that super-cleaning fiber helps rid the body of excess substances it doesn't need, including detoxified hormones.[24] Plus, a plant-based diet can help reverse obesity, which has been linked to fertility challenges like high blood pressure and diabetes,[25] in addition to being an effective answer to polycystic ovary syndrome. According to one study published in the *New England Journal of Medicine*, losing as little as 5 percent of your body weight can improve your body's sensitivity to insulin, lower levels of hormones that mess with fertility, and improve menstrual regularity and ovulation.[26] (Check out "Kind's Beauty Bonus" on page 14 to see why that will be easy peasy!) Women who eat the highest amounts of foods rich in lignans, a type of phytoestrogen found in flaxseed and whole grains, have less than half the risk of fibroids compared with women who generally don't eat these foods.[27] And women who have 14 or more servings of vegetables a week have a *70 percent* lower risk of endometriosis compared with those who ate fewer than 6 servings a week.[28]

So let's recap: lower infertility-causing inflammation! Less risk of hormonal imbalance, obesity, and high blood pressure! Less risk of polycystic ovary syndrome, fibroids, and endometriosis! That's what's in store for your baby house when plants are on the menu. Believe me, when you start making some of the scrumptious veggie dishes I've included in this book, you'll see just how delicious a prescription this is. But before we get there, here are a few more reasons why you and plants are about to become best friends.

Mama to Mama on . . . Getting Healthy

My husband and I both lost a significant amount of weight the year before [we started] trying to conceive. We were both unhappy and chronically tired and thought going vegan would make a difference in our health. In 3 days, we noticed an increase in energy. In 2 weeks, I was able to walk around the block, which was previously impossible due to shin and foot pain. Four months later, I was jogging a 3-K and my husband was running. He lost 70 pounds and I lost 50. When it came time to try to get pregnant, it only took us 4 months!

—Kimberly Taylor, Forest Park, Illinois

KIND HAS FIBER POWER

Of all the amazing gifts of plants, fiber is at the top of the list. When we eat plants, it's like sending a scrubbing-bubble task force through our intestines. Because we don't digest most of the fiber we eat, it not only helps move things along from entrance to exit but also sucks up many chemicals and toxins it encounters on its way out. Not getting enough fiber can cause constipation-based disorders like bloating and hemorrhoids and diseases like large bowel cancer.[29] The more fiber you eat, however, the lower risk you have for gestational diabetes,[30] high blood cholesterol, and rectum and colon cancers.

KIND IS YOUR BEST BODYGUARD
AGAINST DISEASE

Plants have the ability to put up a shield whenever they're under attack from potentially dangerous toxins or "free radicals." These shields—made out of a chemical blend called phytochemicals—soak up the invaders and keep them from harming the plants' tissues. As genius as our bodies are, they can't do that on their own. When free radicals, industrial pollutants, or toxins hiding in animal foods (which we'll talk about in the next chapter) enter our system, they wreak serious havoc. They can cause our tissue to start breaking down, which can lead to Alzheimer's and dementia, cataracts, hardening of the arteries, cancer, emphysema, and arthritis. Luckily, though, when we eat plants, they lend us their power to fight evil. And like any superhero team, each plant comes equipped with its own special antioxidant properties, which is why it's crucial to get a variety of colors on your plate.[31]

Kind's Beauty Bonus

When your insides are working like they should to clean and purify your system, your outside shows it. The same phytochemicals that keep you from getting sick also protect your cells from damage and produce more collagen, which is the ultimate in antiwrinkle technology. Whole grains are packed with B-complex vitamins essential for beautiful, glowing skin. And sea vegetables—a Kind Mama's secret weapon—are so rich in minerals and nutrients that they boost circulation and detoxify the body, giving you firmer, more revitalized skin, stronger nails, and glossier hair.

KIND GIVES BABIES A HEALTHIER START

Believe it or not, nature and nurture aren't the only contestants in the how-will-my-baby-turn-out competition. *We* have control over how our babies' genes will express themselves. This idea is currently being studied in a cutting-edge field called epigenetics, which focuses on the environment around the genes.[32] So while we've given our babies our DNA, everything from what we eat to how we act and feel during pregnancy can affect how those genes are expressed. Think about this crazy fact: When women are obese during their first pregnancy, then lose weight before getting pregnant again, the babies born pre–weight loss are heavier than those born afterward. It's because a less healthy mama's body teaches baby's body things like storing more fat and having a slower metabolism.[33] But if we teach a baby's growing body how to be healthy in our bellies, there's a very good chance that baby will continue to flourish and thrive on the outside.[34] A growing amount of evidence suggests that adult diseases and conditions like high blood pressure, obesity, and diabetes are linked to early nutritional influence on the fetus.[35] After all, the organs we grow in utero are the ones we have for life!

> ## Kind's Eco Bonus
> You'll score major karma points from eating plants because eating kind food is about the greenest thing you can do! It requires less fuel, water, and other precious resources than plants' mooing, oinking, clucking, and bleating counterparts.

You know, I'm not the only one who believes in the amazing healing power of plants. Check this out:

- Harvard researchers have proved that eating a diet rich in whole grains, beans, and vegetables can improve ovulation and your chances of getting pregnant.[36]

- A British study showed that women who eat fruits and vegetables daily were 46 percent less likely to miscarry.[37]

- The Academy of Nutrition and Dietetics (formerly the American Dietetic Association) says that a well-rounded vegetarian diet is not only nutritionally adequate for all stages of pregnancy and lactation (not to mention for infancy, childhood, adolescence, adults, and athletes) but also associated with the treatment and prevention of all kinds of diseases. They confirm that we Kind Mamas tend to have lower rates of hypertension, type 2 diabetes, and cancer and lower cholesterol and body mass than our meat-eating counterparts.[38]

- According to Susan Levin, MS, RD, staff dietician with the Physicians Committee for Responsible Medicine, women who follow vegan diets not only have healthy pregnancies but are often *healthier* than moms who consume meat, thanks to eating lower levels of saturated fat and cholesterol and higher levels of fiber, folate, and cancer-fighting antioxidants and phytochemicals.[39]

- Recent studies point out that without consuming whole grains and legumes, the average American cannot obtain enough nutrients from daily food without supplements.[40]

- Studies of vegetarians' breast milk show that the levels of nasty environmental toxins are much lower than in nonvegetarians.[41]

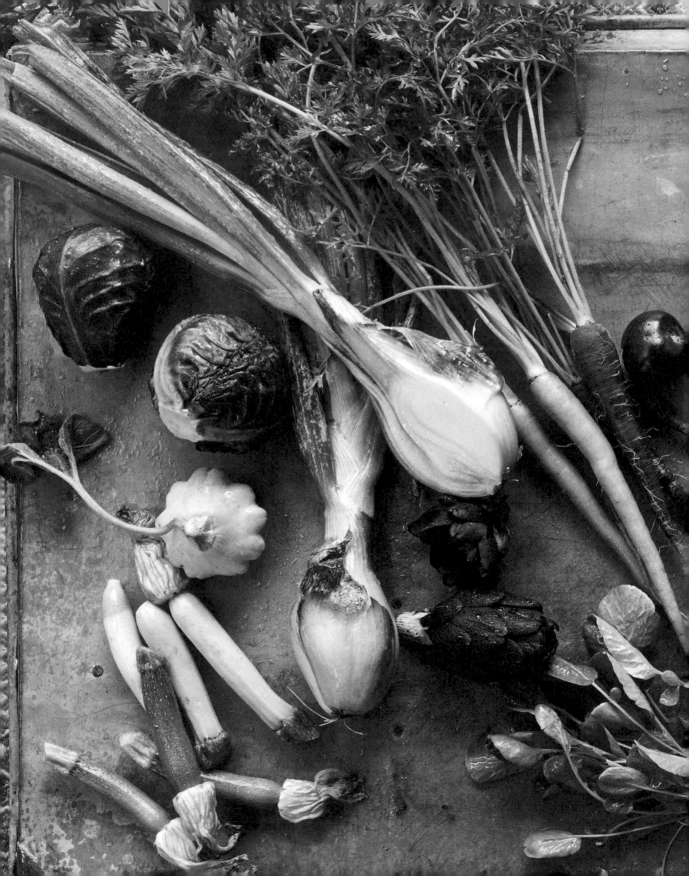

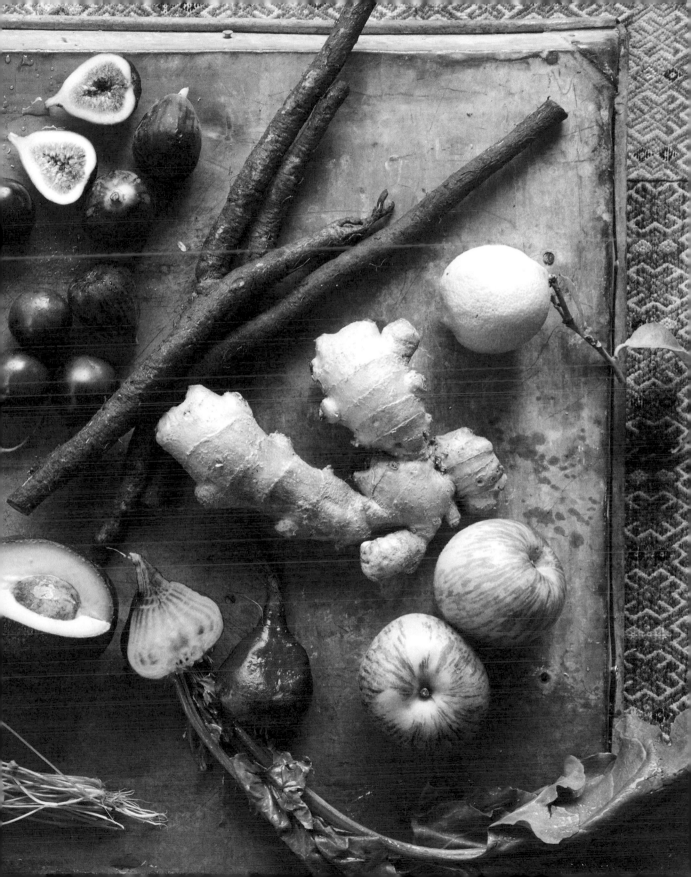

4

Kicking the Nasty Stuff

Kind foods are nature's little miracles. They're the ultimate building blocks for healthy bodies and minds, and they make a huge difference between a pregnant you who unleashes her most radiant self versus one who's swollen, sick, and tired more often than not. Nasty foods, on the other hand, are those that don't do you any favors. They're no good if you're trying to get pregnant, no good if you're already pregnant, and they're no good for your baby.

Most women think of pregnancy as a total departure from normal life, like it's some kind of 9-month-long excuse to wear fat pants. But all those pints of ice cream and pepperoni pizzas will probably come with a side of hemorrhoids, varicose veins, swollen feet, diabetes, and high blood pressure. That's because filling your diet with nasty foods is the quickest way to derail the balance in your body. If your system is busy doing damage control after mealtimes, then it'll be too short staffed to get to the really important stuff like making a cleaner, safer, healthier place for your baby to live.

WHAT'S NASTY?

We've all heard the commandments: Eat meat to be strong! Drink milk for healthy bones! Have fortified cereal and bread for vitamins! But here's the deal: Meat, dairy, and processed foods are tracking toxic sludge through your baby house. They're clogging your arteries, raising your blood pressure, and pumping you full of cholesterol, toxins, hormones, and antibiotics that you don't need. According to the World Health Organization, 80 percent of cardiovascular disease, more than a third of all cancers, and virtually all of the obesity and type 2 diabetes in this country can be linked to a diet high in animal products like meat, dairy, and eggs and in sugar- and fat-laden processed food. These foods increase the acidity in your system, which causes bodywide inflammation. At that point, the body has to borrow minerals like calcium, sodium, potassium, and magnesium from your bones and organs to neutralize the acid. Inflammation also creates the perfect environment for pregnancy complications and other things like obesity, diabetes, cancer, joint pain, fatigue, depression, headaches, immune deficiencies, stroke, osteoporosis, blindness, kidney disease, multiple sclerosis, rheumatoid arthritis, and hyperthyroidism.[42]

NASTY AND YOUR BABY HOUSE

Your placenta, which transfers nutrients and oxygen from you to your little one, isn't a magical filter. It can't make the distinction between harmful and helpful. So long as a particle is the right size to fit through the placenta's front door, it's in for good. That means that all the foul nasties we're about to discuss (like toxic chemicals)—in addition to things like saturated and trans fats, which we'll also get to—can potentially make the cut.[43] Plus, health conditions that are majorly attributed to nasty foods can take an enormous toll on how well you nourish your baby. Heart disease, which is the number one killer of women in the United States, is linked to high amounts of saturated fat in animal products. But sat fat isn't just blocking up the arteries around your heart, it's gunking up *all* your arteries, including the ones that are responsible for bringing fresh, healthy blood to your placenta. Meanwhile, hypertension and diabetes can cause your placenta to calcify and harden, which limits the organ's capabilities. So instead of having a four-lane highway delivering nutrients and immunity to the growing fetus, you might only have an unpaved, single-lane backcountry road.[44] Even though there are skeptics who question the link between saturated fat and these diseases, the overwhelming amount of evidence-based research supporting what makes saturated fat so nasty is why the American Heart Association, the Academy of Nutrition and Dietetics, and the US Departments of Health and Human Services and Agriculture's *Dietary Guidelines for Americans* continue to suggest limiting your intake.[45]

Nasty Food #1: Meat

As a highly evolved and generally sophisticated species, we sport a lengthy intestinal tract to give our bodies more time to break down fiber and absorb all the good stuff from our food. Unlike true carnivores (think big jungle cats with huge pointy teeth), whose short intestinal tracts allow for much faster input–output, when we humans eat meat, it gets to spend time on the 98.6°F lazy river of our insides—up to 72 hours, to be exact. And what's it doing in those 72 hours? It's rotting.[46] That's 3 days that a decomposing piece of flesh is sharing a bunk bed with your baby! Yes, it's being dealt with by your digestive system, but while that meat is taking days and days to break down, it's leaching a noxious cocktail of hormones, antibiotics, pesticides, pollutants, bacteria, and viruses into your body. Animals—us included—are really good at storing some of this muck in their body fat,[47] so it'll only continue to sit and fester once it's been digested.

If you don't eat meat, here's what you're actually saying "no thanks" to:

- **Extra hormones:** The FDA and USDA allow factory farmers to use hormones to promote growth and milk production in their cattle. Two-thirds of all cattle raised for slaughter in the United States are regularly treated with natural and synthetic forms of estrogen and progesterone and other hormones that have been linked to colon and breast cancer in humans.[48] When cows are given these hormones, their fertility drops and their rates of mastitis, an infection of the milk ducts, go up (as does their need for antibiotics, which I'll get to next).[49] When researchers tested fish living downstream from a Nebraska feedlot where hormones were used on livestock, they discovered significant reproductive problems.[50] It's no wonder the European Union banned the import of most American meat from animals treated with hormones![51] The scary side effects go up the food chain, too: Researchers at the University of Rochester found that the more beef a pregnant woman consumed—organic or factory-farmed—the less sperm her sons would go on to produce as adults.[52] While organically raised cows aren't being jacked up on extra hormones, they still have significant levels in their tissues because, like us, it's part of how their bodies work.[53] So you're still getting an extra dose that's (a) more than you need, and (b) meant for a cow.

- **Antibiotic overdose:** Because factory livestock farms are really just huge expanses of crowded animals knee-deep in their own waste, which naturally predisposes them to illness and infection, farmers mix low doses of antibiotics into the feed and water. This isn't just a few random cows we're talking about. Eighty percent of all the antibiotics sold in the United States aren't used on people—they're being used on animals! Cows, chickens, pigs, and other animals raised on conventional farms are often fed these (usually) unnecessary meds to prevent disease in crowded and unsanitary conditions,[54] which are then passed down to you undercover in that nice, juicy steak/chicken breast/pork chop. (Although the FDA recently issued recommendations to curb farmers from using the drugs to boost growth, compliance is voluntary.) Pumping our animals and ourselves full of these drugs makes bacteria resistant to antibiotics,[55] meaning it could be harder to treat both you and your baby if you were to get truly sick.[56]

- **Toxic pesticides:** To ward off insects, kill weeds, and protect their bottom line, conventional farmers spray their crops with a potent mix of pesticides and fertilizers. What does this have to do with meat? Think about what all those cows, pigs, and chickens are eating—grain! While we can sometimes rinse these pesticides off our produce—or buy organic, which is free of synthetic pesticides—animals don't have the same luxury. Most of them are eating the corn, soybeans, wheat, and hay that have gotten the royal nasty treatment, which all ends up on your dinner plate.

- **Dangerous pollutants:** An even more troubling aspect of eating meat is the issue of persistent organic pollutants (POPs)—environmental chemicals from things like industrial processes, pharmaceuticals, and pesticides that have soaked into our soil and water supply. Even organically raised, free range animals lucky enough to graze are munching on grass that may have trace amounts of POPs. It's nasty for them, and it's especially nasty for you, since POPs bioaccumulate. So the more an animal eats over time, the more that animal will have in its body. And the pollutants accumulate as you go up the food chain. That's why meat eaters have much higher levels of these chemicals in their bodies than vegetarians do.[57] Eighty-nine percent of our POP intake comes from meat sources, and when pregnant women are exposed, it can increase the risk of their children having heart defects, delayed cognitive development, behavioral issues, reproductive difficulties, and lower IQ scores.[58]

    Then there's the particularly nasty POP called dioxins (the by-product of some manufacturing processes like herbicide production and paper bleaching). They are classified by the EPA as a serious public health threat and a Group 1 carcinogen, and they make it into our mouths by clinging to animal fats.[59] A May 2001 study found that a person eating a typical American diet will receive 93 percent of his or her dioxin exposure from meat and dairy products, including fish and eggs.[60] Even relatively low levels of exposure have been linked to reproductive and developmental problems, including decreased fertility, reduced sperm count, diabetes, learning disabilities, immune system suppression, and lung problems. The only way dioxins leave a woman's system is through the placenta—and into a growing fetus—or through breast milk.[61]

- **Viruses and bacteria:** According to the USDA, meat is the cause of 70 percent of foodborne illnesses in the United States because it's often contaminated with bacteria like E. coli, listeria, and campylobacter.[62] This is because feedlot cows are fed a grain-based diet instead of the grass-based one they're built for, and this creates more potentially hazardous bacteria in their intestines.[63] Add to that the potential for sloppy slaughtering, which causes these contaminated intestinal contents to splash across the meat. And if you thought turkey was a nice, lean meat alternative, consider this: A recent lab analysis conducted by Consumer Reports found that more than *half* of ground turkey sold in supermarkets is contaminated with fecal bacteria. That means poop, people! And some samples also had germs like salmonella and *Staphylococcus aureus,* two of the leading causes of foodborne illness in the United States.[64] Instead of cracking down on feedlot and slaughterhouse practices, the FDA approved the spraying of live viruses with ammonia and other detoxifiers onto poultry and meat products to kill some of these bacteria. What's even nastier? Meat companies don't have to tell you which products have been treated.[65]

- **Chronic conditions and fatal diseases:** Meat—both factory-farmed and organic—is loaded with saturated fat, which you read about on page 19. It's really bad for your baby house and for the rest of you, too. Eating meat contributes to high blood pressure and heart disease, cancer, osteoporosis, and digestive conditions such as colitis and diverticulitis.

What Would Cavemen Do?

Every time I hear "But aren't we *supposed* to eat meat?" I can confidently answer: Nope! We weren't built for it. According to biologists and anthropologists who know far more about this than I do, humans are and always have been herbivores.[66] Remember when we talked about the jungle cats and their pointy teeth and short intestinal tracts? Compare those maws to our stubby little molars. Not exactly cut out for shredding a water buffalo, right? It's true that early man did eat meat, but it was only to survive in periods when plant foods weren't available.[67] Regardless, that didn't exactly turn on the carnivore instinct. Think about it: When you see fuzzy little lambs or doe-eyed cows, is your first thought to go for the jugular?

Some people—especially those who support the "Paleo" diet—love to say that we started getting sick when we left our nomadic tendencies behind, settled down, and started growing and eating mostly grain. But according to the Physicians Committee for Responsible Medicine, DNA tests show that humans who lived during the Paleolithic era did consume grains and legumes, and they also conclude that many hunter-gatherer tribes were less healthy than we are today, especially because of infections related to eating raw meat! Until recently, only the wealthiest people could afford to feed, raise, and slaughter animals for meat, and the poor folk ate mostly plants. In fact, prior to the 20th century, it was only the rich who were afflicted with things like heart disease and obesity.[68] And they didn't care because it was a sign of their wealth. Gout was cool! I'd argue that's not the case anymore.

FISH ISN'T MUCH BETTER

Most fish have become too toxic to be a part of any diet—let alone a kind diet—regardless of whether or not you're pregnant. The tons of garbage floating in the ocean slowly breaks down into snack-size particles for little plankton-eating fish.[69] And when those little fish become dinner for the big fish—which we in turn eat in our *negitoro-maki*—they're passing on not only the much-talked-about neurotoxin mercury but also organochlorines, polychlorinated biphenyls (PCBs), and other environmental toxins that are known to be major offenders in fertility, increasing the risk of endometriosis and altering hormonal function.[70] They also affect nervous-system development in fetuses, the immune system, heart health, and bone integrity. Researchers at Harvard and Michigan State found that women who delivered preterm were three times as likely to have had mercury levels above the 90th percentile, which they linked directly to more fish consumption.[71]

There are some people who hold up small fry like sardines, anchovies, and mackerel as being super-healthy, uncontaminated, and sustainable. But consider what Susan Levin, MS, RD, director of nutrition education for Physicians Committee for Responsible Medicine, has to say: "Ounce for ounce, sardines and anchovies have the same amount of cholesterol as ground beef. They are also 40 percent fat (beef is 50 percent) and have a sodium content that is higher if not the same as ground beef. If they are canned and packed in oil, then it's a whole other ball game with fat and sodium (as in, much worse). Plus, while they might have less mercury contamination than larger fish, that doesn't mean they don't store toxins, including mercury, in their fat. If it's in the water, it's in the fish."[72]

Yes, omega-3 fatty acids (found in some fish) are good at lowering the risk of heart disease, improving blood vessel function, and improving the overall health of people with diabetes, but we can also get these health benefits from omega-3–rich sources like walnuts, chia, hemp, and flaxseeds, without any of the fishy stuff.

Besides, omega-3 gold mines or not, there's nothing compassionate about eating fish that struggled for air as it died, or about buying fish in the store all wrapped up in plastic and styrofoam. To me, that doesn't seem like the ideal food for sustaining life.

WHAT ABOUT EGGS?

You've probably been told—maybe even by your doctor or midwife—that eggs are the miracle protein quick fix. And they do certainly offer nutritional benefits like lutein and a bunch of other vitamins and minerals. But I'll first point out that all these things can be found in plant foods. Second, these seemingly positive qualities come with a hefty dose of not-so-kind cholesterol: about 200 milligrams per egg, to be precise, which is more than you'll find in 16 tablespoons of lard![73] And what's also scary is that scientists are now finding *lead* in our eggs. This heavy metal is incredibly nasty to both you and baby, and not only does it weasel its way into animal tissue but it also finds its way into every part of an egg—shell and all.[74]

Plus, consider what exactly an egg is: It's the reproductive cell of a chicken. When you make an omelet, you're scrambling up another animal's ovulation. Fried chicken period? No thanks! Let's leave the eggs for the chicks.

Nasty Food #2: Dairy

Dairy, like meat, is full of unwanted surprises. With the approval of the FDA and USDA, many farmers use growth hormones to rev up milk production[75] and antibiotics to treat the frequent infections cows get from being tethered to milking machines three times a day with no fresh air,[76] and feed them livestock grains that are doused with any number of purposely life-killing compounds.

Also like meat, dairy is at the root of a number of life-threatening illnesses. There is strong evidence that autoimmune diseases such as MS, type 1 diabetes, rheumatoid arthritis, hyperthyroidism, and scleroderma are linked to dairy. Milk protein is particularly good at mimicking our own body proteins, and when not digested properly—which is common in humans—can trigger a self-destructive autoimmune attack. This in turn can cause inflammation.[77] Milk is far from being the bone-saving tonic that it's touted to be: The rate of fractures is actually highest in milk-drinking countries.[78] It turns out animal protein might actually *promote* bone loss.[79] Dairy products are also one of our biggest sources of saturated fat and sugar. And according to Neal Barnard, president of the Physicians Committee for Responsible Medicine, sugar in the form of lactose contributes to about 55 percent of milk's calories (including skim). Ounce for ounce, it has the same calorie load as soda.[80]

I know milk seems like a healthy staple of our diet—I mean, most of us grew up drinking a glass with dinner. But the truth is, most humans never tasted any milk besides breast milk for almost all of human history. Cow's milk is a fairly recent addition to a majority of our diets, thanks to industrial production.[81] Besides, no other mammal quenches its thirst on the milk of another species.

Nasty Isn't Good Baby Karma

I've already given you tons of good reasons to stop eating meat, drinking milk, and buying eggs; but here's one more: It's cruel. These animals are kept in waste-filled cages so small they can't stand up, turn around, or lift a leg. They don't see the light of day and have been completely denied the right to express themselves as Earth's creatures. Pigs and cows are beaten, stabbed, and tortured before they're inexpertly slaughtered.[82] Babies are torn away from their mothers right after birth, never to see them again.[83] Egg-laying hens are often sick, abused, and starved until they're thrown—still alive—into wood chippers and meat grinders. ("Free range," cage-free," "hormone-free," and "antibiotic-free" labels don't guarantee humane treatment either.) Sadly, I could go on, but I won't. I'll simply say this: When you don't eat animals, you're making the world a sweeter place for all of nature's beautiful creatures, not just the baby growing in your belly now or one day.

Also, eating animals hurts the planet. The energy required to run these massive livestock operations represents the *number one* cause of global warming in our food system.[84] Methane-filled cow burps alone account for *18 percent* of the world's greenhouse gases.[85] Plus, all the fertilizers and pesticides used to grow feed for these animals is poisoning our soil and water supply. And it's all chipping away at our natural resources one cheeseburger and shake at a time.

YOU DON'T NEED MORE HORMONES!

Pregnancy and birth are hormonal affairs. Not in a manic-panic kind of way, but in a don't-worry-we've-got-this kind of way. Hormones help the body make sure it's doing exactly what it needs to do, when it needs to do it. They help us get pregnant, have a safe delivery, encourage our babies to latch, nurse effectively, prompt our uterus to return to its prepregnancy size, and instill in us that lioness protective instinct.[86] With unnatural amounts, a domino effect happens. Suddenly, we need a boost to get pregnant and another to give birth, which interferes with initial bonding, then breastfeeding. By introducing synthetic hormones or the hormones naturally produced by other animals, you're making it that much more difficult for the home team.

Nasty Food #3: Sugar

Sugar is bad for the baby house and bad for you. It causes inflammation, makes you fat, can lead to diabetes, and is linked to cancer. But let's think about the most obvious point of all: Sugar makes you feel like garbage. When I eat too much of the sweet stuff, my head hurts. I get cranky and moody and depressed.

But don't worry, I'm not going to steal all your treats. I'll actually give you more! When I talk about foods that sustain me, bring me vital energy, and instill a deep sense of contentment and peace, I'm not just referring to vegetables. I'm talking about dessert! For me, there is no better way to maintain some approximation of balance in my life than indulging in a sticky, gooey, plate-licking-good treat every once in a while. Plants are not without their unprocessed sweet rewards, and after you give your poor taste buds a break from the white sugar assault, you won't believe how utterly satisfying something as simple as a bowl of ripe berries can be. Or getting a little wilder with something like my Chocolate-Dunked Coconut Delights (page 319). But we'll get to that a little later.

KICKING SUGAR

If you're caught in the sugar-craving hamster wheel, consider this: Refined sugar is really bad for the baby house. The Nurses' Health Study found that eating too many simple carbohydrates can lower your chance of getting pregnant.[87] And if you do manage to get pregnant, according to a Norwegian study, continuing to consume large amounts of refined sugar puts you at an increased risk for high blood pressure, which can endanger the baby. This study also found that a diet high in fat and sugar can increase your chances of having a larger baby, which ups your risk of needing a cesarean section and can lead to other complications during delivery.[88]

Refined sugar—along with its alter egos dextrose, maltose, evaporated cane juice (organic or otherwise), high-fructose corn syrup, and even honey and agave—takes your body on a roller-coaster ride that taxes all your systems.[89] Your blood sugar skyrockets, which sends your pancreas into an insulin-making frenzy in order to get all that sugar into cells where it can be used as fuel. But if you're chasing your morning latte with a muffin and eating most of your other meals out of a bag or box—even processed food that's dressed up as "all natural" or "organic"—then your blood sugar level is high all the time. Your insulin won't be able to keep up and can stop working altogether, a recipe for type 2 diabetes.[90] These drastic ups and downs can also cause mood swings and depression.[91] What's the first thing you'll reach for? More sugar.

FAKE SWEETENERS

Aspartame, saccharin, and sucralose—otherwise known as NutraSweet, Equal, Sweet'N Low, and Splenda—were not handed to us by nature. They were cooked up in chemistry labs! Saccharin is a coal tar by-product! Aspartame was derived from an antiulcer drug! But their nasty heritage pales in comparison to what they might do to your body. As William Sears, MD, sagely points out, there are no studies on the long-term effects of fake sweeteners on humans—adults or children.[92] When you also consider that a developing fetus is exponentially more sensitive to chemicals than our own full-grown bodies, I think it's a pretty compelling reason to stay away from these sugar wannabes.

Nasty Food #4: Processed Food

Believe me, I know the allure of a quick-and-easy meal or snack snapped off the grocery store shelf. But food that comes in a box or bag, that has a mile-long list of ingredients, and that can sit unrefrigerated for days is not the "kind food" we're talking about. Yes, there might be whole grains or even kale listed on the side of the box. But chances are, during its factory-processed life, those good bits were souped up with hidden sugars and fats and a scary mix of preservatives and additives that are suspected to be carcinogenic, contributors to obesity and heart disease, and seriously detrimental to the health of your developing baby.

While it's not all bad news for quick-and-easy options—like kale chips and Amy's Organic frozen pizzas—there are major pitfalls to watch for. In general, if you can't recognize much less pronounce an ingredient, then there's a good chance it's bad news. Keep an eye out for:

- **Trans fats:** This nasty ingredient (also called "trans fatty acids" or "partially hydrogenated oils") is created in an industrial process that makes vegetable oils more solid.[93] People who sell you food love this ingredient because it helps products—namely cookies, cakes, doughnuts, french fries, shortening, and margarine—stay fresh longer and feel less greasy.[94] Although the FDA has begun to move towards banning trans fats from US food, until they're all gone, know that they're serious trouble for your baby house. Trans fats crank up your cholesterol more than other types of fats,[95] and as the researchers saw in the Nurses' Health Study, the more trans fats you eat, the less likely you are to conceive. The consequences were noted in participants who had as little as 4 grams a day, the equivalent of one doughnut or a medium order of fast-food french fries.[96]

- **Excitotoxins:** Processed foods can contain nasty ingredients called excitotoxins, which include flavorings like MSG and autolyzed yeast—additives that can wreak havoc on our brain chemistry and are especially risky for developing babies and children. Excitotoxins have been linked to asthma, autism,[97] ADD/ADHD, hyperactivity, diabetes, neurodegenerative diseases, and immune problems.[98] Foods that frequently contain these foul ingredients are frozen meals, soups, bouillons, broths, snack foods like chips and crackers, sauces, dressings, candies, chewing gums, beverages, and, most alarmingly, children's snack foods and baby foods. Other excitotoxins to look for on a label include corn protein, glutamate, gelatin, wheat protein, and yeast extract.

- **GMOs:** Genetically modified organisms are basically man-made Frankenfoods. They are plants into which scientists have bred outside genes (from plants, animals, and even bacteria and viruses) in order to fend off pests, resist disease, and withstand cold or drought. GM food crops include corn, soy, cotton (cottonseed oil is in a lot of processed food), and sugar beets and are found in roughly 80 percent of packaged foods in the United States, from cereals to crackers.[99] They are also added to processed foods such as oils, dressings, sweeteners, and processed soy proteins.

  So what's the big deal? According to Robyn O'Brien, a food industry analyst turned mama advocate and author of *The Unhealthy Truth*, a majority of the GMOs on the market are either those that produce their own insecticide (ew) or those that can withstand increasing doses of the pesticide Roundup. (Great—more pesticide residues on our food.) O'Brien notes that according to Charles Benbrook, PhD, and researcher at Washington State University, GMOs have ushered in the use of about 527 million pounds of chemicals since their introduction in 1996 through 2011 and have resulted in "superweeds" that can only be killed with more heavy chemical spraying.[100]

  Few studies exist on the health hazards of GMOs, but think about it: Many of them are designed to attack an insect's brain and nervous system.[101] We know that pesticides can wreak havoc on a tiny developing body: Research indicates that children exposed to these chemicals either in utero or during other critical developmental periods face significant health risks, including a higher incidence of birth defects, cognitive impairment, childhood brain cancers, autism spectrum disorders, and endocrine disruption.[102] But because the FDA doesn't require GM foods to be labeled (makes me crazy mad!), most people don't know they're consuming them, so it's difficult for researchers to study how they're affecting human health. I don't think it should take a scientist to know that messing with Mother Nature's design is not a bright idea, but something must be up if GMOs are restricted or banned in 40 countries, including Russia, China, Japan, and in Europe.

  The only way you can know for sure that your market haul doesn't contain genetically modified ingredients is to buy food that is Certified Organic or bearing the "Non-GMO Verified" seal. Avoiding processed foods is again another way to dodge these nasty culprits.

- **The "all-natural" promise:** Just because you buy crackers and cookies at a health food market doesn't mean they're exempt from the nasty list. "Natural" or "all natural" claims aren't regulated by the FDA in packaged foods, so manufacturers can take artistic license with what they're claiming, i.e., high-fructose corn syrup is from nature![103] This is when the "Do I recognize that ingredient?" rule of thumb comes in handy.

- **BPA:** You won't find this chemical on an ingredient label, but if you're eating out of a can, there's a very good chance it's in your food. Bisphenol A (BPA) is a nasty organic compound that's used to make plastics and prevent metal corrosion in food packaging.

It has the mutantlike ability to mimic estrogen in our bodies[104] and can impair brain development as well as increase risk for brain cancer, prostate cancer, metabolic changes, decreased fertility, early puberty, neurological problems, and immunological changes.[105] A new study published in the *Journal of the American Medical Association* found that ingesting high levels of BPA is likely related to an increased risk of childhood obesity.[106]

A 2010 FDA report warning of BPA's hazards[107] led to a ban on manufacturers using it in baby bottles.[108] Unfortunately, though, our greatest exposure to BPA is from canned foods.[109] And according to a 2013 report by the Breast Cancer Fund, BPA is particularly harmful to babies when they're in utero or perhaps before they're even conceived.[110]

SOME PEACE OF MIND

If you've gotten to the end of this chapter and are freaking out about a lifetime spent eating bacon, egg, and cheese sandwiches for breakfast every day or smoking cigarettes or not eating enough veggies—take a deep breath. Consider this your clean slate. The human body is incredibly resilient. It *wants* to heal and be healthy! By beginning to make cleaner, kinder choices now, you can give your body the opportunity to be the amazing little machine it was meant to be. And if you're fretting about all the tuna salad/cups of coffee/glasses of wine that you might have thrown back before discovering you were pregnant, fear not. Plenty of women inadvertently expose their babies to toxins, and these exposures can be offset if you change course now.[111] So let's get started!

Alcohol, Drugs, and Caffeine

If you smoke, do drugs, or drink too much alcohol and/or caffeine, your chances of getting and staying pregnant plummet.[112] One study found that drinking just two cups of coffee a day— we're talking 8-ounce cups; one monster trough of latte at Starbucks is 20 ounces, or 2½ cups, on its own!—can double a pregnant woman's risk of miscarriage.[113] Alcohol has a tendency to increase estrogen levels and inhibit the body's ability to detoxify and heal.[114] And women who drink alcohol can have a greater incidence of endometriosis.[115] In fact, in a study of nearly 5,000 women, infertility due to endometriosis was 50 percent higher in women who consumed even moderate amounts of alcohol (up to one drink a day) compared to those who didn't.[116]

Once you've gotten knocked up, a little caffeine or sips of alcohol as a treat every once in a while isn't as big a deal. But for cleaning out the baby house, put these things on the naughty list.

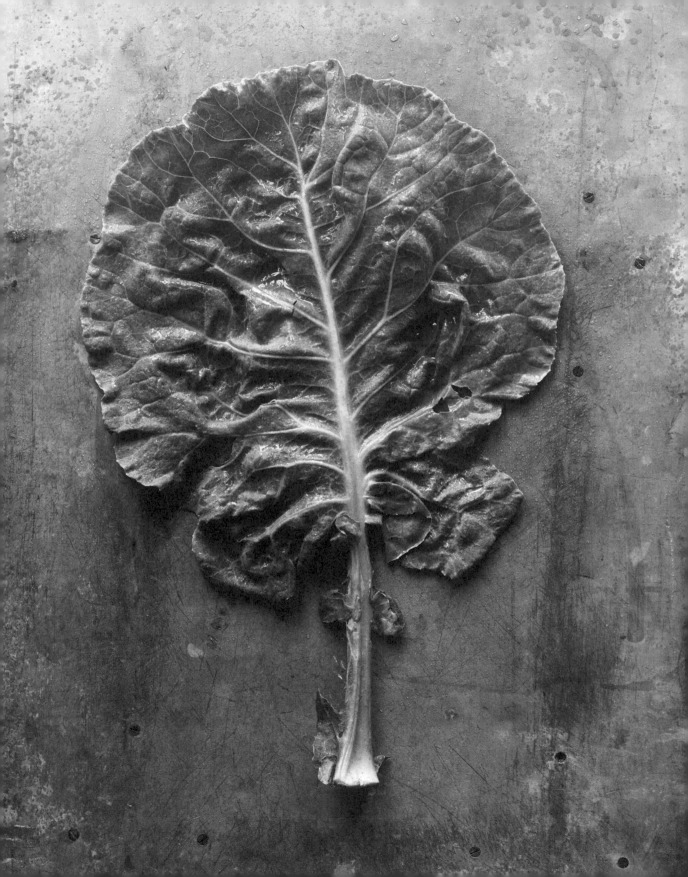

5

Blueprint for Baby:
Adding More Kind

Okay, at this point you've got the basics down: no to animals, yes to plants. While that's a pretty simple equation, I know you still have questions. You—and concerned loved ones—are probably keen to know whether you can get all the vital nutrients you need from a kind diet. Surely it can't be all peace, love, and leafy greens, right? Wrong! If you're heaping your plate with good, clean, kind foods, you are getting everything you and your baby need to be strong and vibrant.

Some care providers are pretty militant about tracking every atom of protein, iron, and folic acid while you're pregnant. But as I've learned, that degree of control is not necessary. Is it good to be mindful? Yes! Do I believe it's important to be covering every single nutritional base and then some? Of course! We'll talk much more about how to tune in to whether your body is being fueled in a balanced way. In the meantime, though, rest assured that these little miracles from the ground have you covered. Macrobiotic educator Diane Avoli sums it up beautifully: "You get everything you need from this diet. If you realize that pregnancy is not an illness and that all you need to do is eat this wide, healthy diet and listen when your body tells you it needs something, you will get everything you need."

During one of my first visits with my midwife, she asked me to start keeping a food diary because she wanted to make sure I was getting all the necessary vitamins and minerals. I knew that the food I was eating was totally, utterly, completely nourishing, but I still couldn't help but wonder whether I was missing something. A week later, I handed over my journal. She took a look and said, "You're on fire!"

Your body gets everything it could possibly want from kind foods, and the body in pregnancy is no exception. These miraculous little plants are what will keep you shiny, bright, and sustained while you're eating for two (and well beyond!). Better yet, they'll be the building blocks for your growing little one. As my good friend Lalanya put it, "It seemed healthier to have an avocado and walnut baby rather than a cheeseburger and bacon one." I couldn't have put it better myself!

The key, though, is getting enough variety. Every plant has its own unique magical properties, so filling your plate with a wide range of veggies, beans, nuts, seeds, and grains is how you make sure your body is completely fortified. Check out "Kind Food from A to Zinc" on page 326 for inspiration for how to get every vitamin and mineral you need from these amazing plants.

YOUR NEW PLATE

Now that you have all these fun new foods to play with, you're probably wondering, "How much of them do I eat?!" The beauty of eating kind foods is that you don't need to worry about boring stuff like portion control and calorie counting. What is helpful, though, is understanding how much real estate on your plate you should give each one.

And don't forget to be inspired by variety! Sometimes, people think they're doomed to a life of sad, bland food when they envision a plant-based diet. I did when I first made the change. But what they don't realize is that so many of the foods we're talking about are already on their plate. And even better—those foods are delicious! So before you think I'm taking away everything that is good and tasty in your life, pause for a minute to consider some of the most scrumptious treats you enjoy. You might be surprised to see what pops up in the kind category. Definitely flip through the recipes starting on page 295 to see just how sexy and inspiring these foods can be.

Grains: Since we first figured out that we can sprinkle little seeds onto the dirt and they'll grow into big, beautiful, tasty plants, whole grains have been at the center of our diet—and they should continue to be the foundation of your meals. It's for good reason: Whole grains are the purest form of energy we can eat. These tiny kernels contain vitamins and minerals that are essential to every function of the body. They help us break down proteins, sweep out waste, protect our cells, release energy from our muscles, and keep our hearts healthy. They're also rich in B-complex vitamins, which are calming and make skin glow. And because whole grains are such a fun project for the body to break down, they keep you feeling fuller and more satisfied longer than their processed counterparts (grains that have been ground up to make flour; stripped down to make white rice; or otherwise mutated to make crackers, chips, and cereals).

Start building your plate with whole grains such as brown rice, wild rice, farro, millet, barley, and whole oats. Cracked grain like bulgur or cracked wheat—quicker-cooking grains—are perfect for adding necessary variety to meals. They're softer than whole grains, easier to digest, and help us feel lighter and more relaxed. Try to mix them up so you're not eating the same ones again and again. Do you love rich, creamy risotto? That's a grain! And you don't need all that butter and cream to make it super-decadent—you can make delicious versions with brown rice and barley. Or how about fried rice? If you crisp up leftover brown rice with diced-up veggies and simple seasonings, you have a much healthier version than the greasy, heavy original. And super-tasty, too.

Some flour products made with whole grains are good to have, like bread, noodles (whole wheat, soba, and rice), and whole grain couscous. But for the most body-scrubbing benefits, stick with whole grains as your foundation. All told, aim to have whole grains 1 or 2 times a day and then feel free to have cracked grains and flour products—1 cup of couscous, some noodles, a slice of bread—2 to 4 times a week. It's just enough to get some variety but not so much that your system will get sluggish.

Vegetables: These are the main event. Each meal is an opportunity to load up on these guys—and lots of them. Be sure to change it up and get plenty of variety. Are steamed greens amazing for your health? Yes. Is that the only option you have in the veg department? No! Think about the most sumptuous vegetable dishes that you love to order in a restaurant. Caramelized, crunchy roasted Brussels sprouts? Creamy braised leeks? Crispy grilled asparagus? Sweet mashed yams? Those are vegetables dressed up in their Sunday best. Instead of thinking of them as sides, let them become the main attraction. Be sure to add a sea vegetable dish into the rotation a couple times a week along with dishes like Nishime (page 299) or a pressed salad (see *The Kind Diet*), and get in those greens at least one or two meals a day.

Beans: Now add a cup of beans to the mix. As you can see from the chart on page 326 there's a ton of legumes out there, and each one has its own special superpower, so variety is essential. These don't always have to be boiled up plain. Do you like hummus? Black bean tacos? Lentil soup? Chili? Those are all loaded with legumes!

Other proteins: Bean products like tofu, tempeh, and wheat gluten–derived seitan (pronounced *say-tan*) are versatile, packed with protein, and give you that toothsome, meaty texture that's perfect for hearty dishes. Aim for two or three servings a week as a replacement for beans.

Soup: Treat yourself to miso soup or some other kind of soup (veggie, bean, grain) as often as you like. Soup is a key part of this way of eating because it relaxes the intestines and prepares them for digestion. It's perfect for starting a meal because it gently awakens the body and prepares it for the food to come. If you can eat soup twice a day, that's even better!

Putting it all together: Don't drive yourself crazy, but aim for a plate that's a quarter full of grain, a quarter full of legume or protein alternative, and half full of vegetables.

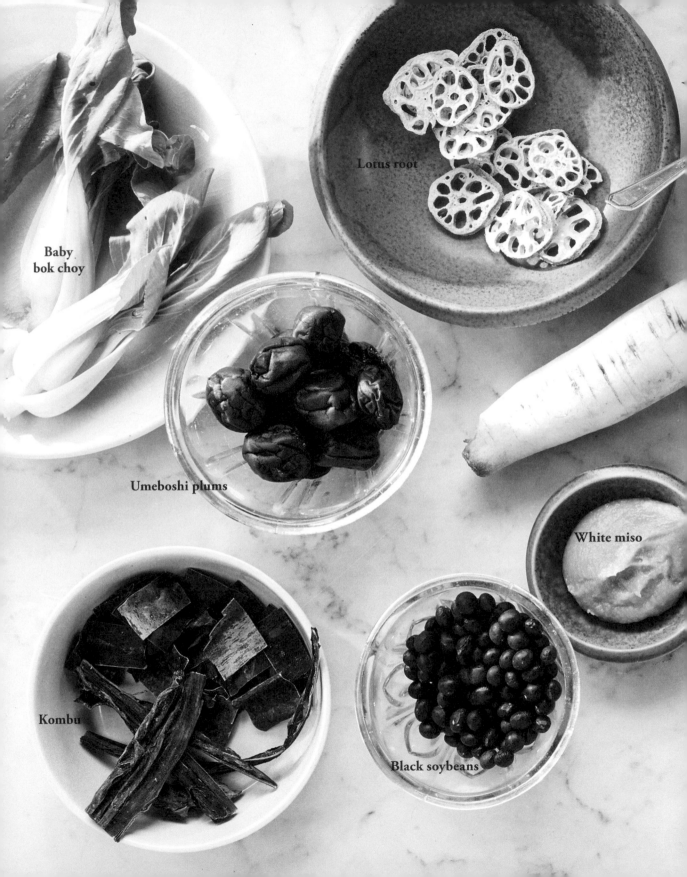

Lotus root

Baby
bok choy

Umeboshi plums

White miso

Kombu

Black soybeans

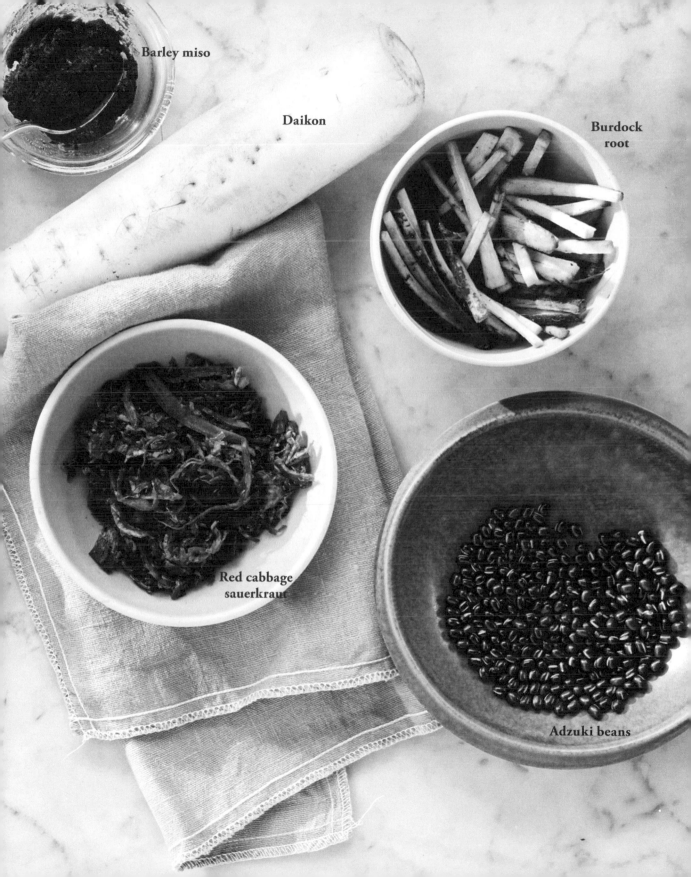

Barley miso

Daikon

Burdock
root

Red cabbage
sauerkraut

Adzuki beans

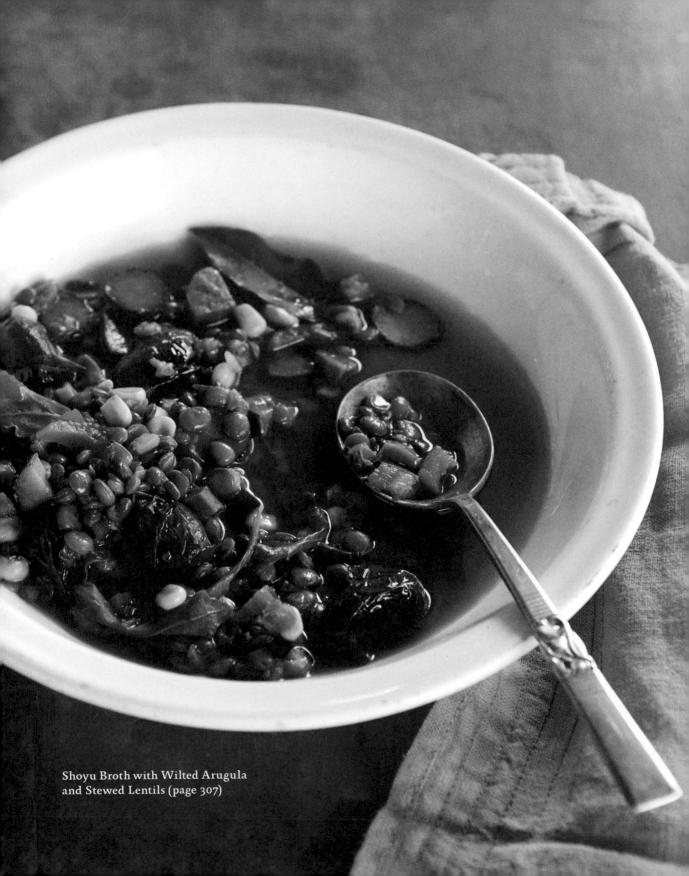

Shoyu Broth with Wilted Arugula
and Stewed Lentils (page 307)

MAGIC FOODS THAT PACK A PUNCH

While all of the foods mentioned are jam-packed with baby-making power, there are a few magical items out there that take acts of kindness to a whole new level. (See the image of all these foods on pages 34–35.)

Miso: This salty paste is made from a bean (usually soy), sometimes a grain, salt, and a bacteria called *koji*. It's fermented, meaning it's full of live probiotics and enzymes. It acts like yogurt, but without the icky problems of dairy. Eating miso in soup—its most powerful, healing form—is great for digestion; is a huge boost for the immune system; is alkalizing to the blood; and packs some protein, iron, vitamins, and minerals. Basically, it keeps your body balanced and happy.

Treat yourself to homemade miso soup every day. (Check out Immune-Boosting Miso Soup on page 295, my go-to recipe.) Just make sure you're buying high-quality miso paste that's made with barley and aged at least 2 years. The powdered stuff isn't going to give you the same benefits, and the same goes for the soup served in Japanese restaurants. That miso's usually pasteurized (so the enzymes aren't alive anymore), and the broth is often super-salty, is made from fish stock, and may even contain MSG.

Pickled veggies: Just like miso, these sour little fermented gems are full of live probiotics and enzymes that help your body absorb nutrients and put them to good use. They're also a boost for the immune system and act as antioxidants. The pickles that will do your body the most justice aren't the jarred dill variety you normally think of. In fact, most supermarket pickles aren't naturally fermented and are made with a lot of preservatives and unnecessary ingredients like sugar. Look instead for unpasteurized pickles or sauerkraut in the refrigerated section of your health food store. Use them to add a tasty, tangy, crunchy, salty punch to any meal. Because these guys are pretty salty, though, don't go overboard and, if you can, rinse them lightly before digging in. You only need about a tablespoon each meal to reap the full benefits.

Mama to Mama on . . . Healthy Conception

I hadn't gotten pregnant in the 6 years that my partner and I had been together, but 3 months after both of us became vegans, we conceived without even trying. The rest of my pregnancy was a vegan one, and now we have a little vegan daughter who is *loving* it.

—Katie Pace, Los Angeles

Umeboshi plums: These super-sour pickled plums are alkalizing to the blood, which means they help counteract acidity in your system—a major bonus if you're just starting to clean house. Eat a quarter of an umeboshi plum with your grains a few times a week and you'll also enhance your digestive health. The great news, too, is that these are pretty easy to find. Check out places like Whole Foods Market or your local natural or Asian market.

Burdock root: This long, brown root has an earthy flavor with just a tiny bit of sweetness. It has unbelievable restorative powers and is used to cleanse and purify the blood, support digestion, scrub away toxins, and even help lower blood sugar. It has more protein, calcium, and phosphorus than carrots and is a great source of potassium. I love adding it to soups, stews, and stir-fries, and dishes like Braised Burdock Root with Hearty Seitan (page 306). Some farmers' markets carry it, but more often you'll find it stocked in Asian markets and health food stores.

Daikon: Though it looks kinda like a huge white carrot, this miraculous veg is actually a member of the radish family. It's a natural diuretic, which is perfect for when you've been a little naughty. It has a spicy, pungent flavor when raw but becomes meaty and sweet when cooked. These have been popping up in more and more regular supermarkets, but your natural market or Asian market should have you covered.

Lotus root: In Chinese medicine, they say that foods that look like certain body parts are extra fortifying for those organs. Lotus root—which looks like a long, white tube—is a breath of fresh air for our bodies. It helps circulate and enrich our blood, gives us more energy, nurtures the heart, quiets digestive issues, supports the stomach, and flushes out toxins. Chopped and steeped in hot water as a tea, it's a curative remedy for a chest cold or phlegmy cough. You'll most likely find lotus root in an Asian market, but make sure that the vegetable is cream colored—white lotus root may have been bleached. You can also order it dried online and reconstitute it with a little hot water before cooking. Chunky Stewed Veggies (page 299) is a great recipe for working in some lotus root.

Sea vegetables: There's something almost mystical about these calcium- and mineral-loaded gifts from the ocean. Sea veggies like nori, *hijiki, arame,* wakame, and kombu are high in protein; alkalize and detoxify the blood; can reduce blood pressure and inhibit tumor growth; have anti-inflammatory properties; and are amazing for your hair, skin, teeth, and bones. Consider these guys an important medicinal food to be eaten a couple of times a week. They'll keep you glowing and beautiful and beyond healthy. Plus, they're so tasty—especially in Arame, Sun-Dried Tomato, and Zucchini Stir-Fry (page 305).

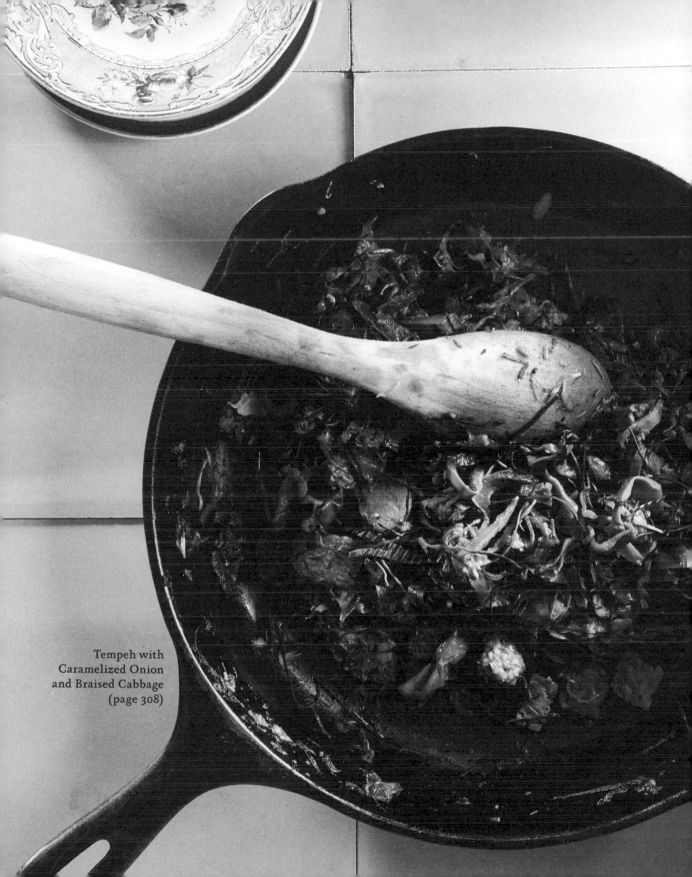

Tempeh with
Caramelized Onion
and Braised Cabbage
(page 308)

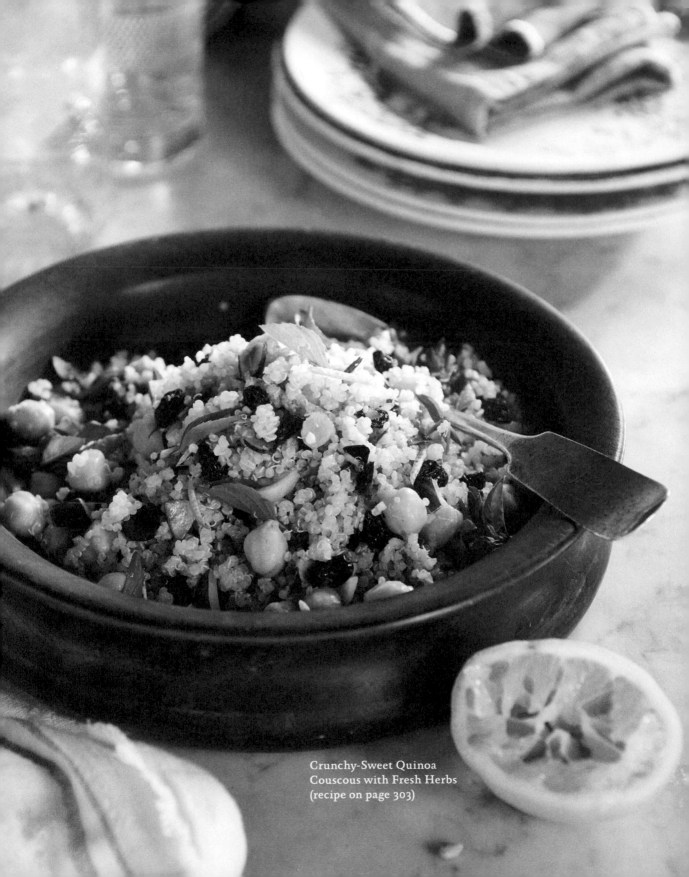

Crunchy-Sweet Quinoa
Couscous with Fresh Herbs
(recipe on page 303)

Green leafies: Kale, collards, turnip greens, mustard greens, watercress, and bok choy are not only loaded with minerals that make the blood strong and energized, but their chlorophyll can help you feel relaxed, open, and happy. They are really, truly a crucial part of your diet if you want to feel amazing. But please don't just throw greens in your smoothie and call it a day. When plants get all ground up before we eat them, we assimilate them differently. Blending is not the same as chewing. Also, when you're adding them to a smoothie, you're probably adding in other sweet treats like fruit and sweeteners. While that's completely kosher every once in a while, it isn't the kind of pure, green loveliness you want to indulge in more often. See my Delicate Steamed Greens with Toasted Sesame Oil Vinaigrette on page 300 for how to get the perfect steamed greens every time.

Adzuki, black beans, and black soybeans: In addition to giving you a leg up in the iron department, these members of the legume tribe are good for the adrenal glands, which in turn can help relieve stress on the body (and help you get pregnant! While all beans are amazingly good for you, these varieties pack an extra punch. Black soybeans can help cleanse your system if up until now you've been overdoing it on animal foods or baked flour goodies. Adzukis are known for their super-charged healing properties, especially for reproductive function, and black beans are the most anti-oxidant rich of the entire legume family. Black Soybean Stew (page 310) and Adzuki Bean Soup with Kabocha Squash (page 312) are two of my favorite bean recipes and are both super-strengthening.

Take Time to Chew

True satisfaction and wellness don't start with just our food; they start with how we eat it. When we take the time to sit with our meals; reflect on all the goodness we're about to lavish on our cells, flesh, bones, veins, skin, and organs; and actually *chew* every mouthful into sweet submission, we're feeding our minds and spirits, too. Eating peacefully and with gratitude ensures that you're giving yourself some quiet space in the world.

When you give your food a good working over—30 to 50 chews per bite—you'll feel less bloated or gassy with undigested food and fuller after eating less. That's because a special enzyme in your saliva called ptyalin breaks it down further into glucose, and this good-for-you sugar travels to your brain and gives you a feeling of satisfaction. Chewing well also helps release all the nutrients and energy from your food so your body can absorb them.

Preparing to Eat Well

The best piece of advice I can give you is to be prepared. If you wait until you're starving and exhausted to go out foraging for food, things can get dicey, and you're not going to make choices in line with your real wishes. The first remedy is planning ahead and filling your house with delicious, nourishing food (and not keeping too tempting foods in the pantry). It will take less time than watching your favorite TV show! Draft your menu for the week so you know exactly what you need from the market to fill your fridge. Play around with new flavors of tempeh. Make a big pot of rice or stew. Snack on soups, leftovers, and mochi! You can eat those things for days and not get bored because you can change things up with fresh veggies and salads.

The second solution is keeping healthy treats on hand. Especially if you're just starting to kick nasty foods, it's important to know that you still have your yummies, but ones that will keep you and your baby house on a wholesome path. When I'm feeling a little frisky, I like to mix Maisie Jane's Almond Butter with a tiny bit of rice syrup and dip apple slices in the "caramel"—a once-in-a-while treat that helps me feel better in the long run than naughtier indulgences. My hope for you is that you'll get as clean as possible first so you can really feel the bliss, but don't think for a second that getting kind means not having any room to play. And remember that snacking is not the answer to boredom, cooking with new foods and flavors is. So keep exploring all the recipes in this book, *The Kind Diet*, and on thekindlife.com.

WHAT ABOUT DESSERT?

I promised I wouldn't take away your sweets! There's no reason why you can't pamper yourself from time to time with treats made from whole grain flours like spelt, whole wheat, barley, and brown rice, or natural sugars that don't tax your system—including brown rice syrup, coconut sugar, barley malt, maple syrup, molasses, and fruit.

If you're just beginning to kick processed sugar out of your life, these kind swaps will make the road a little smoother. Believe it or not, eating balanced, kind meals is one of the best ways to stave off cravings, especially for sweets. Try to have grains, beans, and vegetables for at least two meals a day. Eventually, you'll find that you won't crave sweets as much as you used to.

But you do need *some* sweets: good-quality treats to keep the body happy and nourished without overdoing it—things like sweet veg (squash, onions), amasake, carrot

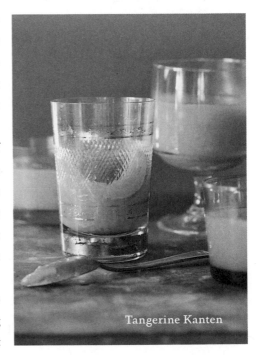

Tangerine Kanten

juice, or warm apple juice. One of my favorites is Tangerine Kanten (page 319). You need things like that almost daily to feel satisfied and relaxed. As for extra-special treats, the fastest route to the healthiest you is limiting them. That's because baked flour goods—while so, so tasty—aren't healing. But I'll also be the first to admit that sometimes you just need something naughty, like a cup of Chocolate Dunked Coconut Delights (page 319). If you're replacing a morning doughnut with a bowl of granola, then you're moving in the right direction. Consider sweets the treats that they are, and don't confuse them with magical, healing foods that nourish us.

Check out the "Conquer Your Cravings" section on page 114 for more advice about how to deal with an I-need-to-have-it emergency, including gentler alternatives to naughtier indulgences. Kind can be decadent and delicious!

Get through the Detox Funk

When you liberate your body from meat, dairy, and processed foods, there can be a small period of time when you'll notice nutty things happening. It could include rashes, headaches, phlegm, sleeplessness, constipation, diarrhea, shakiness, or other gentle—and temporary—discomfort. The amazing news? That means the kind foods are working! Your body is doing a huge spring cleaning and is shoving out the mucky stuff, and what you're feeling is all that built-up nastiness on its way back out. If you're already pregnant, don't worry. Because you're doing this gently by simply introducing new foods (as opposed to fasting, juicing, or more dramatic dietary changes that wouldn't be advisable during pregnancy), it's completely safe for your baby. And it means you're one step closer to not feeling any of these symptoms during pregnancy as well as having better skin, deeper sleep, and a lot more energy. Celebrate this transition to full, luminous wellness.

Kick the "Diet" Mentality

Eating kind is about treating your body to balancing, nourishing, healing, calming foods that help build yourself and your baby. It's not about eating "superfoods" because, innately, all whole, plant-based foods are superfoods. And this isn't by any means a strict regimen; we're *definitely* not taking the joy out of eating! So do your best to switch that part of your brain off. Getting kind is about eating *more* foods, really. Be generous with all these amazing sun-powered, baby house–healing foods, and fill that belly of yours with them until you feel *satisfied*. Is there anything more delicious than that?

Organic: How Important Is It?

Some people say organic is just a big scam to get you to buy fancy produce and that it isn't any healthier than regular fruits and vegetables. But that's just not true. When you buy "Certified Organic," it means you are buying something grown in healthy soil nourished with nothing but organic matter—no petrochemical fertilizers or residues from synthetic pesticides.[117] This is particularly good for your baby house, since exposure to these nasty chemicals can increase the risk of birth defects.[118] According to a report by the American Academy of Pediatrics, food is the number one source of pesticide exposure in children, which is linked to a host of childhood health problems, from reduced birth weight to mental impairment and cancer.[119] Organic offers another bonus to you and your baby, since when plants are grown in rich, fertile soil and have to hold their own against pests and disease, they may even develop more antioxidants than their conventional counterparts.[120]

True, organic can cost a little more than conventionally grown produce, but that doesn't take into account the considerable long-terms costs to you and your baby's health—and our planet's: no nitrogen runoff or growth hormones seeping into the watershed, and no land poisoned for the next generation.[121]

If you're still concerned about the cost of organic food, try to buy as much locally as you can. Since it doesn't have to be shipped halfway across the world, local produce tends to be cheaper, and local small farmers are less likely to spray their crops with heavy-duty industrial chemicals. Fortunately the explosion of local farmers' markets puts more organic and local produce within easy reach of most people. Going to the farmers' market is our little family ritual—it's so much fun to see all the other kids and familiar faces. Another affordable way of going organic is to join a CSA (community supported agriculture), which gets you a weekly box of seasonal fruits and vegetables that have been grown nearby.

Ask your local grocer or health food store to start carrying organic foods that are grown in the area. Encourage your friends and family in the community to ask, too, and the store should respond. The more we support small organic farms, the less conventional farms will hold their monopoly, and the less organic food will eventually cost. And at the very least, steer clear of the following nonorganic fruits and vegetables—identified by the Environmental Working Group as the Dirty Dozen—since they tend to absorb the highest amounts of pesticides.[122] These include: apples, blueberries (domestic), celery, cucumbers, grapes, green beans, kale/leafy greens, lettuce, nectarines (imported), peaches, potatoes, spinach, strawberries, and sweet bell peppers.

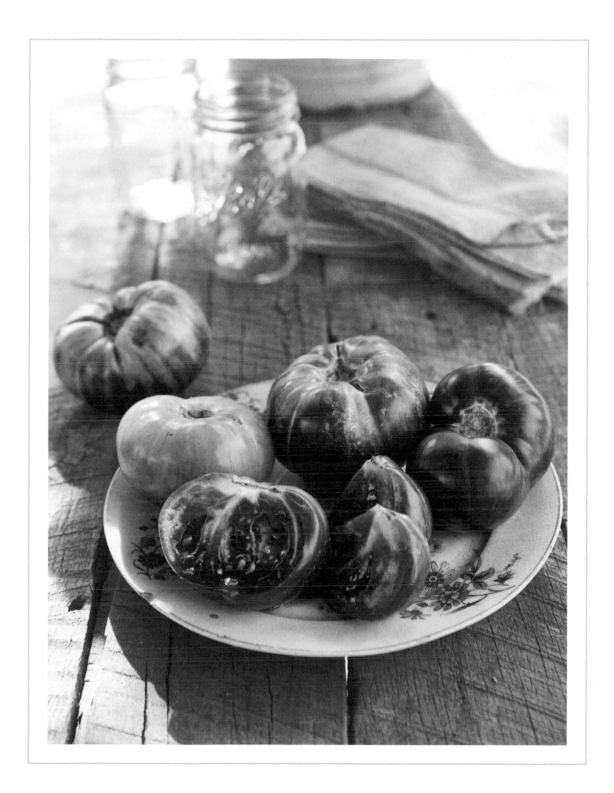

HOW MUCH WATER SHOULD YOU DRINK?

The recommendation for eight glasses a day is for people who are choking down fiber-free meat and processed foods that turn to dry goop in the intestines. Meat, sugar, salt, chemicals, caffeine, and processed food can be so dehydrating that your body needs help getting it all out the other end. A diet composed mainly of grains, veggies, and legumes, however, is rich in fluids and light on toxins, so you won't be so parched. Fruits and veggies are often more than 90 percent water, and grains and legumes contain more than 80 percent water when cooked.[123]

That said, no element is more life-giving than water, and the secret to great health is to get just enough. Dousing your organs and cells with too much water can weaken the energy in your body and cause constriction, which can negatively affect your digestion. Too little H_2O, on the other hand, can cause constipation, tension, dryness, and even inflammation.[124]

Keep in mind that throwing back icy-cold water can slow down your natural healing abilities. According to traditional Chinese medicine, our bodies have little furnaces inside that help break down and absorb the nutrients we're eating. This keeps the metabolism stoked and our organs working at peak performance. But if we douse that fire with drinks that are too cold, our digestive system has to work double time to bring the temperature back up, slowing the metabolism. One of my favorite little treats is to have hot water and lemon (occasionally with a few drops of stevia). So simple, right? My dad used to order this at restaurants at the end of his meals all the time, and I'd think, *How boring!* But it actually hits the spot.

Clean Food Calls for Clean Water

By the time water reaches our tap, it will have snaked its way through bedrock and soil and sopped up all kinds of minerals but also all kinds of industrial and agricultural runoff. According to green-living expert Mary Cordaro, a lot of nasty things can be floating around in our waterways, like pharmaceutical drugs, bacteria, viruses, parasites, fluoride, heavy metals, and petrochemical solvents. Some of these "additives" are filtered out by municipal treatment plants, but then chemicals like chlorine are added back in to kill off potentially harmful bacteria. And when chlorine reacts with organic materials that are already in the water, it can form traces of chemical products called THMs (trihalomethanes), which are carcinogenic.[125] Then the water still has the journey to our faucets, which can expose it to a number of gunky things in our pipes, from pathogens to hard water scale to lead.

But before you consider moving to the nearest glacier, know that there are ways to clean up what's going in your glass and on your skin. The most important thing is to make sure your drinking water is as pure as it can be. Consider installing a reverse-osmosis system under your kitchen sink, which filters nearly all pollutants. A more affordable option (though not as thorough) is the Zero Water Purifier (sold at most big-box stores), which eliminates dissolved solids and nearly all fluoride. Because skin is our largest organ and we absorb so much of what touches it, you might also consider a whole-house carbon filtration system for bathing—or, if that's too pricey (it has to be professionally installed), a simpler filter for your bath like one from Rainshow'r. You can find more info about these and other water gadgets and systems on thekindlife.com. At the very least, you might want to run your cold tap for a minute first thing in the morning, especially if you live in an older house, which can cut down on the lead that has leeched into the water while it sat in the plumbing overnight. (Instead of letting all that valuable water run down the drain, catch it in a pitcher and use it to water plants!)

Finally, try to avoid bottled water. Aside from the 137 million petroleum-based, BPA-riddled plastic bottles dumped into landfills every day that take at least 1,000 years to decompose, the water inside isn't worth it. A 4-year study by the Natural Resources Defense Council found that water from one-third of the 103 bottled waters tested were lower quality than tap water. Bottled water is not required to be tested as frequently as tap water for bacteria and chemical contaminants, and it doesn't have to comply with the same standards.[126]

FREEDOM FROM WORRY: WHY A KIND PREGNANCY IS NOTHING TO BE AFRAID OF

I know how the naysayers in your life can make you feel—as if by not eating meat or dairy, you're going to shrivel up and die. Food manufacturers aren't exactly helping your case by perpetuating that myth. But that's just it: I've never heard of anyone dying because they didn't eat animals! I have, on the other hand, heard of 7.6 million people dying of cancer every year,[127] 3.4 million from diabetes,[128] 17 million from heart disease,[129] and all the other bad things out there that are directly linked to eating nasty foods. So my question to anyone who takes issue with your not partaking in chicken dinner or sushi night is this: If all these foods have been proven to cause these illnesses, then why would you want someone to eat them when she was trying to create precious, delicate new life? (Or eat them at all, for that matter!) By the same token, kind foods cure us of those very illnesses, so why would they suddenly not be as healthy?

All of the vegan (and veganish) pregnancies I have witnessed—mine included—have been way smoother than those of my nonvegan friends. My Kind Mama tribe didn't have to worry about the medications and interventions that our society considers normal. And because we were armed with research backing up our conviction that what we were doing is right, we could shake off the unnecessary fear that the world inevitably threw our way. When I was pregnant and looking for a remedy to my nausea, I went to see an acupuncturist. At first, she treated me like I was wellness personified. But after I mentioned I was a vegan, she starting going on and on about how I was super-anemic and that my liver was *sooo* weak. I suddenly went from being the healthiest girl in the world to what sounded like being just shy of my deathbed. "Really?" I said. "That's weird because I just had my blood tested and everything checked out perfectly." A blood analyst had actually taken pictures of my cells as an example of what beautiful healthy blood cells look like!

Being a Kind Mama is the healthiest thing you can do for yourself and your baby. Period. But it takes a little resolve. Arm yourself with the facts so that no naysayer, no matter how well intentioned, can sway you from your commitment. To help, I've dedicated this section to answering all of the big questions that come up from women on this path.

Your Body Will Get Every Nutrient It Needs

Not only will you be getting all the vitamins, nutrients, and minerals you need from kind foods,* but you'll actually be getting *higher* doses than your animal-eating friends. So the next time your mother-in-law/husband/nosy neighbor gets on your case, point to this chart and say, "Hello! Calcium! Vitamin A! Folate!" They'll see in no uncertain terms that you're superior and awesome in every single way.[130]

The "See, I Told You So" Box of Nutrients

	BEATS THE PANTS OFF MEAT EATERS	A NOSE ABOVE MEAT EATERS
Vitamin A	X	
Vitamin B$_1$, thiamine	X	
Vitamin B$_2$, riboflavin		X
Vitamin B$_3$, niacin	X	
Vitamin B$_6$, pyrodoxine		X
Vitamin B$_9$, folate	X	
Vitamin C	X	
Vitamin E	X	
Vitamin K	X	
Calcium		X
Magnesium	X	

*With just a couple of exceptions (which we'll talk about in a minute)

But I Turned Out Okay! Combating the Most Common Excuse for Unhealthy Behavior during Pregnancy

We've all heard the stories—"My mom smoked during my pregnancy," "I was a formula baby," "My mom was high as a kite during delivery"—and they all end the same way: "But I turned out okay!" My mom supports my vegan diet and is mostly vegan herself (except when she's not at all), but she recently brought up the foods that I'd eaten growing up: meat, potatoes, maybe some vegetables, tons of sugar and dairy, and caffeine. She said, "You ate those foods, and you're fine!" But I was running around like a crackhead most of the time, hopped up on sugar—tea and biscuits, anyone? Plus I needed an inhaler for my asthma and shots for my allergies. I had bronchitis three times a year and got massive migraines until I cleaned up my diet.

What we consider healthy when a child is born is that it's alive, it's breathing, and that it passed some tests. Maybe his mom took every kind of medication for the past year just to make him, and maybe she got the super-deluxe drug cocktail in the hospital to deliver, but if he's breathing and pink, he's good to go. No one's questioning the condition of those little organs or the quality of the blood in that body.

There's certainly no point in looking back at our parents' decisions with any sort of resentment or regret, but what you can do is choose to give the next generation the best start possible, starting with your own kind choices.

Will I Get Enough Protein?

Everything we eat, with the exception of fruit, naturally has it. Grains, beans, nuts, seeds, and even vegetables are rich in the stuff. According to Physicians Committee for Responsible Medicine's Susan Levin, MS, RD, broccoli gets one-third of its calories from protein![131] So if you're eating enough food in general to sustain you and your growing baby, then your needs will be met. Think about it: Gorillas and elephants are two of the strongest animals on the planet, and they don't eat anything but plants! You can rest assured—and readily point out to anyone who might be apprehensive—that your source for protein might not be a slab of cow, but you're still getting the same amount if not more protein, a ton more nutrients, and none of the nasty stuff like chemicals, hormones, and antibiotics. For more concentrated protein, look to lentils, beans, nut butters, and nuts, plus tofu, tempeh, and seitan.

What's Up with Soy and Estrogen?

Okay, so I know what you've heard about soy: It's going to cause your husband's baby maker to go limp and your little boy to grow breasts, and it'll give us all thyroid problems. Then what's up with all the promises that soy is good for us? It seems like every product under the sun is packed with it now—ice cream, cheese, chips, yogurt, milk, you name it. The fact is, soy in its purest, least processed forms has some pretty amazing qualities. In small quantities, its plant-based estrogens, or phytoestrogens, have been shown to protect against breast cancer, can help rebalance hormones in postmenopausal women, and are totally fine for men.[132] And as a major baby house bonus, soy products may reduce the risk of fibroids in the uterine lining.[133]

Take your cue from Asian cultures, which have used soybeans or tofu in moderation for millennia without any problems. They don't have higher rates of birth defects in baby boys relating to phytoestrogens.[134] That's because they're eating tiny bits of high-quality tofu or miso. And they're definitely not indulging every day in products that are made with soy fillers and by-products. The key here is moderation and quality. If you're transitioning to whole, unrefined foods, then give yourself license to savor soy products like soy milk, soy cheese, and soy ice cream once in a while. As you start really cleaning house and getting more balanced, think of these soy products as occasional treats, and opt for purer forms like organic tofu and tempeh instead.

GIVE TOFU A BREAK!

People are so mean to tofu. I definitely get that it has a bad rap. I mean, if someone cut it into blocks, served it raw on top of a salad, and told me to eat it, I, too, would think it was disgusting. Tofu is exactly like vegetables in that way: If you've never eaten it cooked right, you're going to think it's gnarly. You wouldn't just eat a piece of plain boiled chicken. No way! You'd marinate it, season it, grill it, and sauce it until you had something tasty. Tofu makes creamy dips, belly-filling soups, and rich, creamy desserts. Tofu—and seitan and tempeh—is far from being a sad vegan consolation prize; it's one of the most scrumptious things you can have in the fridge.

LET'S TALK ABOUT VITAMINS

The most powerful supplement on the planet is your food. No pill can give you as great a boost as what's packed in your greens, beans, grains, good oils, and fats. That said, no matter how much of the good stuff you're eating every day, there are two vitamins that are difficult to get enough of from a plant-based diet. It's not because that diet is incomplete; it's due to changes in our Western lifestyle and in how we source our food.

Vitamin D: There's been something of a vitamin D craze lately, but the jury's still out on how much you need. This crucial vitamin helps us absorb enough calcium in our bones to keep them strong. Try to get as much as possible from the most natural source—the sun! But it's not always easy to get all you need that way because of pollution, cloud cover, the amount of pigmentation of your skin (darker versus lighter), and the latitude where you live (as in, the entire top half of the United States). There are no reliable food sources—plant or animal—for vitamin D (and the vast majority of fortified cereals and breads contain added isolated, synthetic vitamin D_3). So think of a supplement as a backup plan.

It's best to figure out your ideal dosage in consultation with your health practitioner, who can administer a simple blood test to determine where you are and what you need. Steer clear of that isolated synthetic D_3, which is from lanolin (otherwise known as "wool grease"), a waxy substance secreted by sheepskin to help keep its wool dry. It's certainly not kind. D_2, which is derived from mushrooms, is now available in a USDA Organic Certified form, but according to integrative pediatrician Dr. Lawrence Rosen, D_2 isn't considered as absorbable as D_3. A great new alternative is D_3 that is derived from lichens (remember that stuff from seventh-grade biology?). Make sure the label says vitamin D_3 cholecalciferol from lichen or it's not vegan. No matter which type you take, remember that vitamin D is fat-soluble, so pop it with food containing healthy fats to help boost its absorption.[135]

Vitamin B_{12}: Because this vitamin comes from bacteria that thrive in our soil, you'd think we plant eaters would be getting more than our share. But now that our produce is so squeaky clean when it hits the market—and our soil just isn't as nutrient rich as it used to be—we're no longer able to get as much B_{12} as we need. When cows and other grazing animals munch on grass, they're getting plenty, which is why grass-fed-meat eaters have an easier time getting the B_{12} required (in addition to lots of other junk, so don't be too envious; and this B_{12} benefit *definitely* doesn't apply to people who are eating factory-farmed meat). And some meat-eaters still have to take a supplement because they can't absorb all the B_{12} they need. While people don't need a whole lot of B_{12}—only 2 micrograms a day—it's imperative that we get it. Long-term B_{12} deficiencies are irreversible and can affect the brain and nervous system function.

Even if you're growing your own food and nibbling on the dirty bits, you should still take a supplement at least every other day. (Though, as Susan Levin points out, most B_{12} deficiencies

> ## Mama to Mama on . . . Kind Nutrition
>
> My husband and I were both amazed by the gift of health a vegan diet provided, but we hesitated about a vegan pregnancy. Would I get enough calories and nutrients? We decided to track my protein intake for a week, and on any given day, we both easily consumed above and beyond the RDI's guidelines. We were also worried about calcium and folate, but it turns out that dark leafy greens and even tofu are great sources and are easy to incorporate. We asked our doctor if what we were doing was okay. He said as long as I was meeting nutritional guidelines and taking a B_{12} supplement that it was not just okay but very, very healthy for the baby.
>
> —Kimberly Taylor, Forest Park, Illinois

pop up in the elderly population and not the vegan one.) Make sure that the brand you buy does not contain cyanocobalamin, a cheapo semisynthetic form of the vitamin that manufacturers use to cut costs. It's bound to the cyanide molecule (yes, the poison) and has to be cleaned out of your body by your liver.[136] Look instead for the much higher quality methylcobalamin.

The Scoop on Prenatal Vitamins

As I said before, the most powerful supplement on the planet is your food. And if you're being truly kind, then a prenatal vitamin would be redundant. That said, because growing babies can be little nutrient-sucking vampires—and because overfarmed, nutrient-depleted soil can lead to plants with fewer vitamins than in days of yore—it's sometimes necessary to supplement. Try to get as much as you can through food, and think of the vitamins as backup or, as my midwife, Margo Kennedy, says, as "an insurance clause for the days we don't get everything from our diet."

What's the difference between a prenatal vitamin and a multi? According to Kennedy, prenatals are just more specific nutrient-wise for pregnancy and breastfeeding so you know you're getting plenty of things like folic acid, calcium, and iron. As for how much of each nutrient you'd ideally be getting, it's a good idea to have a discussion with your care provider—especially because you may already be getting enough from your diet (check out the chart on page 326 to see the vitamins and minerals available in all the foods you're eating). This is particularly important when it comes to iron and copper, an imbalance of which can affect brain health and increase the risk of Alzheimer's disease.[137] Iron specifically is associated with risks for heart disease, diabetes, and cancer if taken in too-high amounts. Susan Levin advises that you work with your doctor or midwife to figure out the earliest point you can stop taking these vitamins. "Iron needs actually decrease during lactation," she says, bringing the recommended amount down to 9 milligrams a day, versus 18 milligrams a day during prepregnancy and 27 milligrams a day during pregnancy.

If you do decide to go the vitamin route, make sure you're opting for a high-quality brand that's vegan—which is particularly important when it comes to vitamin A—food-based, and 100% Certified Organic.

What's All the Fuss over DHA and Folate?

DHA: This omega-3 fatty acid helps create your baby's brain.[138] The human body can produce all but two of the essential fatty acids it needs: linoleic acid (LA) and alpha-linoleic acid (ALA).[139] The most common recommendation is to take a fish oil supplement. But these pills can contain high levels of vitamin A, which when derived from an animal and not a plant, has been associated with fetal abnormalities if consumed in excessive doses.[140] Also, fish livers—just like our own—are meant to concentrate toxic materials. So why now, of all times, would you want to be adding those things into your diet? Also because they come from fish, the supplements may contain mercury.[141] While some companies are more transparent about the purity of their products than others, there's still no reason to get animals involved in this plant party.

The great news is that both of these fatty acids are available in plant oils! According to Christina Pirello, we can get what we need from sources like microalgae (chlorella and spirulina), sea plants, and nuts. A super-simple solution is sprinkling a teaspoon of ground flaxseed or flaxseed oil—one of the richest sources of omega-3 fatty acids there is—on your oatmeal, salads, or vegetables. Also, be sure to eat plenty of whole grains like quinoa, dark beans like black beans and adzukis, and dark leafy greens (which are rich sources of zinc, magnesium, calcium, biotin, and vitamins B_6, B_3, and C) to help your body metabolize those fatty acids. Another option is to add a cold-pressed Certified Organic plant oil supplement to your diet. One tablespoon can give you a perfect balance of the two essential fatty acids ALA and LA, plus beauty-promoting omega 7s.

Folate: Folate is probably one of the biggest buzzwords when it comes to pregnant women, as in *Are you getting enough folate?* There's good reason, too. A deficiency can cause serious birth defects. Luckily, plants are packed with the stuff. In fact, the word *folic* is derived from the Latin word *folium,* meaning "leaf." So once again, if you're eating a varied diet of supercharged veggies like leafy greens and some fruits like berries and bananas, then you're most likely getting what you need. Just be mindful of two things: First, folic acid is very sensitive to heat and can be destroyed by cooking, too much sunlight, and even pureeing in the blender.[143] So make sure you're eating your folate-packed foods (like leafy greens, asparagus, and peas) very gently cooked (steamed or lightly sautéed, for example). Second, synthetic folic acid—or molecules that mimic the nature-made version—is not the same superpowered nutrient found in plants. In fact, this knockoff version may carry its own health risks.[144] So when getting your fill, opt for plant-derived sources and steer clear of "fortified" products (yucky processed foods like white flour products and cereals that are stuffed full of synthetic nutrients). If you're still concerned about not getting enough folate, then it's all the more reason to take a prenatal vitamin for peace of mind. Be sure the brand you choose has L-5 methyltetrahydrofolate or 5-formyltetrahydrofolate on the label—the nature-made form of this nutrient—and not "folic acid," which indicates that a synthetic version is being used.[145] These methyl folates are the most active, available form of folic acid for your body to absorb.[146]

Anemia and Pregnancy

If you're eating a varied diet of whole, plant-based foods, then you can absolutely get enough iron! That also goes for when you're pregnant and your body more readily absorbs it. Plants are packed with the stuff, and studies have shown that vegans tend to consume more iron than meat eaters.[147] That also goes for when you're pregnant and your body more readily absorbs it That's because we're heaping our plates with iron-rich foods. Sea vegetables like arame and kombu, adzuki beans, tempeh, dried tofu, sesame seeds, kale, turnip greens, squash, and pumpkin seeds are all packed with iron. Be mindful about chewing these foods really well, since that can help ensure you're absorbing as much as possible. Try to eat more vitamin C–rich foods—parsley, leafy greens, broccoli—which will help your body absorb iron. And because dairy can significantly reduce iron absorption, kind eaters are all-around ahead of the game.

So why all the smack talk about plant-based diets not supplying enough iron? One possible reason is because people who don't eat meat tend to have lower iron stores than those who do. Yet according to the Academy of Nutrition and Dietetics' position paper on vegetarian diets, "Although vegetarian adults have lower iron stores than nonvegetarians, their serum ferritin levels are usually within the normal range."[148]

Before you let someone bully you into eating that burger, know that low iron stores can actually be a *good* thing. According to Christina Pirello, MFN, CCN, levels on the lower side are associated with higher glucose tolerance, which might help prevent diabetes, whereas high levels have been linked to cancer and heart disease.[149] Luckily, plants contain what's called nonheme iron, which is more absorbable when the body is low in iron and less absorbable when the body already has enough. This means that the body can regulate its iron balance. Meat, on the other hand, has heme iron, which slams right into your bloodstream, whether it's needed or not.

If you're feeling sluggish or fatigued, instead of jumping on the meat bandwagon, first take a look at what you're eating. If you're not taking in enough calories or protein, or you're eating too many high-sugar foods, then that could very well be why.[150] That said, you should work with your caregiver to make sure you're maintaining healthy iron levels. Ideally, this person would understand that your iron stores are going to look different than a meat eater's. They also should understand that when it comes to iron, a safe balance is key. Here's what my trusted experts have to say on the topic—including my own midwife, Margo Kennedy, who has been attending births for more than 21 years and stopped counting how many babies she's brought into the world after number 2,000!

WHAT THE DOC SAYS Neal Barnard, MD

It's probably best to have your hemoglobin on the low end of the normal range. If your energy is good and your hemoglobin and hematocrit are at the low end of normal, that is likely the best place to be.[151]

WHAT THE MIDWIFE SAYS Margo Kennedy, CNM, MSN

Every test for iron has normal and ideal ranges, but in general the ideal iron level should be 60 to 170 mcg/dl. Iron in pregnancy normally declines as a result of dilution of the blood volume, but with adequate sources in your diet, your body is quite good at regaining equilibrium.

WHAT THE HEALER SAYS Diane Avoli

Women who eat a plant-based diet have lower iron levels—it's the way it's supposed to be. There are no tests out there specifically for macro women, or in any realm of health, really. People who are eating meat and sugar need more iron because they're eating so many foods that are constantly depleting them. But if you're eating iron-rich foods and grains and chewing your food, your body is going to start assimilating iron well because it's in balance.

Other Ways to Deep Clean Your Baby House

> When women are having a hard time getting pregnant, it's
> generally because they're too contracted energetically—too yang,
> too tight. Too much dairy, too much meat, too much type A, too
> much do do do do do and not enough surrender and relaxation
> and green leafy vegetables and whole grains.
>
> —Angelica Kushi, holistic mentor and granddaughter of macrobiotic trailblazers
> Michio and Aveline Kushi, authors of *Macrobiotic Pregnancy and Care of the Newborn*

FIND SOME PEACE: STRESS AND THE BABY HOUSE

According to integrative gynecologist Katherine Thurer, stress is one of the biggest factors
in infertility. "It plays a huge role in the natural balance of the monthly cycle," she says.
"And if you're super stressed out, which most people in our society are, then that's a crucial
thing to address." Clinical Ayurvedic specialist Dr. Suzanne Gilberg-Lenz agrees and
estimates that 70 percent of her patients' complaints have at least some foundation in
stress.[152] The same building blocks our bodies use to make cortisol (the main stress
hormone) are what we need to make sex hormones like estrogen and testosterone. So if
you're running yourself ragged, your body is putting conception on the back burner.[153]

That said, what we carry around with us emotionally can take a brutal physical toll.
I took the question of stress and fertility to Randine Lewis, PhD, who is a healer and
fertility expert and the author of *The Way of the Fertile Soul*. Here's her wisdom:

> Twenty-first-century living is one of the foremost causes of infertility. We have
> more advances available to us than ever before, but as the ancients say, we have
> "lost our harmony with nature." Most women I work with (as I did myself) pursue
> a child as if it is a mental goal. Rarely is it successful, however, because when one is
> "in pursuit" of anything, the reproductive hormones take a backseat to the adrenal
> (stress) hormones, which block conception at multiple levels. A baby is not a goal—
> it is a process of becoming receptive. Allowing. That's why so many women finally
> succeed when they "let go." And as we age, the consequences of a stressful lifestyle
> are compounded. The adrenal glands divert the blood supply away from the ovaries
> and uterus and make the tissues unresponsive to the reproductive hormones.

To invite a softer flow into your life, try these prescriptions for peace:

Prioritize. Do you have any relationships that aren't fulfilling you? Is your job out of sync with who you are and what you want? What makes you feel most alive? Most feminine? "Use this as an opportunity to improve the life you're inviting your child into," Dr. Lewis says.

Let go of the effort. Channel the kind of receptivity that mirrors how our reproductive systems work. Forget eggs and sperm and ovulation for a minute and instead melt into the things that you most enjoy. "Treat yourself as you would a new child," says Dr. Lewis.

Dr. Gilberg-Lenz also reinforces the importance of relaxation and balance. She advocates hands-on therapies, such as massage, acupuncture, or Ayurvedic bodywork like Panchakarma therapy, to help you let go. She also loves when her patients meditate. As she says, "Decades of solid and widely reproduced data demonstrate how meditation lowers blood pressure, increases oxygen consumption, decreases stress hormones, and positively effects a multitude of health challenges from depression to heart disease."[154] To find a little more Zen harmony with super-simple exercises (seriously, you can do some of these in under a minute), check out the meditation section on page 79.

Get some exercise. Exercise doesn't mean having to run a marathon or spending hours (or any time, really) at the gym. It can be a fast-paced walk outside or a yoga class—something you enjoy that gets your blood pumping. A nice sweat does wonders for your heart and your circulation and your digestive system, and it gives your skin the most gorgeous glow. It's no surprise that, as part of the Nurses' Health Study, Harvard researchers saw that regular moderate exercise was correlated with higher fertility.[155]

Sometimes, I forget how powerful exercising is for relieving stress. Just think about those big, deep breaths that you take; it's like *whoosh!* You let go of all the stuff that will otherwise sit in your body if you don't get it out. If we don't do it, then we get stagnant. And stagnation breeds mosquitoes. So no matter how hard it is to sometimes get your butt in motion, get out there. You'll remember how sublime it feels.

INVIGORATE WITH A SCRUB DOWN

To give your body a boost while it cleans itself out, try this simple technique that magically refreshes your whole body while increasing circulation, opening pores to release toxins, and circulating lymph fluid. It gives you better energy for the whole day and then helps you settle down in the evening. Try it first thing when you wake up and again before bed.

Fill the sink with just enough hot water to dampen a washcloth. Remove the cloth from the water, wring it out, and—starting with your face—scrub yourself silly, moving

Other Ways to Deep Clean Your Baby House—*continued*

in the direction of the heart (up from the feet, down from the face), continually dunking and wringing out the washcloth as it cools off. Scrub your face, chest, pits, arms, and hands. Avoid your breasts and chichi, but do make sure to cover the entire groin area around your lady parts to stimulate the lymph nodes there. When the water in the sink gets cool, add a touch more hot. Instead of thinking about the day's to-do list while you scrub, use the time to send yourself the same compassion, love, and positivity you'll soon shower on your little one. The whole practice should take 5 to 8 minutes.

If you can't seem to find the time for this full-on scrub down, try a simple dry brush instead. Or use an exfoliating mitt, loofah, or washcloth without soap when you bathe.

GET YOUR BOX IN CHECK

Good female health starts with the period. A regular period is a sure indication that all your lady gears are working like they should. The more out of balance your plumbing—or according to macrobiotic wisdom, the more foods like meat and dairy you eat—the heavier and less regular your period will become. Conversely, when you clean out the baby house, you can expect more stable, shorter, lighter, and less crampy, cranky periods.[156] It's worth noting that when some women start cleaning up their diet, their period stops or becomes irregular. Don't worry, it'll come back, even better than before.

Another benefit of a predictable cycle is knowing when you're most fertile. It's a great way to get back in touch with your body's natural rhythms so you can relax into the baby love flow.

This super-simple three-part method is expertly outlined in Margaret Nofziger's *A Cooperative Method of Natural Birth Control,* which I highly recommend adding to your reading list. It's so empowering. Here's the basic idea:

- **Track your basal body temperature.** By taking this reading every morning and recording it (in a diary or using one of the very handy apps out there that'll keep track of it for you), you'll be able to see when your BBT peaks. These tiny tenths-of-a-degree spikes indicate when you're ovulating.
- **Chart cervical mucus.** Okay, so the idea of checking your own southbound mucus might sound strange. But don't feel squeamish about getting to know more about a very basic function that defines your baby-making abilities. Plus, if your goal is childbirth, bodily fluid should be low on your list of concerns. Checking your

mucus every morning for changes, along with tracking your temperature, is a straightforward way of knowing when you're most fertile.

■ **Put it all together.** After charting at least one go-round of your cycle, you'll have a much better idea of when you're about to ovulate, or are most fertile. You'll also know exactly when to have your partner save his swimmers and when to have him make a dash for your Grade A eggs.

Coming Off the Pill

If you think you have regular periods but have been on the Pill, think again. When you take birth control pills, you don't get a true period. It's what's called "withdrawal bleeding" caused by stopping the Pill each month for a few days.[157] Plus, taking the Pill can mask that there might be an underlying baby house problem in the first place. Here's what integrative gynecologist Dr. Thurer has to say about it:

"Some young women are put on the Pill when they're 15 for cramps, and they have no idea what their bodies would be doing otherwise. So issues that would have been addressed, especially with ovulation, aren't addressed until later in life. I tell patients that they should stop whatever form of hormonal birth control they're taking a whole year before starting to try to get pregnant because it gives the body more time to figure things out."

If you're just now going off the Pill, be extra mindful of your basal body temperature, since calendar and mucus cues can be slightly off for a few months.

Why Your Tampon Sucks (and We're Not Talking Absorbency)

Your sensitive, precious lady bits are not only the gateway to fertility and new life; they're also kind of like your body's front door. In fact, your chichi is the most absorbent part of your body.[158] Unfortunately, feminine-care manufacturers aren't required to tell you what's in their products, which means that no one's talking about the potential pesticide residues from nonorganic cotton and the "fragrances" containing hormone-upsetting, fertility-knocking phthalates that are snuggling up to your hoo-ha.[159] For a kinder period, choose a tampon or pad that's made with organic cotton or another unbleached and completely natural material. Or better yet, if you don't want your monthly discards to join the seven billion disposable tampons that we throw away every year[160] (it's estimated that those plastic applicators take anywhere from 300 to 500 years to break down![161]), try a reusable option like Lunapads (which I've been using for years and love), the DivaCup, or the Keeper.

> ## Mama to Mama on . . . Staying True to Your Path
>
> I've been a vegan for about 2 years (after reading *The Kind Diet*!) and am currently 35 weeks
> pregnant. But because I lost a lot of weight at the beginning of my pregnancy from severe
> morning sickness, I was naturally concerned about my baby's nutritional needs. I could also
> sense my parents and relatives were worried, and though they didn't really push me into eating
> meat, I still felt vulnerable enough to give in to trying some animal products for a week or two.
> However, I started getting pains in my hips and legs. It got to the point where I could hardly
> move or walk and became so unbearable that it finally convinced me to stop eating animal
> products for good. Within a week, I was completely pain free! Now I embrace my diet with
> confidence and am sure it will sustain me and my baby with perfect health.
>
> —Tomoko Abe, Kashiwashi, Chiba Prefecture, Japan

WHAT ABOUT THE PAPAS?

If you're doing all this work to clean yourself out, tune in to your intuition, and eat all kinds of yummy
kind foods, it raises a great question: What about the papas? I know there's a bit of a duh factor to this,
but the papas are as much a part of the fertility foundation as you are. In a third of all cases, the cause
of infertility can be traced to the father.[162] Even though deep down all papas know how important
they are, sometimes we need to nudge them to get involved—or at least point them in the right direction so they can start to see pregnancy, birth, and parenting through the same lens that we do. It can
be overwhelming, and we need to be gentle with our men, so I'm including sections just for them: "For
Gentlemen Only." Simply hand over the book to your partner, point to the sections, and say, "Read."*

He'll learn how he can get his body in the best shape for conception (nasty foods can wreak
all kinds of havoc on sperm), be your support system (and official back rub specialist) during
pregnancy and birth, and get in touch with his proud papa–ness.

BABY-MAKING REALITY CHECK

Even though I deeply believe that we can make baby making easier, I'm not promising one-and-
done success. Even when all your parts are doing what they're supposed to, conceiving can still
take time. According to Michael Roizen, MD, and Mehmet Oz, MD, the average person has a

---

*Plumbing-related issues aside, this information isn't just for dudes and dads. If you have a female partner, share it with her, too!

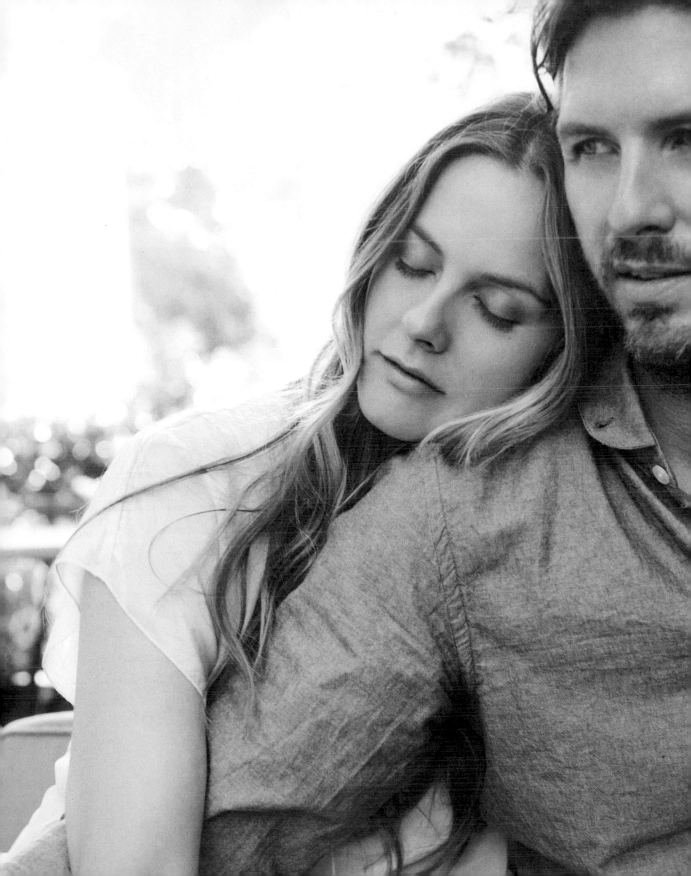

35 percent chance of getting pregnant within the first month of actively trying, an 80 percent chance of conceiving after 6 months, and a 90 percent chance within the first year.[163] But keep in mind that this stat includes some of the not-so-immaculate baby houses out there. As you've heard from the mamas sharing their stories here—including me!—eating a kind diet is like a baby magnet. And bringing in that fresh, clean energy means the whole affair will feel more like a breezy, gooey love fest than a scheduled project.

For Gentlemen Only: Getting Your Equipment in Shape

Whether you're on your way to becoming a daddy or trying to be, you'll benefit from a few Kind Mama insights, too. When you're eating plants, they get your blood flowing to all the right places. Your whole body surges with cell-throbbing, pulse-thumping virility and strength. And by not eating fatty, greasy meat that can clog major highways in your body—including the one in your pants[164]—you're getting the kind of bedroom superpowers that put little blue pills to shame. After a little kind loving, I promise you'll never look at kale the same way again.

But there's more to making babies than inserting part A into part B. Yeah, I'm talking about love and intimacy and all that, but at the end of the day, if you want to get pregnant, all the equipment needs to be in top shape. Right now, your partner is doing her best to get knocked up. The least you can do is give her the very best superpowered baby-making sperm you can. The way to do this is to look at how you're fueling. If your diet is high in meat and dairy-rich foods, soft drinks, sweets, and coffee, your swimmers may be more *Slackers* than *Superman*. Add in being overweight or a smoker, and you're drastically inhibiting your sperm production and the strength of those guys that do actually make the trip.[165] Take a look at the foods that I outline in this chapter as powerful, totally delicious alternatives. They're great not only for boosting your baby-making powers but also for fighting off illnesses like cancer and heart disease, which means a long, happy life of being a proud papa. If you want more information about how you can become a total rock star dad, check out this whole chapter, Dr. T. Colin Campbell's *The China Study,* John Joseph's *Meat Is for Pussies,* Rip Esselstyn's *Engine 2 Diet,* or *The Kind Diet* by yours truly.

Remember Love

A very groovy doula named Lisa Jacobson once shared an inspiring bit of wisdom about a better way to bring babies into our lives. She said that the Buddhists believe the way women get pregnant is when a soul has passed on and then looks for a loving relationship it wants to be part of. These spirits can see how connected the woman and her partner are, and how warm and intimate and gooey their relationship is. These babies-to-be don't want to cozy up with someone who's too busy or stressed or anxious. They want warmth and peace and gentleness. Isn't that what you'd want if you were a baby? So be sure you're making space for a baby to enter your life. Make your body and the body between you and your partner a place that a baby wants to call home.

Eat well, get healthy, then ditch all the planning and *trying* and just let it flow. There's no better way to make a baby than with yummy, soulful sex!

For More Information

For more great recipes, stats, and advice about getting kind, check out my first book, *The Kind Diet*, and my Web site, thekindlife.com. The Kind Life is a community where amazing mamas, mamas-to-be, and otherwise awesome ladies come together to share questions, discoveries, support, and inspiration. You can find posts and discussions on topics like living the green life, kind fashion, and healthy tips; my personal updates on life and being a mom; and best of all, recipes for delicious food.

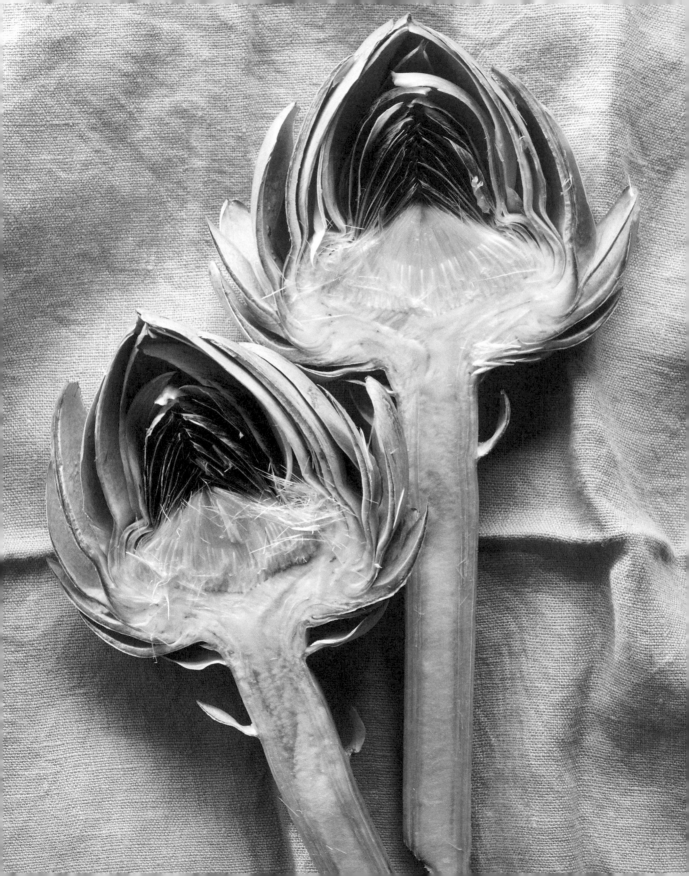

i'm pregnant!
now what?

A Trimester-by-Trimester Guide

6

First Trimester

Pregnancy defined is getting company inside one's skin.
—Maggie Scarf, author of *Intimate Partners*

Woo-hoo! You're having a baby! Don't you feel amazing? All right, so maybe you're actually feeling a little nauseated and food might be insanely unappealing and the second you sit down to tie your shoes you fall asleep—but I promise, you are *about* to feel amazing. Believe me when I say that in just a short while, we'll have you back to feeling like a goddess. In the meantime, embrace this new sluggish you. It's totally okay if life needs to go at a slower pace right now. After all, you're growing a whole new organ—the placenta, which will connect to your baby's house for the next 9 months—*from scratch*. On top of that, you're creating and nourishing an *actual human being*. Anyone in their right mind should celebrate you just for that, and you should, too.

So no matter how much you might want to puke now, remember that you are about to have a miraculous, beautiful journey. Once your body adjusts to its new tenant, you'll feel more vibrant and full of life than ever before. I'm going to show you the path that will make these next 9 months so incredibly delicious. Because you'll be giving your body everything it needs, it will be humming with health. You'll be able to stave off the icky things that are preventable and build a stronger foundation to sail through the things that aren't. And all that effervescent energy will be infusing the happiest, healthiest, shiniest, brightest little one. So let's get started!

WHAT YOU MIGHT BE FEELING

The Big Nauseous Box: Morning Sickness

Shortly after I conceived, I felt like I'd been hit by a giant truck of nauseous. Suddenly, all of my kind go-tos were gone. Veggies? No way. Beans? Gag. If I even *saw* a piece of brown rice, my stomach would turn. I was miserable—I couldn't eat, I couldn't go to yoga. I was working on a movie and shooting 15 hours a day, mainly at night, playing a vampire. So this took exhaustion and nausea to a whole new level. Any time I had away from work I would use to call my friends to ask, "*Why would you have another kid after going through this?!* Are you insane?!" I felt like everyone had kept this a secret from me! Okay, so I was being a little melodramatic. But there I was, extoller of all that is kind and leafy, and not interested in a single bite. I tried *everything*— cereal seemed grainy and fortifying, but then didn't sit well. Soup and toast did the trick, but then didn't. Peanut butter and jelly was good for a few days; OJ was okay for a minute. Ginger tea, mint tea, Sea-Band wristbands, juices, smoothies, acupuncture, crackers, even french fries. Nothing helped. But I gave my body permission to work out what it needed and took solace in the fact that everything I was going through was completely normal.

Morning sickness—though you may beg to differ—is not really sickness at all but rather your body adjusting to its rapidly changing condition. In fact, about 80 percent of pregnant women report feeling nauseated during some point of their pregnancy, and as many as 20 percent are too sick to work![1] While there's not a ton of insight as to why only some women experience this, according to Drs. Mehmet Oz and Michael Roizen, women who have more intense nausea throughout the day are less likely to miscarry than those who don't.[2] Or as my midwife said, the stronger the nausea, the stronger the pregnancy. And the Chinese medicine POV is that pregnancy is a stagnation of our energy. It's a beautiful stagnation but a pretty dramatic one that can throw off the body's balance. Studies have also shown that it can be our bodies' overcautious way of protecting the developing embryo.[3] And it's possible you can make your morning sickness *worse* by eating nasty foods such as meat, fish, poultry, eggs, fried and fatty treats, and coffee.[4]

There's a theory that the reason greens suddenly sound so barfy now is because it was once difficult to discern the good roughage from potentially poisonous plants in the wild. And it's also possible that our cravings for bland, dry, starchy food are designed to help relieve nausea.[5] (Not that it worked for me!) It's why some midwives call the first trimester "the beige period."

Luckily, morning sickness—or let's just be honest and call it all-day sickness—often disappears by your third month, though if you're like me, it can extend well into your sixth. But as much as I hated feeling crummy, I embraced my morning sickness. I liked to think that it was reassuring, like my body was telling me that everything was working exactly as it should. Or maybe it's humbling preparation for becoming a mother—a reminder that life is hard but also beautiful. And while we are powerful, there are larger forces at play in this universe.

Remember that one day you'll be able to eat all your favorite kind foods again. But in the meantime, here are some things you can try to get a little comfort. There's no one-size-fits-all solution, so keep experimenting until you find something that works. If you're not feeling the urge to eat, don't force it, though getting something in your stomach could make you feel better.

However, this is not the time to let yourself go. Giving in to an Oreo craving isn't going to help you feel good, it's not going to help you create a healthy baby, and it's not going to help you give birth. I'm not saying you can't make yourself feel a little better with some comforting yumminess, but make those treats as kind as possible. And if you fall off the wagon, don't beat yourself up. Just get right back on again. Here are a few things to help you through those first months:

Ginger tea: Ginger is a natural digestive aid and can soothe the stomach. Grate 2 teaspoons of peeled fresh ginger and add 1 cup of boiling water. Let the tea steep for 10 minutes before you drink it. It's nice plain, but if you want to sweeten it, add a few drops of stevia, brown rice syrup, or maple syrup.

Peppermint tea: Calming for the tummy and digestive system.

Sweet Vegetable Drink: This macrobiotic remedy settles nausea and combats cravings for sweets. See the recipe on page 296.

B-complex vitamins: Medical studies have shown that taking 25 milligrams of pyridoxine (vitamin B_6) every 8 hours for 3 days can bring significant relief from morning sickness.[6] You could try incorporating more of the foods that are

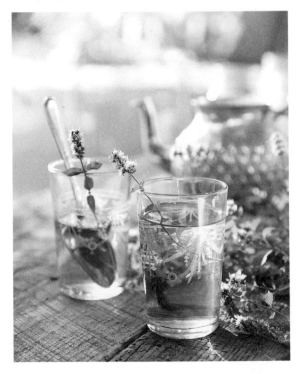

rich in this vitamin, like molasses, brown rice, wheat germ, bran, corn, or yellow bell peppers. A small spoonful of molasses stirred into your oatmeal in the morning is a tasty way to get B vitamins *and* iron, so you're already ahead of the game!

Soft-cooked rice or oatmeal: Some women find that porridge is calming for the stomach.

Mochi: Made out of pounded sweet rice—a fattier cousin of brown rice—this yummy, chewy treat puffs up like a waffle and can be fortifying while settling the stomach.

Umeboshi plums: Sucking on the pit of one of these sour pickles helps quell nausea and restores the appetite.

Gentle movement: Activity can ease morning sickness.[7] Be tender and patient with yourself, but try greeting each day with your usual chores and rituals instead of giving in to the nausea. Walks in the fresh air can also help.

Meditation: Morning sickness is more common in women under a lot of stress, which I can vouch for firsthand. Fifteen-hour days, shooting nights, *and* a baby? Hello, stress! I know it's hard sometimes, but try to take a little time to unplug—even if it's 15 seconds of deep belly breathing. See page 79 for more ways to Zen out.

Bigger (and More Tender) Pregnancy Boobs

As your breasts—or boobies, as we've come to call them in my house—make the transition from cute decoration to baby-feeding apparatus, they'll most likely start feeling a little tender. One tactic that may ease discomfort is cutting back on mushrooms. Even though these meaty, succulent fungi can be delicious, they may cause painful soreness and swelling in breast tissue.[8] Or feel free to get your freak on and ditch the bra. Embrace the new earth mama you!

WHAT YOU MIGHT BE WONDERING

What Are My Chances of Miscarriage?

There are so many women out there who have had miscarriages. Miscarriage is not at all uncommon. The American Pregnancy Association says 10 to 25 percent of all "clinically recognized" pregnancies will end in miscarriage, and that number is higher if you include very early pregnancies where women may not have even known they were expecting.[9] I know that doesn't necessarily make it easier if you do miscarry, but hopefully this insight from the experts will help you remember that it is normal and natural.

WHAT THE OB/GYN SAYS: Suzanne Gilberg-Lenz, MD

A vast majority of miscarriages occur because of some kind of chromosomal abnormality. It's nature's way of saying, "This embryo isn't healthy." Occasionally, hormonal imbalances need to be corrected, and things like thyroid problems, polycystic ovarian syndrome, and insulin resistance can increase risk. But most miscarriages happen because genetically the embryo isn't normal, not because you went on that trip or got in that fight or went running. As women, we want to explain this loss to ourselves. Blaming ourselves is usually the first thing we do. We want to be in control. But pregnancy is a big opportunity to realize that if you let go of the illusion that you can control everything, you'll have a better pregnancy, birth, and parenting experience. It's also important to note that if you've had one or more miscarriages, you should consult with a doctor to make sure there isn't something else going on that needs to be treated.

WHAT THE HEALER SAYS: Diane Avoli, macrobiotic counselor

The thing I see most often is that women's bodies and reproductive systems are just too weak to hold on to a pregnancy. Either they're taking in too much sugar and dairy, or they're going through some kind of trauma—medical, emotional, etc. It could even be the stress of someone who is exercising too much or working too hard or coping with the illness of a loved one. So either the body can't handle the birth or the baby itself is malformed in some way and the body naturally has to let it go.

WHAT THE MIDWIFE SAYS: Margo Kennedy

A majority of miscarriages are caused by something genetically wrong with the developing embryo. The body recognizes it and stops the pregnancy. I find that it's reassuring for people to know that the body knows what's right and takes care of it. It's completely out of our control, even though women always want to know what they did wrong. I like to remind women of how many different chromosomal combinations have to occur—and just right—for a pregnancy to be successful. It's pretty amazing that there are as many pregnancies as there are! Nonetheless, miscarriage is a quiet and lonely experience that women don't talk about. Once they experience it and bring it up, that's when they discover how common it is. I always encourage them to talk about their feelings and make sure their partners get to also. It's a grief they must go through, and time is their best friend.

Do I Need That Test? (Ultrasounds, Sonograms, and Blood Tests)

Modern medicine can offer a ton of tests nowadays, from screening for genetic diseases and Down syndrome to anatomy scans that can point to developmental problems. And that's on top of all the ultrasounds and sonograms that some doctors hand out at regular checkups like some kind of free-with-purchase prize. So what's really essential? And do you need all of the tests? Ultimately, this is an educated decision you should make with your trusted caregiver. There are different philosophies about whether these tests are safe and/or necessary. To make a decision that feels right for you, consider these points of view:

WHAT THE OB/GYN SAYS: Suzanne Gilberg-Lenz, MD

When it comes to prenatal testing, I see my role as an educator. I give the latest information on what testing is available and appropriate. I do this because patients can't make an informed decision without it, and I personally believe that that information should come from a trusted source. And by that I mean someone who knows the patient and her values.

I find it's best to be direct: I ask my patients what they hope to gain by doing this testing or not. Some people would never terminate a pregnancy for any reason, but they would still want advance notice so they could prepare for a special-needs child or maybe have a surgeon available at the birth to correct something treatable like a heart defect. Some genetic tests are for lethal anomalies, but some are for conditions that are easily treatable if we know in advance. So I try to help tailor the testing to my patients' views.

WHAT THE HEALER SAYS: Diane Avoli, macrobiotic counselor

Anything that's invasive to the body is going to affect the mother and child because it changes the flow of energy to the body. If a doctor puts a needle into your abdomen to get amniotic fluid, then that's definitely affecting the flow of energy. Unfortunately, many women are afraid to stand up for themselves and say, "This IS what I want; this is what I don't want." What you should ask yourself before having any test is, "What difference would the outcome make to me?" If you're going to carry the baby to term no matter what, then why put your body and baby through more stress?

It used to be that we'd only screen women over the age of 35, but things have changed and these tests are now typically offered to everyone. Most people don't know that they have the option to decline particular tests. I like to tell all my moms about the tests and explain the different components. But to me, the most important thing is what you're going to do with that information. Some couples are going to carry the child to term and take care of that child no matter what. In that case, they figure why go through with the screening? Why risk an amniocentesis or worry about false positives? Most of these tests are screening tools but not diagnostic, which means they can tell you that there's, say, a 1 in 600 chance that your baby has Down syndrome, but without an amniocentesis, they can't give you a diagnosis with more certainty than that. So if it wouldn't change your course of action, or it would only create nervous anxiety, then perhaps it's not worth it. However, there are some newer blood tests for women with increased risk of chromosomal abnormality. They are available privately and provide noninvasive testing with the use of cell-free fetal DNA.

I know not everyone will be on the same page on this issue, but ultimately you should do what feels best to you. I had three ultrasounds my entire pregnancy, and I wrestled with whether to have them. I mean, if a baby was supposed to be seen in utero, we could do it without all kinds of crazy machines, right? Something didn't feel right to me about the whole thing, so I chose to have as few as possible but still confirm that everything was healthy and normal. By the 5-month mark, Christopher begged me to have the third ultrasound so I'd stop asking him—half-kidding—if he thought the baby was alive. The relief that we got from that confirmation outweighed my concern that my little one wouldn't love having all those funky rays disturbing his home. But otherwise, I wanted to go with my gut and my heart and my knowledge that I was in the best of health, which made me believe that everything was okay.

Can I Have *Any* Alcohol?

The US surgeon general says that pregnant women should lay off the booze altogether. But what about the occasional glass of wine? There have been only a few clinical trials and long-range studies looking at moderate drinking during pregnancy,[10] and some of them have found that it might be okay. A recent study in the *Journal of Epidemiology and Community Health* reported no negative effects of drinking one glass of wine per week.[11] And a study out of Denmark found that low to moderate weekly drinking (one to eight drinks a week) had no effect on the brain development of the children of the participants, who were tested at 5 years old.[12] That said, American doctors are still skeptical about these findings.

I say before you channel your inner French girl and chill some rosé, keep one thing in mind: Western medicine can test quantifiable facts like how your baby is developing and whether he has a strong heartbeat, but it doesn't tell you about *true* health. Everything you eat and drink during the next 9 months is building your baby. Every single choice you make affects how that baby will grow and live for the rest of his or her life. While I'm no teetotaler—I'd take a teeny tiny sip out of a friend's glass if I was feeling frisky—I didn't want to grow my baby out of wine. Is wine a plant food? Sure. Is it health food? No. I wish it were! But it's not. I've never had a glass of wine and not felt the effects of it. I don't feel nourished and vibrant afterward, the way I'd feel after eating a healthy Kind Mama meal. So I chose to avoid alcohol during my pregnancy and for a long time after I had Bear, with the exception of the occasional sip, and never really missed it.

If you choose to have a glass of wine here or there, don't go thinking that it's some kind of medicine to prevent heart disease. (Seriously, it's not doing anything that all those other plants you're eating aren't already handling.) Let's call it what it is: party food, fun food. Don't beat yourself up over the occasional indulgence; just be present when making that choice. For a kinder, gentler buzz, choose a small amount of high-quality organic beer or sake (brown rice, if you can find it) over wine, and certainly over stronger spirits. Unlike wine, which is a fermented fruit and has a lot of unbalancing sugar, beer and sake are fermented grains. But the same moderation and mindfulness are still key.

Which Beauty Treatments and Products Are Safe?

Cleaning house isn't just about getting your insides in order; it includes your outside, too. Your skin is an organ! And it's a biggie—it can absorb as much as 60 percent of what we put on it.[13] Unfortunately, a skimpy 11 percent of the 10,500 chemical ingredients floating around out there in our shampoos, conditioners, nail polishes, scrubs, masks, lotions, perfumes, etc., have been tested for safety by a publicly accountable agency,[14] and many are less than ideal.

Luckily, it's easy to spot nasty chemicals lurking in your beauty standbys and to replace those products with kinder ones. Plus, thanks to your amazing diet—and a boost from pregnancy hormones—you won't need much more than Mother Nature. You'll have more luminous, delicious skin and longer, silkier locks than any bottle could give you.

When going through your cabinet, keep an eye out for these major offenders:

Parabens: These are the most popular synthetic preservatives in products like shampoos, makeup, lotions, scrubs, and deodorants[15] and are estimated to be in 75 to 90 percent of all products on the market.[16] Studies have shown that parabens mimic estrogen, which can interfere with the functioning of our own natural hormones. They can be listed as methyl/ethyl/butyl/isobutyl/propyl paraben or variations including those prefixes, hydroxybenzoic acid, hydroxybenzoate, or ester.

Phthalates (pronounced *thal-ates*): These chemical compounds are used in many conventional beauty products—nail polish, hair spray, eyelash glue, lotion, perfume, cosmetics. Pretty much everything that has a scent.[17] They're a class of chemicals that include suspected carcinogens and known hormone disruptors and that can interfere with fetal development, especially in our little boys. Phthalates have been shown to mess with the development of their genitalia[18] and have links to other problems like autism spectrum disorders,[19] testicular cancer, and lowered sperm counts.[20] They can be listed as DBP, DEHP, DMP, DEP, with variations like dibutyl/diethyl ester, or 1,2-benzenedicarboxylate. Or they can be disguised simply as "fragrance," so you'll want to choose products that are labeled "fragrance free" or that are scented only with essential oils. (Just keep in mind that some oils can still be allergens, so if you or your little one has a reaction to a product you're using, know that the oil could be the culprit.)

If you're totally overwhelmed by the alphabet soup on the back of your beauty products, go to thekindlife.com and search for my list of favorite yummy, natural products.

Other nasties to watch out for include:

Hair dye: While some studies have shown no detrimental effect to a fetus if a mother dyes her hair during pregnancy, a 2005 examination found a link between women who used hair dye and neuroblastoma, a rare childhood cancer, in their offspring.[21] But largely the jury is out. Because it's not crystal clear if getting a touch-up can be risky, it's safest to at least wait until the end of your first trimester, when your baby isn't quite so vulnerable.

Ideally, though, you should try to hold off until you're done growing your tiny babe, and even until you're done breastfeeding. If you absolutely must get those roots or that gray attended to, choose natural, vegetable-based dyes versus conventional ones made with nasty junk like lead acetate, coal tar dyes, and heavy metals.[22] Be sure to read packages and ingredients lists, because even those colorings labeled "natural" can still contain questionable ingredients along with plant-based ones. Also, the less the dye comes into contact with your scalp—which is skin!—the better.

Electrolysis: Your bikini area is essentially your baby house's front porch, and we don't know for sure how the electric current from electrolysis can affect your baby. For that reason, many health care providers recommend skipping that electrolysis during pregnancy.[23] Plus, any zapping or waxing in this area can be super-painful because it's more sensitive during pregnancy. If that's the case, try embracing a more natural downtown—your chichi might enjoy the break!

Synthetic vitamin A and retinols: Studies have shown that excess synthetic vitamin A from animal-derived sources, also called retinol, can be harmful to babies and has been linked to things like facial and palate abnormalities, heart defects, nervous system anomalies, and cleft lip in fetuses.[24] Though Retin-A is the only topical form that's been linked to severe birth defects,[25] it's certainly better to be safe than sorry when it comes to your beauty regimen. Even if that retinol-containing product was your miracle skin cure for years, you should hands-down stop using it while you're pregnant . . . and forever, while you're at it.

Am I Frying My Baby? (Computers, Cell Phones, Appliances, and EMFs)

I've always had a weird feeling about technological devices like my laptop and cell phone and whether all those EMFs (electromagnetic fields) were scrambling up my insides. Especially after I got pregnant, I'd think, *Oh, my God—my laptop is sitting right on top of my pelvis . . . and it's hot.* My friend Woody said he put a lizard from the garden on his laptop because the little guy loved the warmth. But he came back later and the lizard was dead! It made me take a closer look at EMFs—which are created through our energy use and are emitted by outlets, appliances, and electronic gadgets—and their effect on our health. It turns out that more and more experts are suspecting our out-of-control device dependency is linked to some serious issues.

According to Devra Davis, PhD, president of the Environmental Health Trust, emerging evidence is raising "significant questions" about these health risks.[26] In 2007, the Bioinitiative Working Group released a report citing more than 2,000 studies that detail just how toxic EMFs can be. They concluded that chronic exposure can cause a variety of cancers, impair immunity, and contribute to Alzheimer's disease, dementia, and heart disease.[27] In May 2011, an expert committee of the International Agency for Research on Cancer of the World Health Organization classified cell phone radiation as potentially carcinogenic to humans.[28] And studies from Yale School of Medicine and the UCLA School of Public Health have raised concerns that exposure to cell phone radiation during pregnancy could be linked with developmental and behavioral problems.[29]

The conclusion I've come to—as backed up by EMF expert Marilee Nelson—is that being intuitive and mindful about how much you're using your devices is essential.

Here are a few handy tips from Nelson for cutting down on your EMF exposure:

- Use a desk when working on a laptop instead of keeping it on your lap. Better yet, use a separate plug-in keyboard and mouse so you're not resting your hands on the laptop. Save recharging for when you're not using it.

- Whenever possible, use a landline instead of your cell phone. Opt for the good old-fashioned plug-in models instead of a cordless, which is the same as being on a cell, EMF-wise. If you're out and about, use an air tube earphone with your cell, a metalless earpiece that helps deflect harmful frequencies from your brain. Texting and using regular earbuds or speakerphone are also better options than holding that thing right up to your head. Keep in mind, too, that your phone is still receiving signals even if you're not actively using it. So stash it in your bag rather than your pocket.

- At night before bed, unplug all electric devices and disable your Wi-Fi router. Your body heals and restores itself while you sleep, but these frequencies can inhibit it from doing all the work it needs to accomplish. Creating an EMF-free zone during the night means you'll wake up feeling fresher, better rested, and best of all, healthier. You can also turn off the Wi-Fi on your computer and switch your cell to the "airplane" or "off-line" mode.

- Get grounded: Walking outside barefoot in the grass, dirt, or wet sand is the ultimate recharge for your body. Some studies have even connected grounding, or "earthing," with balancing the nervous system, improving inflammation, and relieving stress.[30] Whenever you can, spend a few minutes letting your toes soak up that powerful goodness.

KIND ACTION

Get Some Rest

I know how hard it can be to take time away from what seems most important, things like work, e-mail, phone calls, appointments, so on. But if you're going to give your body exactly what it needs over the next 9 months, you have to get some rest. Right now, every single one of your organs, bones, and tissues is scrambling to keep up with all the changes in your system. Give yourself permission to take it easy. It's nature's will! If you have the luxury to lie around and daydream all day, do it. Meditate, journal, nap, garden, breathe into your belly, take a bath—do whatever it takes to feel nurtured.

You might be tempted to think that feeling a little sluggish means there's something wrong with your diet. But if you continue to eat well, what you're experiencing is completely normal.

To help boost your energy during the day, get your circulation going with gentle movement like stretching or walking, and be sure you're drinking enough water. Try to keep travel to a minimum. Distance yourself from anything or anyone who zaps your energy. See if you can cut back on your hours at work. You need rest and joy more than money. I know there's pressure to earn a living, but what about living your life? I realize that you can't pay bills with hopes and dreams, but I want you to dig really, really deep and ask yourself if the additional stress of your job is truly worth it. And if it is absolutely necessary or you are head-over-heels in love with what you do, then at least try to be mindful of the fact that you can't continually work 12 hours a day and expect your body to do what it needs to do. It needs all the love and attention it can get. Chronic stress depletes your immune system, and right now your priority is to preserve your vitality so that you and your body are up for the rest of this amazing, crazy ride.

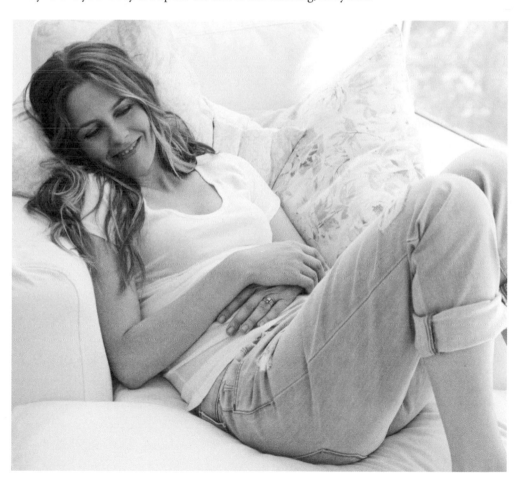

Set Your Intentions

To create a strong foundation as a Kind Mama, it's important to reconnect with why you're on this journey in the first place. Getting clear on why and how you want to parent is essential for raising your baby in the most loving, substantial, and purposeful way possible.

ASK YOURSELF WHY YOU WANT TO BE A MOM

I've always wanted to have a baby. My mom would tell me about how when I was as young as 2, I would carry around other little ones, saying, "My baby! My baby!" Once I had Bear in my arms, I said, "You are going to feel loved so deeply that you'll feel it in your skin, in your tummy, in your toes. You are going to feel comfortable and safe and supported when you're with me, and when you go out into the world, you will do it with confidence and ease. You can trust me, baby. Because I see you. I see your heart and your soul and your magical elf-angel self. And what you need matters to me."

To me, that seemed like fundamental care that every child should have and any parent should feel honored to give. Reflecting on what your needs were as a child and whether they were met can inform your actions going forward. Did you feel heard, seen, validated, loved? How did your parents help you feel that way? And if you didn't feel any of those things, what might you do differently? What do you want to protect her from, and how will you protect her?

IF APPROPRIATE, SEEK COUNSELING

The same way you need to actively heal your body with nourishing foods, your emotions also need TLC—especially if not all is at peace when it comes to your relationship, your family, etc. While I think you'll be pleasantly surprised at how calm and clear you'll feel after cleaning out your body, getting some quality sleep, and channeling your thoughts through journaling and/or meditating, we all benefit from learning and growing, and therapy can be a wonderful way to do that. It doesn't mean there's something wrong with you; counseling is just another way to reach way down inside and create the best version of yourself.

Now more than ever, it's crucial that you get in touch with your truth—what you need and want in your life—so you have the tools to cope with the things you don't love and to reach for the things you do—like having more exciting sexy time with your partner or conquering anxiety. This will not only make you happier in the long run, but it will make you a better parent. If you and/or your partner aren't in a good place, that's going to manifest in how you're able to care for your child. So think of this work as putting down strong roots the way big, tall trees plant themselves deeply in the soil. The sturdier your foundation, the better you can support your family. I highly recommend checking out two books that I found helpful a long time ago. *Finding Your Own North Star,* by Martha Beck, and *Organizing from the Inside Out,* by Julie Morgenstern, are great inspirations for living life the way you truly want to live it, or at least getting pretty darn close.

Meditate

One of the best ways to channel your intentions is through a meditation practice. The more connected you are to your body and your breath, the more you can tune in to your truest self. Meditation doesn't necessarily have to be an all-out affair with incense and candles. It's any practice that allows you to be completely present. It can be washing the dishes, taking a shower, or vacuuming the house. So long as you are mindful and contemplative and watching your breath and the moment instead of the day's agenda, it counts as meditation. But now and then, I also like to set aside special time to fully submit to mindfulness exercise. Here are a few of my favorite techniques:

ENERGY BALANCE

Close your eyes and begin to breathe deeply from your belly. Visualize sending a grounding anchor deep into the earth. As your anchor drops, imagine the earth's warm, strong energy grounding your body. Then extend your awareness up to the sky and let that energy bring you into your heart. Savor these sensations for a few breaths.

When you feel complete, bring your thoughts back to your body and sit until you're ready to resume your day. Try to hold on to that feeling of anchoring and connectedness.

QUICKIE CALM

Close your eyes and notice your breath. Don't try to change it, just watch what it's doing. If you notice you're holding your breath, let it out. By opening your mouth a tad wider than what feels normal, your jaw will release and your tummy can make room for more breath to fill it. Let yourself completely relax and breathe naturally, waiting until you have an impulse to inhale and then allowing breath to come in and out. Inhabit this lovely, present space for as long as you can, doing nothing but breathing and observing. Congratulations—you just meditated! If you can go for 10 minutes, great. But just 1 minute or even 30 seconds a day is certainly better than nothing.

For a little peace on the go, pay more attention to how you're breathing throughout the day. It's a trippy thing, but most of us don't open our mouths when we breathe. When you relax your jaw, though, breath comes into the body in a much deeper way.

HYPNOSIS

Hypnotherapy can be truly life-changing work, and I highly recommend it. It's particularly helpful for post-traumatic stress (or stress in general), insomnia, fears, and phobias. It's a powerful way to reset the little tape recorder in your brain that plays negative messages over and over. Hypnosis helps replace those nasty thoughts with new, positive ideas while allowing you to kick any of your bad habits. It's loving and healing and all-around wonderful. Check out Ida Kendall's Web site at idakendallswordsofwonder.vpweb.com for her CDs. She has the most soothing voice in the world!

JOURNALING

Another way I calm my mind is by writing down my thoughts. Instead of letting my fears, worries, and hang-ups slosh around in my head, I channel them onto paper. That way, I can get a little distance and ask myself things like, "What's really the problem?" or "What do I really want?" We all have inner gurus who are sometimes the wisest guides of all, and journaling helps them be heard. A brain imaging study by UCLA psychologists showed that when we put our feelings into words, it can make negative emotions feel less intense.[31]

Start a Movement Practice

Exercise is super-important for a healthy pregnancy and natural birth. But that doesn't mean crazy sweat sessions at the gym—though the American College of Obstetricians and Gynecologists confirms that it's generally safe to participate in a wide range of activities.[32] The rule of thumb is to not do something that you haven't already been doing. So if you weren't a sprinter before you got pregnant, don't start sprinting now. If you loved cycling, yoga, or martial arts before baby, then feel free to keep it up. Just make sure you're talking to your instructors and caregiver so they can guide you away from any exercises or movements that can be potentially risky.

What's most essential, though, is listening to your body. If you're exhausted, honor that. Maybe just go for a gentle walk or lie in bed and hug a pillow. Or if something doesn't feel good, don't do it! Your body will be going through so many changes—your ligaments and joints are loosening to help your pelvis become more flexible for birth, your growing belly will be changing your center of gravity, and the extra weight means your body will be working harder to carry you around. If there's one gift that pregnancy gives you, it's the lesson of how to be gentle and kind to yourself in normal life, too. We should always treat ourselves as nicely as we do during pregnancy!

DAILY WALKS

I stayed active through my pregnancy by walking some 3 miles a day, which my friend Lalayna couldn't recommend enough. She and our midwife swore that it was her walking regimen that made her pregnancy and birth experience so smooth. She said the key was getting out there and walking as though she were training for a marathon—the marathon of birth! Depending on how I was feeling, I would either take a charged-up hike through the hills or a more leisurely paced path through my neighborhood.

For company, walk your rescued dog, meet your friends, or ask your husband or partner to take you. Or better yet, use walking as an opportunity to soak up as much alone time as possible. Because once that baby's born, spending just a few minutes with your own thoughts becomes a precious commodity. The fresh air and view of sky and trees will do wonders for calming your spirit, fill you and your baby with lots of much-needed oxygen, and help get the baby into the right place for delivery, which is crucial for a natural birth.

PRENATAL YOGA

When I finally got to a prenatal yoga class, it was like coming home again. This gentle practice can sometimes help with morning sickness and connect you more deeply with your body. It slows down your brain waves so you can escape from the chatter in your mind, and it helps you tap into your deepest intuition. It's empowering, humbling, and strengthening—in its way, a preparation for birth. You don't have to be able to touch your toes or even your knees—but it's a way to *practice* opening up and finding space in your body. It helps you walk taller, feel better, and clear out all the cobwebs, physically and emotionally. All I can say is please go at least once.

STAY STRONG

Even though now isn't the time to be getting super-buff, it's important that you find *something* you like to do to keep your muscles strong. Light resistance training, yoga, and other simple exercises can help muscle maintenance, which in turn can keep your metabolism stoked, eat up surplus blood sugar,[33] and get you prepared for not only labor but all the lifting, carrying, swinging, and snuggling that come afterward.

Protect Yourself from Naysayers

I've said it before, but it bears repeating: There are going to be people—well meaning and otherwise—who will want to butt in, ask snoopy questions, and bring negativity where it's not welcome. I've found the best way to deal with naysayers, as hard as it can be, is *not* to engage. Most of those people aren't looking to have a calm, educated, two-sided conversation. Trying to extol the virtues of eating plants and all other choices regarding your baby, sharing even the most mind-blowing statistics will only waste your energy if the person on the other end isn't open and receptive. And that energy is already at a premium. It helped me to think of it as practice for protecting my baby. Here are great ways to deflect the doubters:

FOR THE GENUINELY CONCERNED BUT CLEARLY UNINFORMED

Refer the interested party to any one of the resources mentioned in this book and say, "Here are books I recommend you read about how we've chosen to parent and why. We'd love to discuss them at any time." We did this with my mother-in-law, and she was completely blown away. The information itself was far more powerful than my trying to play social scientist. And we were blown away by her positive response.

FOR THE UNSOLICITED ADVISOR

Listen, nod, and keep your mouth shut (nearly impossible for me!). Breathe deeply and when the verbal drive-by is over, simply say, "Thank you for sharing your opinion." Promptly walk away.

FOR THE PERSISTENT CYNIC

Put your feelings on paper. You'll be able to express yourself calmly and rationally without having to worry about being heard. Try something like this: "Thank you for your concern about our child's well-being. We've gone to great lengths to ensure that he/she is cared for and nourished in every way, and that all his/her needs will be attended to. Our beliefs are supported by reliable research, which we invite you to explore. I've included some recommendations for books that helped inform our choices. I think you'll find that we're all on the same page for wanting the

Mama to Mama on . . . Handling the Skeptics

Because I hadn't gained a lot of weight early on, my husband, doctor, and friends all tried convincing me to "eat some eggs" to beef up my protein intake. I begrudgingly acquiesced, but it made me feel so miserable. Luckily, I had science on my side. I knew I could get appropriate levels of fat and protein from plant-based sources. But it was hard to convince concerned loved ones that it wasn't about the number on the scale, rather the whole picture of health: rate of fetal growth, fetal activity, my blood levels—all of which looked good. I asked for time. I asked for patience. I asked them to read! After a while, they understood that I was actually very, very healthy, and my doctor defended me tooth and nail on that point! And they also realized that I wasn't just doing this to be stubborn; rather, I was doing it for the health of my sweet, unborn baby and for myself. I'm so glad I stuck to my guns on this one. Though I didn't gain much weight, my baby did—when she was born at 39 weeks, she weighed a healthy 7.49 pounds and had a magnificently strong cry. I know I made the right call.

—Krissy MacQueen, Sherman Oaks, California

My family supported me but was still concerned about my baby being too small and not getting enough nutrients. He was born a healthy 9.9 pounds and is now a thriving 16-month-old vegan. Not enough protein? I don't think so! I felt amazing throughout my 9 months of pregnancy, and with each blood test and ultrasound, my doctors began to realize how my diet was only affecting my son positively. Oh, and did I mention how quickly I lost the baby weight? Another bonus! I know that by following *The Kind Diet,* I prepared my body to be the ultimate home for a growing baby.

—Jessica Royston, Waldwick, New Jersey

I think most people knew not to give me a hard time about being vegan during my pregnancy. I was fit, joyful, and visibly thriving. My mother-in-law had friends who expressed their concern about my being vegan, but she stood by me, declaring her trust in my choices. Even today, she quells her naysaying friends by telling them that Olivia is the healthiest person she knows. At 6 years old, she's never had an antibiotic or an earache, rarely gets colds, and eats more vegetables and healthy foods than most adults!

—Allison Rivers Samson, Nevada City, California

happiest, healthiest baby possible." Referring cynics to this book is a great start. Also check out the Resources section on page 332 for books on topics that might be of particular concern.

FOR THE HORROR-STORY PEDDLER

Every woman deserves to tell her birth story—even if it's someone who had her baby ages ago. It's a deep, primal thing to want to share. That said, sometimes women overstep the bounds of what's helpful and what's downright scary. Try to take these terrible tales with a grain of salt. Most naysayers really do think that they're offering you valuable advice. Breathe, give them the benefit of the doubt, then end the conversation as quickly as possible.

Build Your Tribe: Find a Group of Like-Minded Women Who Can Support You

Before mommy groups and pregnancy books existed, women learned how to become mamas from other women. You would watch fellow tribe members carry, birth, and parent their babies. If you needed help, the tribe was there to lend a hand. Nowadays, most of us don't have a tribe. We live in our own homes with only our partner (maybe), sometimes across the country from our parents, and are lucky if we even say hello to the neighbors. But when we lost our tribes, we also lost the support system that was so key in helping mothers stay strong and sane while raising their babies. Having other women to turn to was considered normal, not trying to go at it alone.

Now that you're about to become a mama and start a little tribe of your own, it's crucial to surround yourself with people you really like and, more important, trust. My mama tribe is made up of women who I consider to be my wisest confidantes. I admired the way they birthed and raised their own children, so I knew I could rely on them to help me with mine. They're the ladies I can e-mail day or night with any number of crazy questions and end up the next day with an inbox full of helpful responses—or, in one case, a mailbox full of lifesaving boobie pads. They helped me with their generous insight through my pregnancy and once I gave birth.

How do you know whether you want someone to be a member of your tribe? Once you have an idea of the path you aspire to, think about the people in your life who will be able to relate. Is there someone whose pregnancy experience you admire? Do you love the way someone is with her kids? Know someone who keeps herself healthy with a clean diet (and maybe whips up amazing healthy, kind treats)? Those are definitely tribe-material mamas.

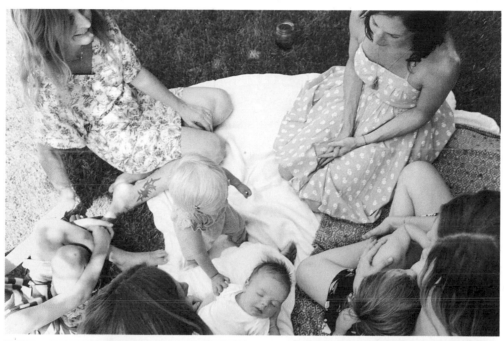

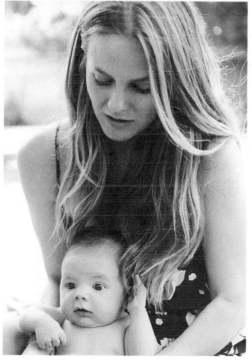

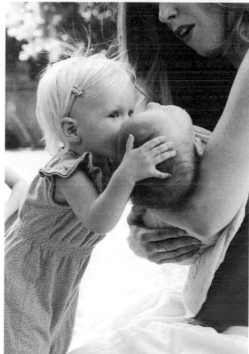

For Gentlemen Only: Becoming Big Papa

Look at your partner's belly. It might not be big and round just yet, but there, below her belly button, is your very own son- or daughter-to-be. Right now you are a daddy. Not in a few months, not after the baby is born, but *right now.*

So, in the time before your baby gets here, think about how amazing being a papa is going to be. Think about the unique way that only you can show your son or daughter the world, and how confident and secure you're going to make him or her feel simply by giving all the love you have. Ask yourself, *What didn't I get from my parents growing up that I wish I had?* Or *What did my parents do that was so special?* Then get clear on how you want to be there for your kid.

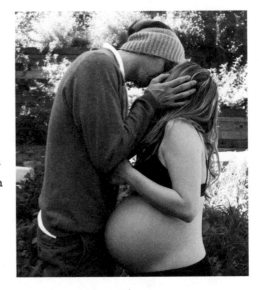

Your partner will definitely feel the power of that, too. Seeing my man holding our baby is such a turn-on. He's so grounded and in his power with his child, and to us mamas, that's just so sexy.

Wow, do I love being a father. Seeing my boy smile, play, and laugh is just the greatest thing in the world. Our boy is a traveling man. He wants me to keep movin' so he can see the world. I can't wait to start playing sports and games with him. I can't wait to teach him all kinds of things . . . . I can't wait to bore him with my stories of how Daddy used to be in a band. When I carry him around, I feel so grounded and wonderful. I love taking him places with me in my sling. And when my head hits the pillow at night, I'm usually exhausted. But to be exhausted over something you love to do is one of the great feelings in life.

—Christopher

You don't have to be related to your tribe member, and they don't even have to live nearby. My tribe is a mix—I have my virtual tribe of mamas who live in all different places and support me through e-mail and phone calls, and then I have friends with babies whom I like to hang out with. They parent in all different ways, but they're smart and fun and always there to lend a hand when needed. You can, of course, turn to your family, as well as to healers, neighbors, yoga instructors, even your midwife and doula. You can also include me! I'm here to help you and to give you strength so you can be confident in your choices. If at any moment on this journey you feel uncomfortable or sad or weird because you're the only one you know doing things in such a groovy way, then use this book as a reminder of why you're taking this path—and that you're not the only one! And definitely check out my Web site, the Kind Life (thekindlife.com), to connect with other mamas who are doing things the kind way.

7

The Case for Kind Birth:

Why Natural Birth Is Normal, Healthy, and Beautiful in Every Way

Having a medicated birth is like going to the Grand Canyon with a blindfold on. You were there, but you missed the majesty.
—Anonymous

Giving birth has an amazing way of connecting us not only with all the mamas who have ever given birth on this planet but also with all the bears, wolves, lions, tigers, and other mammalian mamas who have brought their babies into this world. Regardless of the fancy technology and mind-boggling science we've developed over the past hundreds of years, giving birth is still at its core an act of pure animal impulse. I don't just mean how we give birth, either. When and where are just as big a part of our body's innate instincts. Honoring this age-old wisdom, along with some helpful advance planning, can make your birth the miraculous, transcendent, life-changing experience it's meant to be.

Now is the time to start thinking about how you'll choose to bring your baby into the world. That's right, *choose*. Giving birth doesn't have to be what you see on TV. It doesn't have to be scary or horrible. It doesn't have to be full of machines, IVs, or doctors passing out drugs like it's happy hour, and it certainly doesn't have to be in a hospital. What if I told you that giving birth can be empowering? That you could feel strong, beautiful, and completely tuned in to your body? That you could give birth in a soothing space that's quiet and soft and feels completely your own? Did you know that you can do yoga during parts of labor? Walk around outside to get some fresh air? Swim in a warm, soothing tub? Maybe even lie in that warm, cozy tub with your partner while someone else rubs your feet or temples or shoulders or administers calming acupuncture or aromatherapy? And because you'd be working with a health care practitioner who has a deep understanding of you, your body, and what you're both capable of doing, you'll feel relaxed and safe with total ownership over this experience. You'd be completely prepared and supported to take on what women have been doing since pretty much the beginning of time in caves, mud huts, forests, and fields. They've had beautiful baby after beautiful, healthy baby because that's what their bodies were built to do. And guess what? Yours is, too.

This isn't some New Age fantasy, and it's not some newfangled way we hippies are trying to recruit new members. This isn't yogalates. This is old-school stuff! It's the way birth used to be—a magical, Mother Nature–given experience that hasn't changed physiologically in 200,000 years! And you have every right to honor that. Choosing how your baby comes into the world is sacred. It should be a decision made with love and confidence and trust, not fear or resignation to "This is just the way things are." This experience is way too important!

YOUR KIND BIRTH: HOW TO BUILD A PLAN THAT'S RIGHT FOR YOU

Regardless of how, where, and with whom you ultimately decide to have your baby, a kind birth is one that's in line with your deepest convictions. It's built on the faith that you're in a safe, secure space and that you can completely surrender to your labor. It's free of unnecessary interventions that interfere with your body's innate abilities. It is about feeling strong and capable because this experience is wholly and completely your own. Kind birth is the first step toward becoming a compassionate mother and a confident parent. Kind birth is powerful. Kind birth is your right. Don't let anyone take that away from you.

How do you shape the experience that you want? You begin by understanding the two different models of care during childbirth. The first is the medical model, where labor is usually treated like an emergency and technological interventions lie at every turn. But there is nothing wrong with you when you give birth. It's the exact opposite—everything's *right*. The second model—the holistic path—reflects that rightness in its philosophy. You aren't considered a patient; instead, you are a participant. You are the ultimate authority on your well-being, not your caregiver. Your care is based on education, empowerment, and the trust that you are also doing your part to keep yourself healthy and strong. And when it's time to give birth, you'll be in an environment that truly allows you to perform the most natural, obvious, godly miracle on the planet. How groovy is that?! And if you're wondering how you can get in on all of this, I'll tell you.

Bringing Birth Home

If you were living with your tribe, you would most likely start feeling the surges of labor at night. Like any other mammal, you'd make your way to a dark, quiet, safe place where you wouldn't be interrupted. And then, using the power nature gave you, you'd labor until your baby was born. I'm not suggesting you go out to your backyard and deliver your own baby. But there is a very real reason why women historically gave birth where they felt most comfortable and safe. It's an instinct that Mother Nature gave us because, ultimately, she wants us to survive! Call it greedy, but it is in her best interest for our species to continue to multiply and thrive. And it's why—if we had to—many of us could very well head out back, pop a squat, and bring our babies into this world with our own two hands. Women all over the world do it all the time. In fact, a friend of mine did just that. Am I advocating that? No. Did I do that? No. But let it illustrate that most of us are perfectly capable of having babies without medical intervention.

I know the idea of home birth sometimes makes people nervous. *Why risk it?* is the most common thing I hear. *It's reckless*, they say, or, worst of all, *It's selfish*. And yet I made the decision to give birth at home *because* I care so adamantly about my child's health and well-being and safety. I chose to have a home birth because to me, nothing about a hospital sounds safe or like a natural place where a baby was meant to be born. The only time I'd choose to go to a hospital is if there were some kind of emergency, like if my appendix burst or my arm was broken. And to me, birth isn't an emergency. It's a miracle! I wouldn't go to the hospital if I were simply sick, because chances are a doctor there would send me away with a prescription for pills instead of asking me about my lifestyle and getting to the root of the problem. So if I wouldn't trust my own health to a hospital, why then would I trust this most fundamental goddess-given right to one? I'm not alone, either. According to the Centers for Disease Control and Prevention, the number of women in this country choosing home birth has jumped 50 percent between 2004 and 2011![34]

To understand what makes home birth so divine, let's first take a look at the alternative. These days, 99 percent of women in the United States give birth in a hospital.[35] But according to the 2013 edition of the *State of the World's Mothers* report, out of 186 countries, American maternal health only rates 46th.[36] In fact, our maternal mortality rate is among the highest of any industrialized nation.[37] Are you hearing me on this?! A woman in the States is 10 times more likely than one in Estonia, Greece, or Singapore to die from pregnancy-related causes.[38] In fact, according to a 2010 report by the United Nations, American women today face at least double the chance of dying from pregnancy or birth-related complications than their mothers did.[39] And yet the CDC estimates that more than half of the maternal deaths that occur every year could be prevented.[40] What's going on here?

If you give birth in a hospital, your experience may look something like this: For starters, you'll be hooked up to a fetal monitor, so you won't be able to stand up and move around as easily, which would otherwise help you dilate more quickly and get the baby into a beneficial position for birth. And according to the American College of Obstetricians and Gynecologists, being constantly monitored can lead to a high rate of false positives for fetal distress, causing doctors to call for unwarranted cesareans.[41]

Another obstacle is that you most likely won't be eating or drinking, except for perhaps clear liquids. Standard practice prohibits food and beverages because, whether or not you are high risk, doctors prefer your stomach to be empty in case you'll need anesthesia for a C-section. But dehydration can cause painful contractions that are close together and create no progress.[42] And because birth requires that you be well fed and strong (it's called labor for a reason!), not having any fortifying food during early labor may leave you without enough calories to meet the physical demands of active labor. You'll start burning fat reserves, which can change the acidity in your blood, which can then lead to ketoacidosis. Your blood becomes more acidic and carries less oxygen, which can cause fetal distress and also make your uterus less efficient.[43] The first intervention your doctor or nurse might offer is an IV with some nutrients. That might resolve the ketoacidosis, but now you have a needle in your arm, which means much more restricted movement and, in turn, slows contractions. That means you might not progress quickly enough (which isn't dictated by biological need as much as a hospital's need), so you'll be hooked up with some Pitocin, which is synthetic oxytocin that can lead to particularly fast and hard contractions. (In May 2013, the American College of Obstetricians and Gynecologists conceded that the drug may not be as safe as previously believed, thanks to new research illustrating that Pitocin may be a risk factor for babies being admitted to the NICU and having lower Apgar scores.[44]) At this point, you might start craving those tasty-sounding pain meds. So now you'll get an epidural. After an anesthesiologist has jabbed your spine with a ginormous needle, you'll probably be feeling pretty good. That is, until your blood pressure takes a nosedive, a possible side effect that occurs in a fifth of women,[45] which can cut off oxygen to your baby and lead to a C-section. Or it might dull your contractions or stall labor, so you'll need even more Pitocin. At this point, you may need additional pain meds just to handle these more intense sensations. Or they'll be so powerful that your baby won't be able to handle them, leading you at long last to be wheeled in for a cesarean.

A 2013 national survey titled *Listening to Mothers III* asked 2,400 women about their experiences with hospital-based perinatal care. The questionnaire was part of the Childbirth Foundation's initiative to understand how they can improve maternal care policy, practice, education, and research. Here's what they found:

- **41 percent** indicated that their care provider tried to induce labor.

- **32 percent** of mothers without a prior cesarean reported they were told as they neared the end of pregnancy that their baby might be too getting large. Of those, **62 percent** had a discussion with their provider about inducing labor, despite this not being supported by evidence as a reason to do so. And **44 percent** had discussed a scheduled cesarean.

- Of women with a previous cesarean, **48 percent** were interested in the option of a vaginal birth after Cesarean (VBAC), but many of them (**46 percent**) were denied that option.

- Of those mothers who indicated that they asked for a planned cesarean, a substantial majority (**60 percent**) indicated the idea was initially suggested by their provider, a figure that was similar whether or not mothers had had a prior cesarean. When mothers did raise the issue of a planned cesarean, they overwhelmingly did so out of a belief that having a cesarean would offer a health benefit to her or her baby (**87 percent**).

- **47 percent** of women planning to deliver vaginally experienced an induction. Of those having an induction, **78 percent** had an epidural. And of those who had both an attempted induction and an epidural, the unplanned cesarean rate was **31 percent**.

- **83 percent** of women used one or more types of medication for pain relief during labor.

- One out of six women (**16 percent**) were given narcotics such as Demerol or Stadol.

- **67 percent** received an epidural or spinal analgesia.

- **67 percent** of mothers reported being on an IV.

- **47 percent** had bladder catheters.

- **31 percent** were given synthetic oxytocin (Pitocin) to speed up labor.

- **68 percent** of women who gave birth vaginally pushed on their backs.

- Of those mothers who intended to exclusively breastfeed, **49 percent** were given free formula samples or offers.[46]

Just Say No, for Baby's Sake

Drugs for managing pain during labor aren't just risky for you, they're risky for your baby. Think about it: A substance strong enough to dull the sensations of childbirth is too powerful not to affect your little one.[47]

Opiates, or the class of meds that are considered the gentler, "less invasive" alternative to an epidural,[48] can affect your baby's health. They can cause things like central nervous system depression, respiratory depression, impaired breastfeeding, altered neurological behavior, and decreased ability to regulate body temperature. In fact, your baby might need medication just to counteract the effects of the opiate or to "wake the baby up."[49] Even if your baby isn't given those meds, she still might be taking in whatever you were given. Some of these drugs can take as long as 60+ hours to clear your body, and they are passed through breast milk.[50]

Epidurals aren't much rosier. These megashots can cause things like an elevated heart rate in your baby and difficulty latching on to the breast.[51] In a fifth of women, they can cause a fever during labor, which can also cause a fever in the baby, leading you two to be separated during the first crucial moments of life, with a detrimental effect on breastfeeding.[52]

Now consider the numbers collected on home birth by Kenneth Johnson, PhD, and Betty-Anne Daviss, MSc, RM, and published in 2005 as the largest and most reputable study of home birth in North America by the prestigious and selective *British Medical Journal*. Of the 5,418 planned home births assisted by certified professional midwives, only 12 percent of them were ultimately transferred to the hospital. And of those 650 women, only 4.7 percent had epidural anesthesia, 2.1 percent had an episiotomy, and 3.7 percent gave birth by cesarean section.[53] (Compare that to the national cesarean rate of 32 percent!) No mothers died, and the neonatal mortality rate was only 1.7 in 1,000—far lower than the national average of 6.05.[54]

And a 5-year study comparing outcomes of home births attended by midwives with those of planned hospital births with a midwife or physician found that women in the home-birth group were significantly less likely to have obstetric interventions, electronic fetal monitoring, medically assisted vaginal delivery, and adverse outcomes like third- or fourth-degree perineal tearing or postpartum hemorrhage. Also, newborns in the home-birth group were less likely to need resuscitation at birth and less likely to have meconium aspiration.[55]

(continued on page 96)

A Section on C-Sections

Unfortunately, history shows that advances in the practice of medicine and surgery are rarely attained in a thoroughly rational manner, but that a period of undue enthusiasm, or even of almost reckless abuse, usually precedes the establishment of the actual value of a given procedure. [Cesarean section] requires only a few minutes of time and a modicum of operative experience; while [vaginal birth] often implies active mental exertion, many hours of patient observation, and frequently very considerable technical dexterity.

—Read before the Clinical Congress of Surgeons of North America, Philadelphia, on October 23–27, 1916, by John Whitridge Williams, MD, pioneer of academic obstetrics

The nature of our care is changing. Especially when it comes to childbirth, the threshold to green-light medical interventions is getting lower and lower. And it's largely to blame for the dismal statistics in our country for both moms and babies. Right now, the United States has a C-section rate that is one of the highest in the world, about 32 percent. But the World Health Organization recommends it stay closer to *15 percent*.[56] Why so much lower? Because while these procedures can be absolutely lifesaving when used appropriately, they can do more harm than good when performed on low-risk mothers.[57]

A 2006 study examined 5,762,037 live births and found that neonatal mortality rates were three times higher for babies born via C-section than those born vaginally. (The researchers ruled out any variables that would have affected this rate aside from the mode of delivery, like inherent medical conditions in the baby.[58]) And a paper published in the *Journal of Obstetrics and Gynecology* outlined a clear increase in severe injuries to women during birth between 1998 and 2005, including kidney failure, pulmonary embolisms, respiratory failure, and more. The study, which adjusted for things like hypertension, diabetes, age, and multiple births, found that the most significant influencing factor was the increasing rate of cesarean delivery.[59] Right now, only about 5 percent of C-sections are true emergencies, estimates George Macones, MD, chairman of the department of obstetrics and gynecology at the Washington University in St. Louis School of

Medicine.[60] A vast majority fall into a medical gray zone—past her due date, a previous C-section, labor isn't progressing "quickly enough," or the baby looks "too big."[61]

When it is not absolutely necessary for a mother to receive a C-section, she is exposed to all the risks of major surgery, including anesthesia mishaps like paralysis; hemorrhage requiring transfusion or hysterectomy; accidental cutting of the bowel or uterine artery; surgical trauma to the bladder and uterus; and postpartum infection.[62] And there are also risks that can affect future pregnancies, such as scarring of the uterus, decreased fertility, and increased likelihood of a high-risk pregnancy or uterine rupture.[63] After all, a cesarean is major abdominal surgery, and any surgical procedure carries risk.

And consider this amazing fact: When you give birth vaginally, your child's gut is colonized by all the good flora in your vagina. A child delivered by C-section, on the other hand, is often colonized by hospital bacteria, not the good home-team stuff.[64]

VAGINAL BIRTH AFTER CESAREAN (VBAC) AND SUPERSIZE BABIES

Two of the most common reasons doctors give for administering cesareans are because a woman has already had a C-section and is therefore at risk for rupturing the scarring during a vaginal birth, and because a woman's baby is too large to make it out the natural way. But in 2010, the American Congress of Obstetricians and Gynecologists stated the following: "Attempting VBAC is a safe and appropriate choice for most women who have had a prior cesarean delivery, including for some women who have had two previous cesareans." Richard N. Waldman, MD, then president of the college, went on to say, "The current cesarean rate is undeniably high and absolutely concerns us as ob-gyns. These VBAC guidelines emphasize the need for thorough counseling of benefits and risks, shared patient-doctor decision-making, and the importance of patient autonomy. Moving forward, we need to work collaboratively with our patients and our colleagues, hospitals, and insurers to swing the pendulum back to fewer cesareans and a more reasonable VBAC rate."[65] And as for the situation of a baby being too big to fit through its mother's pelvis, the actual incidence is less than 1 percent.[66] Even the ACOG acknowledges that ultrasounds aren't a rock-solid way to measure a baby's true size, and current evidence supports that in most cases it's safe to allow for a trial of labor.[67] So wait a second—as you already heard, a *third* of mothers surveyed were told their babes were "too large" and almost half of those were asked to at least consider a cesarean. Are you as confused as I am? The numbers just aren't adding up.

This goes to show—along with testimony from all kinds of experts—that giving birth in the security of your home, assisted by a skilled health practitioner, is way better than the mainstream alternative. For us, our bodies, and our babies. Check it out:

Natural birth makes for smoother delivery. The more relaxed we are and the more we can let go, the less difficult giving birth will be. According to Ina May Gaskin, founder and director of the Farm Midwifery Center near Summertown, Tennessee, and the fairy godmother of home birth and midwifery in this country, all our openings—cervical, vaginal, anal—work best when we feel comfortable and secure.[68] It's why it might be easier to go to the bathroom when you know the door is locked or when no one else is nearby. The same thing goes for delivery. Your baby's exit route cannot be opened at will, and it certainly doesn't do well with being yelled at (Push! Relax!). If you feel at all frightened, upset, or self-conscious, then your cervix and vagina won't be able to release as smoothly and completely as they need to.

Natural birth helps us bond with our babies. During delivery, huge bursts of oxytocin are running through your brain. This feel-good hormone is primarily responsible for the "baby lust" we feel when our baby is placed in our arms for the first time. But if you've introduced drugs that interfere with that, then your initial bonding could be restricted. Pitocin, a synthetic version of oxytocin, inhibits the production of the real thing,[69] and as I mentioned a little earlier, babies whose mothers have had epidurals frequently have trouble latching on to the breast.[70] If you've undergone surgery, which is incredibly taxing on your body, then the attention you would normally be spending on bonding with your baby is diverted to look after your own healing.

Plus, when you give birth at home, there's no team of nurses waiting to take that baby away and administer all kinds of unnecessary treatments (more on that in Chapter 9). When you can finally hold your baby in your arms, gaze at his face, and feel his teeny tiny heartbeat next to yours, it's hard to imagine life being more right. What's even more beautiful is that if you're given the space to just *be* together after giving birth, you're also helping each other's bodies cope with the enormous feat they just accomplished. Your warmth keeps your newborn snug since he can't yet regulate his own temperature, and your newborn—who will instinctively wriggle toward your breasts—will jump-start your body's oxytocin production when he starts suckling. Oxytocin, or the "love hormone," will seal your bond forever more, help the uterus contract so that the placenta can detach and be delivered, and close off any blood vessels the placenta was attached to.

You Don't Know Squat: The Original Birth Position

After Queen Victoria blazed the trail for using anesthesia for labor—she got zonked out with chloroform for the birth of her eighth child[71]—lying down during birth became all the fashion. By the end of the 19th century, it was considered low class to give birth in a squatting position. But being trendy didn't exactly pay off. While it was more convenient for a male birth attendant to check in on things if a woman was on her back, it made it that much harder and more painful for women to give birth.[72]

There's a reason why women in traditional societies all over the world have almost always chosen squatting and other upright positions during labor. They knew intuitively that using gravity in their favor would help move things along. It increased cervical dilation, put the baby in the best position to come out, and made contractions more effective.[73] And they figured all that out without a medical degree.

> When you set up a system that focuses on the 1 percent of problems that might occur, you undermine the care of the 99 percent of mothers who don't need those services.
>
> —Eugene Declercq, PhD, professor of maternal and child health, Boston University School of Public Health

PLANNING A NATURAL BIRTH IN A HOSPITAL

So many moms-to-be say they're planning for a natural birth, that they don't want the drugs, that a C-section is totally out—but they're delivering in a hospital. And when push comes to shove (or should I say contraction comes to push?), those plans aren't being realized. So what's happening? Why the good intentions and no results? It's certainly not the women who are to blame!

Here's the thing: When you tour a hospital, you're being pitched. They want you to give birth there because your insurance company is going to shell out. Big time. A vaginal delivery can cost in the neighborhood of $9,280, and it's a whopping $14,374 for a cesarean.[74] A hospital, whether you'd like to think of it this way or not, is a business. And unfortunately, the moneymaking mind-set can influence just how rosy a picture you get as a potential client. You'll most likely be shown their most beautiful birthing suite—outfitted with a big, gleaming tub, lots of comfy chairs, maybe even a garden view—and be given all kinds of reassurances about how natural their birthing protocol is. What you might *not* see in the tour is the actual room where you'll be giving birth, which may be far less lovely. You might not be told up front that even if you labor in a birthing center attached to the hospital, where you could have access to amenities that make the experience a little more homey, the center still has to follow hospital protocols. If your labor is deemed not to be progressing quickly enough, or the staff has decided your baby is "too large," or any number of "red flags" pop up, you'll be whisked out of the birthing center and into the regular delivery unit.[75]

That all said, it is still possible to have a hospital birth that is in line with your core beliefs. But you will need to be vigilant. I'm telling you all these things so you know how best to protect yourself and your choices if you feel more comfortable giving birth in a hospital setting. First, get all the information you can about each hospital you visit. The answers to these questions will paint a much clearer picture of their approach to childbirth than any romantic tour of their quaint birthing suites:

- What is your C-section rate?
- What percentage of moms get epidurals?
- Is continuous monitoring standard, or can I be monitored intermittently?
- Will I be allowed to move around?
- Will I be allowed to eat and drink during labor?
- Can I hold my baby right away, or will you be testing and examining her?
- Do you allow newborns to room-in with their moms?

There are only two states—New York and Massachusetts—where hospitals are required to publish brochures with this information, so in most cases, you'll need to ask for these statistics. If the hospital isn't accommodating, note that the CDC requires these numbers be routinely collected by local departments of public health.[76] I'd argue, though, that if a hospital isn't being forthright about any of these things, then it's not the ideal partnership.

In addition, it will be even more crucial that you find a caregiver who's going to be your advocate. Read the "Choosing a Caregiver" section on page 101 for some great questions to ask potential obstetricians to assess whether they're the right partner for you on this journey.

Birthing Babies: Women's Work?

Sheila Kitzinger, one of the foremost voices for women and their childbirth rights, once asked this amazing question: Want to know the most shocking thing about Jesus's birth? It wasn't that he was the Son of God or born in a pile of hay, it's that Mary gave birth without any women![77] Not to get all *Red Tent* on you (juicy novel, if you haven't read it), but there's a reason why for centuries it was the women who handled baby business. The simplest explanation was that it's what was traditionally done. If you were living in a tribe, you'd most likely have seen your mom, aunts, sisters, and just about every other lady in the tribe give birth. With that experience came knowledge—which, with the intuition of whichever tribe elder was deemed to have the healing "touch"—made a powerful combination. I mean, think about it. How else would the species have survived?!

Now it turns out that there's good physiological reason to this tradition. According to birth studies by John H. Kennell, MD, a pediatrician, and Marshall H. Klaus, MD, a neonatologist, babies and mothers do better when women—in this case, professional labor assistants like midwives and doulas—help them through birth. Of the births included in their studies, there was only an 8 percent C-section rate, versus the 18 percent in the group not attended by women. There were shorter labors and less medical intervention. And only 10 percent of the babies required an extended hospital stay, versus 25 percent of the control group.[78]

Midwives: Not Just for Pioneers and Hippies!

One of the best ways to take control of your birth experience is to work with a care provider who has a profound respect for your body and everything that it's capable of doing without intervention. Someone who honors birth as the wonderful, natural act that it is. And most important, someone who isn't going to treat you like you're sick or an emergency waiting to happen. Welcome to midwifery.

Midwifery is a holistic blend of art and science. It combines obstetric medicine with innate and natural wisdom honed through centuries of practice. Midwives traditionally presided over births but, come the 1700s, were being burned as witches. By the early 1900s, when medicine became a for-profit profession requiring a university education that all but barred women, midwives nearly disappeared from mainstream health care. But now, midwives are specialists in low-risk pregnancy and birth. They tailor their care to each woman's needs; offer a less clinical approach to pregnancy and labor; tend to give longer appointments than doctors (about an hour versus 20 minutes); and can provide emotional, nutritional, and sometimes even spiritual support.

But that doesn't necessarily make them touchy-feely mystical medicine women. Your midwife's medical education means she could do anything a physician can, except for major surgeries. She could arrange—if necessary—for an epidural, give you pain medication, induce labor, give an episiotomy or repair a natural vaginal tear.[79] While they are trained to identify the small percentage of births in which there might be complications and will refer those cases to an obstetrician, midwives more often than not work to minimize the amount of medical intervention. But it's not as though they're showing up to your labor with nothing but their purse and some hard candies. Midwives come prepared to administer things like IV and fluids, suturing materials and local anesthetics, oxygen, and Pitocin (but not to speed things up, rather to prompt the uterus to contract if there's a lot of bleeding after labor). For more information about some of the most-wondered-about scenarios your midwife is equipped to handle, check out the section "Could It Happen To Me?" in Chapter 9.

Also, unlike a lot of other traditional caregivers, the midwives' support doesn't stop once the baby is born. They make sure you and your baby are breastfeeding like pros, then come back to check on you a few days later. Some midwives even help transition you into well-woman care by coming back at the 6-week mark to ensure all your bits have healed. Midwives, like people in any other profession, come in all flavors. Some are warm and fuzzy and nurturing, and some are assertive alpha females. Some work in private practices, some work in birthing centers, and some work in hospitals. But what they all have in common is that they are in a unique position to help you shape a pregnancy and birth that is distinctively and honestly yours.

What about Obstetricians?

In most other countries, healthy pregnant women don't see an OB for their care. That's because obstetricians are trained to detect and treat pathological problems of pregnancy, labor, and birth; their more specialized skills, including performing surgery, are reserved for complicated or high-risk cases. Unfortunately, in our health care system, OBs are applying these interventions much more liberally than necessary.[80]

But that doesn't mean there aren't obstetricians out there who favor a more holistic approach. My backup doctor, Dr. Ronald Wu, was totally old school and had years and years and years of experience delivering babies naturally. There are even OBs who are combining Eastern healing practices with their medicine (Dr. Suzanne Gilberg-Lenz, for example, whom I interviewed for this book). These practitioners won't perform a home birth, but if you are still intent on delivering in a hospital, it's certainly one more way to protect your wishes. Check out "Choosing a Caregiver" (below) for questions you can ask to decide whether working with a particular obstetrician is for you.

PLANNING A BIRTH THAT FEELS RIGHT

If you are questioning whether home birth is the right choice for you, try to get more connected to why. What's standing in your way? Are you afraid? Nervous about what other people will think? A little meditation and journaling can go a long way toward finding some clarity. There are also wonderful birth counselors who can help you work through any blocks that might be unnecessarily keeping you from an experience that could add to your life in significant and unexpected ways. Or best of all, check out the amazing books and have a little film festival with the fascinating documentaries listed in the Resources on page 332. You'll be able to see firsthand how many women are choosing to go this route and why. But ultimately, honor the voice that feels truest. Giving birth in a place where you feel safest and are most able to relax is what's really important.

CHOOSING A CAREGIVER

It's too difficult to tell from someone's impressive credentials or fancy office whether he or she is the health care professional who suits you best. Some midwives have a no-nonsense demeanor with conservative views on nutrition or intervention. Some obstetricians have a warm, holistic approach to birth; value diet as a cornerstone of medicine; and don't believe in unnecessary interventions. Some midwives work in hospitals, and some obstetricians work in birthing centers. The person you choose to be your advocate in birth should be someone you implicitly trust and feel comfortable with. Interview several practitioners and really listen to your gut. Your brain might say, "She* went to Harvard!" but your instincts may be saying, "She's the last person I'd want in a room when I'm in labor." Go with what feels good.

For a great list of questions to ask your caregiver candidates, check out *Ina May's Guide to Childbirth* by Ina May Gaskin. Be especially sure to ask your doctor or midwife what her philosophy is about "overdue" babies. Steer clear of anyone who's going to put pressure on you to

---

*Even though I've chosen the pronouns "she" and "her," there are many, many wonderful male doctors out there who have as much of a knack for bringing babies into this world naturally as women do.

induce just because it's been more than 280 days. In Asian countries, it's considered fortunate for a baby to spend more time in the womb. Babies born several days to a week later are traditionally thought to be stronger and more developed than those born on time or early.[81] Most midwives will monitor you closely, and so long as mama and baby aren't exhibiting any risky signs, they're typically comfortable letting nature take its course. Working with someone who will let you experience this entire process will be rewarding.

What to Ask OBs

Ask potential OBs about how often they perform elective induction of labor, their C-section rates, medical interventions they favor (if any), and their views on a woman's natural ability to give birth. Determine how likely it is that you'll be working with this particular doctor in the practice come delivery time, and not with a more conservative colleague because of the schedule rotation. And most important, pay attention to how each doctor honors your questions. If you find yourself being dismissed, talked over, or the slightest bit bulldozed, keep looking. That way, you'll have a better sense of whether you've found a good fit or if it's smooth-talking lip service.

What to Ask Family Doctors

About 30 percent of the family doctors practicing in the United States provide maternity care. While these general practitioners, like midwives, do not have surgical privileges, studies have shown that family doctors tend to have lower rates of obstetrical intervention than obstetricians.[82] Ask a family doctor the same questions you might ask a prospective obstetrician to be sure you share the same values when it comes to natural birth.

MIDWIVES UNDER FIRE: IF YOU LIVE IN A STATE WHERE MIDWIVES AREN'T LICENSED TO PERFORM HOME BIRTHS

After midwives were witch-hunted out of the medical field in the beginning of the 20th century by a smear campaign launched by obstetricians, their work continued to be vilified by the medical community. Until the 1950s, midwifery was banned in nearly all 50 states.[83] Unfortunately, even though the number of certified nurse-midwives (CNMs) in the country has grown significantly over the last 30 years, the residual effects of the medical community's distrust still has an effect on how they can practice, as some state laws make them work under doctor supervision.[84]

To see what the deal is with your state—and to get much more fascinating information about midwife-related advocacy—check out mana.org and pushformidwives.org. You can try to find a CNM who offers home birth care through midwife.org, the official Web site of the American College of Nurse-Midwives, and you can also join the "friends of midwives" group in your state or other home-birth communities on sites like Facebook and Yahoo. These are generally meeting places where like-minded people can connect and share ideas and resources, including midwife services.

DO I NEED TO FIND A BACKUP DOCTOR?

One of the first things you and your midwife will talk about is what will happen if you need to be transferred to the hospital. It's not a test to make sure you're resolved enough to have a home birth; it's to address the very real possibility that hospital transfers can and do happen. During this conversation, she'll explain which hospital she works with and whether she recommends seeking out a backup doctor. This isn't because she isn't completely trustworthy or because you're inviting unnecessary risk by having a home birth. It's simply one more way of protecting your choices during birth. After all, if you do end up being transferred, wouldn't you rather be in the care of a doctor who understands and respects all the beautiful preparations you'd done for a natural birth and who will do everything in her power to facilitate that—and not just some doc who happens to be on call?

When it comes to finding a backup OB, don't simply settle because you may not ever have to see this person again. Stand by your beliefs! I went to interview one doctor, and right off the bat, he wanted to do an ultrasound to make sure the baby was okay. I assured him that I had just met with my midwife and that everything had checked out. But he was insistent on hearing the baby's heartbeat. "Can't you check with a stethoscope?" I asked him. It was what my midwife had been doing for most of my pregnancy, and what I much preferred—no freaky Frankenwaves! His response? "I always use the ultrasound." But I encouraged him to try the stethoscope. "You know you can hear fine with one, right?" He wasn't sure. Then he put the stethoscope to my belly and goes, "Oh, yeah! I can hear it!" Big fat duh. But then he said he needed the ultrasound to confirm the baby was head down. I asked why, adding that my midwife had done that just last week, and she'd done it by *feeling with her hands*. "Why don't you try that?" I asked. And sure enough, he did. I asked him why he always defaulted to the ultrasound, and he said, "I'm an old guy and it's a toy. I used to practice without these things because we didn't have them, but now we do, and it's fun." It was a fair answer, I suppose. But, to make matters worse, he kept knocking home birth, even though he was a backup doctor for midwives! We ultimately found a wonderful obstetrician—kind, quiet Dr. Wu—who didn't believe in medical intervention during birth as a first response. And even though he was also trained to administer more medical or surgical treatments in case of an emergency, he believed that birth is best left to nature.

If the doctor who is potentially going to become your caretaker—especially in the case of an emergency—doesn't share your beliefs, then he or she can't truly advocate for you.

DO I NEED TO LIVE IN A NICE HOUSE TO HAVE A HOME BIRTH?

No! I hear from women all the time that their main hang-up about giving birth at home is that they don't have the "right kind of space." But believe me, there are no rules about how much square footage you need to have a baby. Remember all those tribal women we've been talking about? I'm pretty sure they didn't have a special wing in their huts or caves just for giving birth. Even if you went to a hospital, do you think that delivery room is going to be bigger than your apartment? No way. The fact is, natural birth doesn't take up a lot of space. And it definitely doesn't say anywhere on your lease that having babies isn't allowed.

Mama to Mama on . . . Finding a Birth Team

My advice is to have a birth team you feel comfortable with. Discuss with them what you want for your birth and make sure they know your goals. This birth is yours and your baby's, not your doctor's or midwife's. *You* hold the power, but only if you're well informed.

—Kim Brenner, Southern Pines, North Carolina

My advice for expecting moms is to do your research. Some people spend more time searching for a car than they do finding the right fit for a birthing experience! Do what feels right for you and your body. Follow your gut and intuition, then relax and let it happen, knowing that you're ready for whatever comes.

—Nita Pettibone, Knoxville, Tennessee

"High-Risk" Pregnancy

There is no uniformly accepted definition of what constitutes risk in a pregnancy. There are, however, some conditions that are commonly classified as "high risk." These include diabetes, heart disease, high blood pressure, HIV and AIDS, placenta previa, and VBAC.[85] The great news is that if you've really cleaned house, you can most likely knock the first three off your list. As for the rest, different caregivers have different opinions. Whereas one might immediately sign you up for a C-section, another might be comfortable monitoring you closely with the hope of letting you have an intervention-free birth. And in many of these scenarios, a midwife can work collaboratively with your doctor.[86]

IS A KIND BIRTH REALISTIC ON A BUDGET?

Not only is a natural home birth less expensive than a hospital birth, but you save money in the long run, too. Having a healthier kid—and a healthier you—means fewer trips to the doctor and virtually no medical bills otherwise. If money is an issue, some midwives will reduce their fees or assist pro bono in certain circumstances. To learn how to get insurance coverage if your plan doesn't cover home birth, visit homebirth-usa.org/choosing/insurance.html.

To get even more inspired about planning a natural or home birth, check out the amazing books, films, and Web sites in the Resources on page 332.

8

Second Trimester

I loved when my wife was pregnant. It was a magical time when
Bear was growing in her. To see and feel Bear kick around was
amazing. Alicia was the cutest thing ever, and she started to really
glow after 3 or 4 months. She became a tired lioness moving
slowly but looking curvy and sexy. Sometimes she would get
nauseated and couldn't find any food that satisfied her—this made
for a cranky lioness at times. So every night, I would heat up some
organic raw shea butter and rub it all over her belly and hips.
(Good work if you can get it!)

—Christopher

WHAT YOU MIGHT BE FEELING

A Big Belly

Being pregnant made me feel so comfortable in my skin. That's one of the incredible gifts of
pregnancy—it allows you to love yourself in a whole new way. The confidence and sensuality of
it all is absolutely amazing! Every moment of these 9 months is precious and only yours for a brief
amount of time. Try to appreciate how beautiful the journey—and you!—can be.

If you're worried about stretch marks, know that they can be hereditary. But according to my midwife, Margo Kennedy, good, clean eating goes a long way in building beautiful, supple, elastic skin. So keep up the kind work in the diet department to help your little belly blossom into a smooth, radiant bump. As a fun bonus, slather on some super-hydrating vitamin E oil, shea butter, coconut oil, or even olive oil from the get-go (including on your soon-to-be upgraded boobies), all of which are great for your skin. Try the Lucky Mama Massage Oil (page 124) or the Beautiful Belly Balm (page 109). Even better, ask your partner to give you a hand for a sexy little rubdown. Try it even if you're not feeling frisky—it might help!

Amazing!

When I was pregnant, it seemed like everyone Christopher ran into wanted to know how moody and awful I was being. They'd look at him with pity—assuming because I was knocked up that I had turned into some kind of raging, prenatal beast—and ask, "Is she *so* ready for this to be over?" But his answer was, "Not at all!" I loved being pregnant. I wholly credit the foods that were nourishing me and believe they made all the difference between a miserable, uncomfortable 9 months and total (well, mostly) idyllic delight.

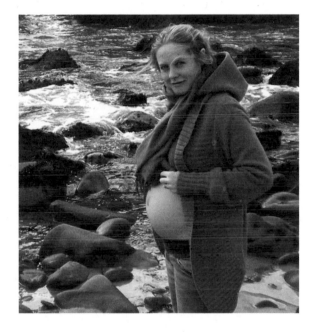

As your body starts to change dramatically both inside and out, it's more important than ever to embrace the kind foods that have kept you glowing and healthy so far. Nourishing whole grains, legumes, and veggies will ensure that every single organ and cell in your body is getting exactly what it needs. So as your physiology changes over the next 6 months, your body can keep right in step. You'll be able to heal more quickly; fend off aches and pains; keep your circulation pumping with strong, clean blood; and prevent swelling and bloating. And all that superpowered fiber will keep things moving and grooving. You won't just feel amazing— you'll look amazing! I can't think of a better way to spend this precious time.

Less Than Amazing

The more squeaky-clean your diet, the more in balance your body will be. And the more balance you achieve in your body, the less it will be thrown off by all the new hormones surging through it. Or to state it more simply: Eat kind and you won't feel crummy. That said, imbalance can happen. Sometimes, it's because we've lost touch with the core magical foods in our diet or maybe snuck in a few too many treats.

If you do happen to experience what way too many women consider "common" maladies, the best fix isn't in your medicine cabinet, it's in your kitchen. The remedies below are tips I've picked up from a variety of healers, macrobiotic experts, and traditional Chinese medicine practitioners. They're all rooted in restoring balance in the body using the astounding power of what we eat.

As you use the following methods to feel well again, think, too, of your unpleasant symptoms as a gentle nudge back toward eating the kindest, most healing foods possible at every meal. Revisit Chapter 5 for a reminder of what that looks like. Also keep in mind that I haven't even mentioned foods like meat, dairy, and processed sugar as the possible culprits behind these conditions. That's because it should be assumed that these offenders—with all their intestine-clogging, inflammation-causing, circulation-inhibiting, mucus-making nastiness—will only cause not-so-fun pregnancy side effects or make them worse.

BACKACHES

As your belly grows, your spinal cord shifts to counterbalance its weight. This postural change, along with more pressure on your lower back and sciatic nerves, can be a recipe for an achy back.

Acidic foods like honey, sugar, fruit, fruit juice, and tea can make your discomfort worse. It's important to eat foods that are gentler on your kidneys, since those organs are working overtime to discharge not only your own waste but also your baby's, and a tired kidney can cause backaches. If you've been overdoing the salt—maybe treating yourself to too much soy sauce (more than a few teaspoons throughout the day) or heaping too much miso into your soup—this may also contribute. Make sure you're loading up on leafy greens, root vegetables, and beans, which nourish and strengthen the kidneys.

Mild movement like yoga and stretching can help relieve back pain, and massage can be a miracle cure. Even simply having your partner rub you for 5 minutes goes a long way. (See "Get Rubbed the Right Way" on page 123 for some of my tips and a homemade massage oil recipe.) It's also safe for you to see a chiropractor, which can further help your body adapt. Just make sure you're seeing someone you trust who has experience working with prenatal patients or, even better, specializes in them. The chiropractor should be able to determine if you're a good candidate for adjustments without using x-rays.

BLEEDING GUMS AND NOSEBLEEDS

As your baby grows, your circulation increases (thanks to your hormone-enhanced superhighway arteries[87]) and your blood volume creeps higher and higher so that your body can get more of your exceptionally divine blood to the placenta. If you're taking in too many foods like simple sugars, fruits, and fruit juices, this can lead to bleeding in your nose and gums. These naughtier treats can cause the lining of your nose and airways to swell and your gums to soften. The first remedy is to honor your body's request for balance and eat these foods in moderation (or cut them out completely, if you're still not getting relief).

To immediately relieve a nosebleed, moisten a piece of tissue paper with saliva or water, dip it into a bit of salt, and hold it in the affected nostril for several minutes. Salt causes the ruptured capillaries to contract. Eating a small piece of umeboshi plum every 10 minutes for about a half hour can also help.

To soothe irritated gums, try a cup of kombu tea: Simmer a strip of kombu in about 1 cup of water until the water turns light brown. Or add 15 drops of calendula or myrrh to 2 ounces of water and swish the solution in your mouth.

CONSTIPATION

During pregnancy, your intestines slow down so your body has more time to absorb the nutrients from food passing through. If you're eating a balanced diet of whole, kind foods, all that fiber will keep the trains running on time. However, if you're indulging in a few too many flour-based foods like bread or white noodles, or in too many nuts and nut butters, then you could be sludging things up. Remember to get most of your grains in their whole form, and don't skimp on the veggies. Chewing really, really well also helps, as can drizzling a little olive or hemp seed oil over salads and sautéed vegetables to ease things down and out. Other remedies include exercise (which can speed up your food's intestinal transit time) and shoulder and neck massage (the large and small intestine meridians run along the shoulders, and stimulating them can help get things moving).

EDEMA (SWELLING)

Just as your body loves to soak up nutrients when you're pregnant, it also wants to hold on to fluid. But once again, if you're staying true to the kind habits we talked about in Chapter 5, then uncomfortable swelling won't be your lot.

If you're feeling more than just a little puffy and have swollen hands, legs, and/or feet, mention it to your doctor and midwife. It's a good idea to rule out nastier possibilities like high blood pressure and toxemia, which can also cause you to retain fluid. But more often than not it's a case of good old-fashioned bloating.

The first thing to do is to make sure you're not taking in more salt and baked flour products than is recommended in a kind diet. Fluid retention is related to kidney function, so make sure you get enough kidney-supporting foods like leafy greens, root veggies, and beans. Dandelion leaf, a natural diuretic, has a strong peppery flavor like arugula and is great as a garnish on soups or chopped up into salads—a little goes a long way. Garlic, a natural anti-inflammatory, is great for releasing excess fluids. So is daikon-kombu tea: Boil ½ cup of grated daikon with a strip of kombu in a cup of water and add 2 drops of shoyu. Drink it every day for several days until you feel better. It'll stimulate the kidneys to discharge water and salt.

Giving your circulation a boost—important whether you're bloated or not!—will also help flush out excess fluids. Keep up your movement practice, elevate your feet whenever you're lying down, and give yourself a daily scrub down (see page 57). Warm baths also offer soothing relief because the pressure from the water helps push the fluids from your tissues back to your veins and then back out through your kidneys.

GAS

While most people eating a kind diet don't experience gas regularly, aside from the normal ½ liter we all expel on the average day, these foods and their fiber turboboost can cause gas if they need to clean house. Indulging in less-than-kind treats, which cause their own gas, and then following them up with cleaner meals can cause extra fartiness while your body rids itself of the nasty. Make sure you're chewing really, really well— which helps the body digest fibrous veggies and cuts down on gas—and that you're cooking your legumes properly.

The reason why legumes are called "the musical fruit" is because they contain special sugars that the bacteria in your gut love to eat. When they metabolize those sugars, it creates farty, burpy gas. But breaking down those sugars during the cooking process means no more toots. To learn how, read "Taking the Fartiness Out of Beans" on page 310.

HEADACHES

Assuming it's not part of your detox transition, a headache is more often than not a reflection of some kind of dietary imbalance. According to macrobiotic wisdom, where your headache radiates from says a lot about where the hitch is and the best remedy.

- **The front of the head, just above the eyes:** Sugary foods like fruit, honey, and chocolate are the culprits. Bring harmony back with lots of healing grains, legumes, and veggies. Try sucking on the pit of an umeboshi plum for a quick fix and apply a cold compress to your forehead as needed. While you're lying down, have your partner vigorously massage your second toe, then your third toe (both are pressure points linked to the stomach), then both toes together by pulling on them forcefully. Repeat this for about 5 minutes, then do the other foot. Such a fun way to get rid of that headache!

- **The sides of the head:** Make sure you're not overdoing it on oily, greasy foods, potatoes, or dried and fresh fruits. Revisit the magical foods in Chapter 5 that will help your body rebalance and heal. The umeboshi plum solution will also work here, as can a cold compress. Or have your partner briskly massage your fourth toe (the gallbladder pressure point), alternating between rubbing and pulling with enough force to move your entire body. Have him do this on one foot for about 5 minutes, then the other foot.

HEARTBURN

The good news is that a kind diet is rich in alkalizing—or acidity-balancing—foods, which means your chances of developing heartburn are super low. That said, sometimes even the kindest mamas-to-be can get that fire-breathing sensation after a meal. That's often because they've eaten too much and the baby is pressing on the stomach, causing whatever's in the belly to come up again. This isn't helped by the fact that pregnancy hormones soften the doorway between the esophagus and stomach, which makes heartburn much more likely.

The best remedy is prevention, which means eating smaller, more frequent meals; chewing them really well; not lying down right after eating; and making sure you're consuming plenty of soothing, inflammation-fighting foods. Fatty animal foods like meat and dairy are a recipe for heartburn since they take much longer to digest. If you do have a flare-up, try munching on fennel seeds, sipping a mug of peppermint or fennel tea, drinking ume sho kuzu (page 297) once or twice a day, or downing a teaspoon of baking soda mixed with a cup of water.

HEMORRHOIDS

The pressure of your uterus on your colon can make it more difficult for food to pass on its way out. And since your body is reabsorbing a lot of its fluid, it can be that much harder for waste to make a smooth exit. Plus, all your veins are dilated because of pregnancy's circulation boost, and that includes those in your bottom.

Eating lots of fiber-rich lightly cooked greens and grains is the first line of defense against this not-so-pretty symptom, as is making extra sure to avoid nasty foods at all costs. Remember, animal foods and sugar cause inflammation and sluggish digestion, which can literally be a pain in the butt. If you've developed hemorrhoids, witch hazel cream is an amazing topical herbal remedy, and one that's kinder than any of the chemical-laden over-the-counter (and up-the-rear) stuff.

VARICOSE VEINS

These can be hereditary, but diet can go a long way in preventing them. Luckily, kind foods are naturally high in things like fiber, vitamin E, and bioflavonoids, so your prevention plan is already in place! But if you start to develop varicose veins, you may be eating too many inflammatory foods, which can increase the pressure in your veins. Pregnancy-related varicose veins often improve after delivery, but if you don't tweak your diet now, they may not go away completely.

WHAT YOU MIGHT BE WONDERING

How Much Weight Is Healthy to Gain?

We've talked about how pregnancy is not an excuse for a dietary free-for-all. That's because as your organs, veins, fluids, ducts, and glands transform into a little baby garden, you will naturally gain weight. Everyone's gain will be different, but the American College of Obstetricians and Gynecologists says that if you're already at a healthy weight, then 25 to 35 pounds is optimal, or about 3 to 4 new pounds a month.[88] Just the baby house gear—your uterus, placenta, blood volume, and boobs, *plus* your baby—can weigh as much as 27.6 pounds.[89] The amazing news is that when you're eating whole, kind foods, you'll maintain a perfect, healthy weight without having to take a single glance at the scale.

What Do I Wear?!

I know I'm stating the obvious when I say that you're not going to fit into most of your regular clothes, but I found that to be surprisingly frustrating. Suddenly, I had nothing to wear, and because I was trying to squeeze into clearly too-small items, I didn't feel my cutest. I was reluctant to buy a bunch of maternity clothes because it seemed wasteful to fill a closet with new things. So I figured out how to use a mix of hand-me-downs, a few newish items, and some of my regular clothes (be forewarned that your tops might get stretched out—just recycle those for your next pregnancy!). I basically lived in a pair of boyfriend-style jeans my friend lent me with a nice big shirt and a cardigan or, if I had to dress up, a black baby doll dress with flats and tights.

Here are a few great tips for how to build a wardrobe that is kind to your confidence, your wallet, and the planet:

Buy "vintage." Hit up your local thrift shops and buy secondhand—or as I like to say, vintage. I shop for almost everything I need at thrift stores and secondhand shops because it means less waste for the planet and more cool, one-of-a kind finds for me. Plus, it's easier on the wallet, and I don't feel bad when I don't get enough wear out of something and end up giving it away.

Hit up your mama tribe. Ask your friends if they have anything you could borrow or possibly hand down to your next friend in need. Or see if your community has an online network for mamas and expecting mamas where you can score everything you need from women looking to clean out their dressers and closets.

Buy smart. You don't need a big wardrobe, just a few well-fitting basics like a great pair of pants or a loose-fitting dress that you can style in different ways. I made it through my entire third trimester with that pair of hand-me-down jeans. Seriously, thank God for those jeans.

What about Sex?

You may have found that thanks to your supercharged circulation—a boon to your lady parts—you have a whole new appetite. Add to that your free-flowing oxytocin, and you could be downright insatiable. This is the time when most women find themselves at their friskiest. It's also when they are at their emotional peak, feeling positive and courageous. Allowing yourself to really open up is beneficial for your relationship with your partner and an important first step toward a deeply satisfying birth. And no, your husband's penis is not going to make a dent in the baby's head. Be creative! You'll figure out what's comfy. For more insight, check out *Your Orgasmic Pregnancy* by Danielle Cavallucci and Yvonne K. Fulbright, PhD.

It's also possible you won't feel like such a seductress, and that's okay, too. There's no real *should* when it comes to your sex life at this point in your pregnancy; everyone will enjoy intimacy on her own terms. Sometimes, it's hard to feel like a sex kitten when you're adjusting to your new life and completely pooped. Try to honor where you are and find the sexy in ways that are right for you. That said, if you're completely disinterested, that could signal an imbalance in either your diet or your emotional life. Make sure you're not eating too many "cold" foods like ice cream, sugar, fruits, fruit juice, raw salads, or even too much salt, which can cause your body's energy to tighten instead of soften and flow. Meditate on where those feelings come from. If you suspect it's a result of your relationship with your partner or unresolved personal issues, seek counseling to investigate how to find some peace *before* the baby comes.

KIND ACTION

Conquer Your Cravings

This wouldn't be a book about pregnancy without a section on cravings. It's beyond cliché at this point that if you're pregnant, you have license to eat pints of ice cream washed down with pickles chased with a brick of cheese. It's somehow totally okay to indulge every culinary whim that crosses your mind. I mean, you're eating for two, right? Or it's what your body is asking for! But here's the deal: When your body is in balance and you're giving it every nutritional boost it requires, that naggy, whiny voice begging for a treat isn't asking for something it *needs*. It's asking for something it *wants*.

Believe me, I'm like most people—I want to dive headfirst into something unbelievably wicked every now and then. We all have those moments where our inner spoiled brat throws a tantrum for something she just *has* to have. But whenever I start itching for something naughty, I take stock: Am I getting every single nutrient, vitamin, and mineral that I need? Yep. So does my body really *need* a full cup of sugar from the vegan brownies I'm staring at while in line at the store? I'm pretty sure it doesn't. And I can guarantee that your blood, veins, tissues, and organs aren't requesting a double cheeseburger. In fact, according to A. Christine Harris, PhD, we only crave things because of our new sensitivity to taste and smell, not because of physiological needs. But as much as you're eating with purpose now and are working so hard to have the most luminous, healthy pregnancy and birth, I know how tough it is to ignore that little (or sometimes not so little) voice whining for a treat.

EVEN GOOD GIRLS GO BAD: IT'S NORMAL TO BE A LITTLE NAUGHTY

Food and I were not friends during pregnancy. Everything I used to love was unappealing. To even want to *try* to eat something, I'd have to really think about it. At work, I'd lie on the floor between takes, desperate to eat something good and yet totally grossed out and tired. Sometimes, I couldn't think of a single thing on earth I wanted to eat, so I'd mentally go through food from different countries—*Anything Japanese? No. Italian? No way. American? Maybe . . .*—trying to come up with something that sounded edible. One of my most vivid memories from labor was hanging the entire weight of my body from my husband's shoulders while squatting and trying to push the baby out, and deliriously asking my midwife, "After the baby comes out, will I like food again?" It's no wonder my mind started drifting to foods I ate when I was a kid. Back then I ate a lot of deli roast beef sandwiches, eggs, and frozen yogurt. Not exactly kind fare.

I was curious. What would happen if I did eat some of these things? Was there any chance I would suddenly feel better? What if all the naysayers were right that animal food was the answer? I doubted it. I wasn't missing anything nutritionally. But 1 percent of me was curious about it. And the rest of me was having a selfish, lazy moment because I was at a restaurant. I just wanted to eat something that finally sounded good! So instead of going home and making any of the scrumptious, satisfying dishes I'm going to suggest you try, I scratched the itch.

I had a few bites of someone's fish. I had an egg. I had a tiny affair with frozen yogurt. And at first it was fun to be a little naughty when I was eating out and not at home with my usual healthy food. But after a minute, it didn't feel so great. It wasn't nourishing my body *or* my soul. Did it stop my nausea and give me more energy? No! Did I feel like I was finally eating foods we humans are "supposed" to eat? No! All I felt was guilty—and nauseated and bloated and sick. If only I'd known about So Delicious Purely Decadent Turtle Trails frozen dessert—or taken the time to make any one of the delicious recipes I've included in this book—that would in those moments have done the trick! But I made my choices, and while I'm not proud, I forgive them.

So there you go—I'm human. And it's important that you realize that the goal here isn't to be perfect—who really is?!—but to be *resolved*. Believe me, trying to be perfect all the time is exhausting and soul dimming. This journey is about doing your best and also being flexible and compassionate with yourself if you fall off the path. You're not going to get kicked out of the Kind Mama club, I promise. Just get right back on your sweet vegan way!

A KINDER DELICIOUS

Instead of ignoring your cravings or giving in completely to them, try seeing them as an opportunity to play with new flavors and textures in the kind world. You'd be surprised just how scrumptious and decadent these foods can be. Whether you're after meaty, sweet, chewy, creamy, salty, crunchy, so on, there's no shortage of amazingly kind *and* delectable dishes out there. Check out the section ahead for some great options and substitutes for common cravings. I've

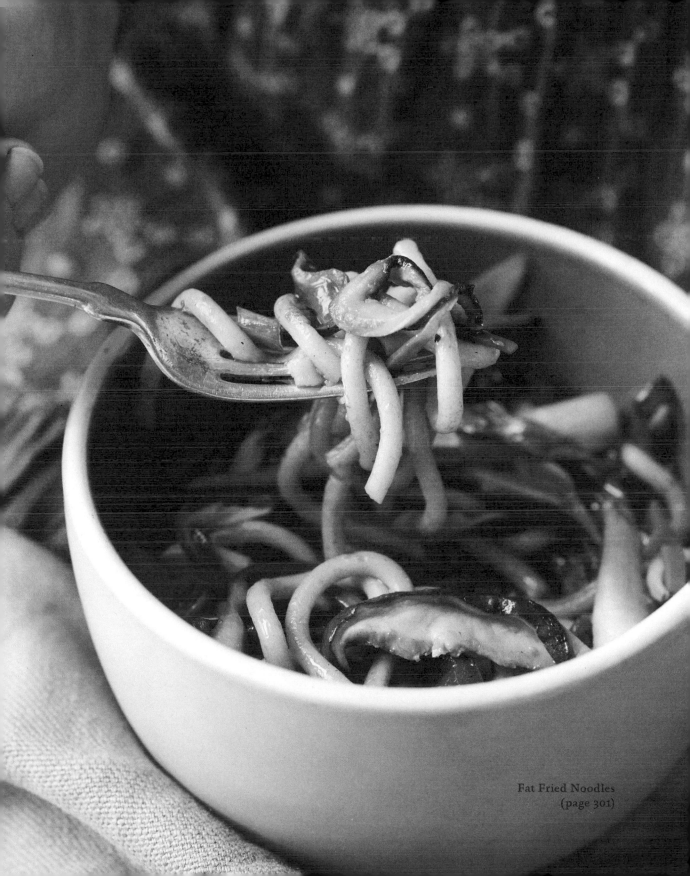

Fat Fried Noodles
(page 301)

divided them into two categories: Goody-Goodies, or more gentle indulgences; and Naughty-but-Nice, treats that are still kind but not exactly health food. Either way, if you treat yourself to these yummies instead of giving in to nastier temptations, then you've done yourself a real solid. You'll still be protecting yourself from an uncomfortable pregnancy and birth and potentially dangerous complications like high blood pressure and gestational diabetes. And you'll be guard-

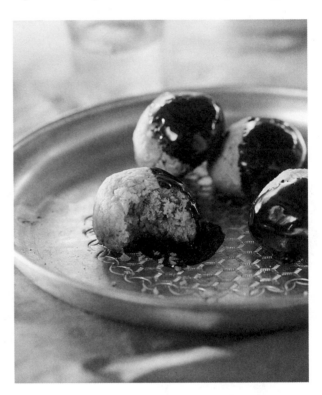

ing your baby from complications during birth and all kinds of harmful illnesses and developmental setbacks. But if you do happen to fall off the wagon, just hop right back on. Make your next meal a super-clean one. Some greens and rice will set you straight.

Also keep in mind that "too much of a good thing" can still apply to kind yet naughty-fun foods. Keep the frisky business under control and watch how you feel after you eat. If you get hungover or puffy, can't sleep, or start developing icky pregnancy-related symptoms, then it's definitely not worth it to indulge quite as much.

IF YOU'RE CRAVING . . .

MEATY: Your magic ingredients are going to be rich and hearty like beans, tempeh, seitan, and tofu that's all dressed up with a ton of flavor.

Goody-Goodies: Fat Fried Noodles (page 301); Braised Burdock Root with Hearty Seitan (page 306); Strengthening Daikon, Carrots, and Tofu (page 314); Tempeh with Caramelized Onion and Braised Cabbage (page 308).

Naughty-but-Nice: Heirloom Tomato Saucy Toasts (page 313); Sausage and Sweet Potato Hash (page 316); Pan-Fried Tempeh with Garlic and Chiles (page 317); as well as commercially available products like Lightlife Organic Smoky Tempeh Strips; It's All Good Veggie Chick'n Good Stuff; VegeUSA Vegetarian Fish Fillets; Tofurky Jurky in teriyaki, hickory, and smoked flavors; Tofurky hickory-smoked deli slices; MorningStar Farms Hickory BBQ Riblets, and VegeUSA Vegan Citrus Sparerib Cutlets.

SWEET: Whether you want fruity, creamy, nutty, or chocolatey, these treats have you covered. I've also included some amazing veggie dishes, because when steamed or roasted, they, too, can really hit the spot.

Goody-Goodies: Sweet Vegetable Drink (page 296); Tangerine Kanten (page 319); Sweetly Glazed Carrots (page 317); Baked Peaches with Gooey Nut Crumble (page 320); Sweet Rice, Amaranth, and Apricot Breakfast Porridge (page 301); or this quickie dessert: Mix 2 tablespoons almond butter with 1 teaspoon brown rice syrup to make a scrumptious caramel that you can drizzle over fruit or just eat like a wild woman!

Naughty-but-Nice: Chocolate-Dunked Coconut Delights (page 319); a fruit smoothie; and commercially available products like So Delicious Purely Decadent Turtle Trails frozen dessert, Rice Dream frozen bars and pies, and Luna Chocolate Peppermint Stick bars.

CREAMY: Sometimes eating a dish with tempeh, seitan, or tofu can help satisfy a craving for dairy. Scramble some tofu with your favorite veggies, a little shoyu, then add scallions on top. It's like eating scrambled eggs, but better for you! (Check out the full recipe in *The Kind Diet*.) Dips made with tofu or tahini might also take the edge off, as might rich and fatty (but healthy!) foods like avocados, nut butters, olives, and oils.

Goody-Goodies: Avocado on sourdough drizzled with olive oil; pureed squash or root vegetable soup; Watercress with Creamy Tahini Dressing and Toasted Sesame Seeds (page 298); Millet Mashed "Potatoes" with Mushroom Gravy (page 304); Seitan and Veggie Mochi Melt (page 313).

Naughty-but-Nice: Heirloom Tomato Saucy Toasts (page 315); Cheesy, Oozy Guacamole Bean Dip (page 318); a fruit smoothie; as well as commercially available products like whole soy yogurt; KiteHill nut-based cheese; Follow Your Heart Cheddar, mozzarella, or Fiesta Blend cheese alternatives; Parmela Parmesan-style cheese; Daiya Shreds; Annie's Goddess Dressing; and Tofutti Better Than Cream Cheese or Better Than Sour Cream.

WHAT YOUR CRAVING MIGHT BE SAYING

Sometimes your cravings can be a signal that your body needs more of a certain nutrient. If you've been hanging out a bit too much on the naughty train—especially during pregnancy when all your systems are in flux—you don't want to ignore these messages. While your body would never ask you for something as unhealthy as a steak or french fries, it might feel a lot like it. But here's what it's really requesting:

What you want: Meat

What you might need: More protein and fat (the kind varieties!) are the obvious answers, but it could also mean your body's asking for vitamin B_{12}. Be sure you're regularly taking a supplement so your nutritional needs are in check and then satisfy the urge with one of the hearty, meaty dishes from the "Protein! Protein!" section on page 305.

What you want: Salty food

What you might need: Less salt. If your body is retaining too much fluid— usually as a response to taking in too much salt in the first place—then it might be asking for even more salt to help balance it out. Reread the "Edema (Swelling)" section (page 110) for easy fixes. Or sometimes, if you've been indulging in a lot of sweet, your taste buds might crave salty for balance.

If you want to scratch the itch without sticking your face in a carton

of greasy Chinese, these are much nicer but naughty-tasting options like Fat Fried Noodles (page 301) or Arame, Sun-Dried Tomato, and Zucchini Stir-Fry (page 305).

What you want: Sweet food

What you might need: Protein. Sometimes the body craves sweet things when it needs energy. The body uses protein to make carbohydrates, which is what we use for energy. So if you're not getting enough protein, your body could be asking for a quick carbohydrate energy boost in the form of something sweet. You might also be off balance from eating too much salt or maybe even too stressed or worn out. Before you go to town on Chocolate-Dunked Coconut Delights (page 319), have some Sweet Vegetable Drink (page 296) to help curb the craving, or maybe even some Tangerine Kanten (page 319), to make sure you are getting enough of the good, fortifying stuff.

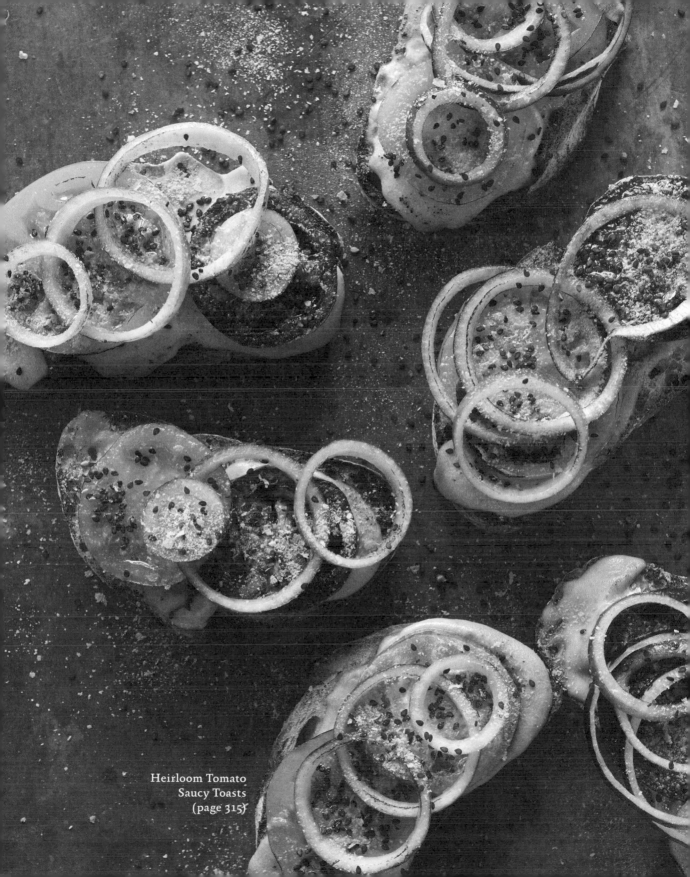

Heirloom Tomato
Saucy Toasts
(page 315)

Get a Good Night's Sleep

Quality sleep is essential for feeling your best. Sure, rest is vital to having a happy, healthy pregnancy, but here's the most important thing to know: Come baby time, sleep is survival! Cherish these sweet, relatively uninterrupted sleep moments now while you don't have a tiny creature to care for. If I could go back and be pregnant all over again, I would try to sleep all day and night for many days in a row! I know it sounds insane, but going into labor and being a well-rested mama is so, so important. I promise you'll thank me later!

Here's the golden rule that kept me sane and rested from my pregnancy well into mamahood: Eat well, sleep well. The cleaner you eat, the better you'll feel. The better you feel, the more restorative your sleep will be. And the more rested you are, the stronger, more resilient, more tuned-in mama warrior you can be during the day. Kind foods allow the body to rest and repair at night, instead of forcing the body to work around the clock to break down things it has no clue what to do with. You'll wake up feeling fresh and bright and have the energy to take care of yourself *and* your family. To get sweeter sleep, try some of these tips:

CHOOSE SIDES: SLEEPING POSITIONS

Getting a good night's sleep can be tricky as your belly grows. Some doctors will tell you to preemptively stop sleeping on your back and right side, even if it's still comfortable. That's because the weight of your uterus can compress a big vein called the vena cava, which is responsible for getting blood to your heart, the uterus, and the placenta. But don't you think you'd be the first one to know if your body was gasping for air?! Without a doubt. That's why the new wisdom, which I heard from midwives, yoga instructors, and childbirth educators, is this: If you can lie on your back or right side without feeling nauseated, light-headed, sweaty, or otherwise uncomfortable—signs that your body needs to change things up—then there's no reason to stop. If these positions aren't comfy, then switch to sleeping on your left side.

MAKE A NEST

If you're having a hard time getting comfortable, or you are waking up achy, try using your pillows to support your belly, hips, and back. Wedging one pillow between your knees and one beneath your belly is sometimes enough. Or you can invest in a pregnancy pillow that tackles both of these at once. Choose one that's made with natural, healthy, and animal-friendly materials like natural latex, kapok, buckwheat hull, or organic cotton. For more handy info on how to buy the kindest, most eco bedding, check out "Cleaner, Sweeter Dreams" on page 257. As a calming bonus, spritz a couple of drops of lavender oil or clary sage mixed with water on your sheets. Or, before bedtime, sip a cup of camomile tea.

FIND SOME FLOW

A prenatal yoga instructor once told me that the reason pregnant women toss and turn at night is because their bodies are trying to keep the blood circulating. She recommended doing some gentle stretches and poses before bed, and sure enough—a few Cat-Cows, Downward-Facing Dogs, and Ankle-to-Knees later, along with a rebalancing couple of minutes of legs up the wall, I got a full night's sleep. The stretches also helped with the occasional leg cramps that aren't uncommon in the second and third trimesters. If you happen to get attacked by a

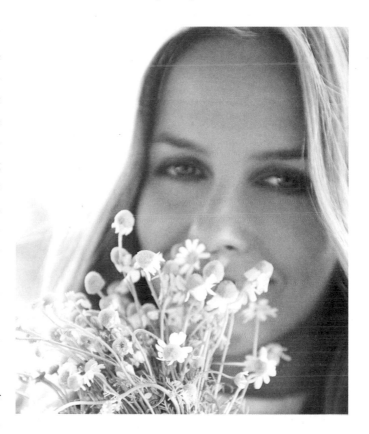

vicious charley horse that feels like an alien monster is turning your calf muscles inside out—which happened to me a few times—all you have to do is jump out of bed and flex your foot as strongly as you can with your heel pushing into the floor. It should be gone in a flash.

GET RUBBED THE RIGHT WAY

I'm grateful that I had massage during my pregnancy. It helped soothe any aches and pains, and every time I felt my husband's strong, capable hands on my skin, I was reminded of what an incredible partner he is. In addition to being a totally sumptuous, decadent treat, massage has all

> ## Lucky Mama Massage Oil
> Start with a yummy emollient base like jojoba oil, almond oil, shea butter, or olive oil. Then add a few drops of your favorite essential oil, like lavender, tangerine, eucalyptus, rose, or ylang-ylang. A good rule-of-thumb ratio is about 1 teaspoon of base oil to 5 drops of essential oil. That's usually enough for one decadent rubdown.

kinds of healthy benefits. It boosts feel-good hormones like serotonin and dopamine, which can help prevent premature birth and too low a birth weight.[90] It keeps your circulation moving, your muscles strong, your joints and ligaments supple, and relaxes the mind—excellent prep for labor! Gentle touch can help you fall into deep, restful sleep. While conventional wisdom suggests that massage therapists handle pregnant ladies like live grenades, there's absolutely nothing wrong with or dangerous about having a head-to-toe massage while pregnant. Here's what super doula and massage therapist Lisa Jacobson has to say about it:

> First of all, if your massage therapist is educated, then she should be able to safely give a massage to pregnant women. There are some acupoints on your heels, inner ankle, bottom of the foot, top of the shoulders, and the webbing between your thumb and index finger that are considered off-limits during pregnancy. That's because strong, deliberate stimulation of these points can cause uterine contractions. But as long as you're not working very deep there—assuming your aim isn't to stimulate labor—it's fine. I work more gently in these areas, but I by no means avoid them.

Check out greenspanetwork.org to find spas in your area that offer eco-friendly treatments. Or whip up a batch of yummy Lucky Mama Massage Oil and enlist your partner for a rubdown. He'll love helping you and your baby feel good.

Start Your Kegels

If I never heard the word *kegel* again I'd be totally thrilled, but because this technique is one of the best ways to maintain good tone in your pelvic floor while your belly gets bigger and to regain tone after you give birth, we're talking about kegels now. Basically, all of your bottom's bits are interconnected by a sling of muscles that make up your pelvic floor. It's a good idea to take care of these muscles because they help you do great things like not pee in your pants when

(continued on page 128)

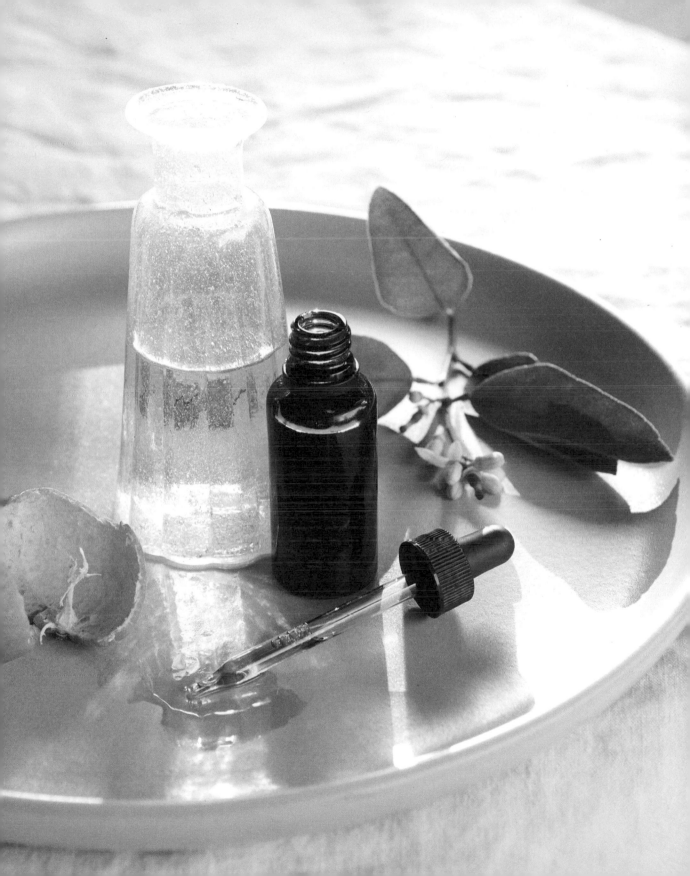

For Gentlemen Only: Make Mama Feel Good

You've probably noticed that your woman's body has changed quite a bit since she became pregnant. If you're like most guys, then her softer, curvier shape—bigger boobs and butt included—is a real bonus. But it might take her some time to fully appreciate this new voluptuousness. Be sure to remind your partner just how radiant and gorgeous she is. Aside from telling her how hot she looks, a great way to show your appreciation and love is to offer the occasional massage. A man who uses his hands is super-sexy, and more likely than not it's *exactly* what she needs to feel good, inside and out.

Another way to capture this time in her life is to take a lot of pictures. Don't make her feel self-conscious about it—and don't post them all to Facebook!—but start documenting this special, sacred time. It will help her know how sexy and beautiful you think she is and that you, too, are savoring her new divine shape. Plus, she's probably secretly hoping you'll do this but feels like too big of a dork to ask. She'll love to be able to look back at herself in her full, glowing, fertile glory.

Gentlemen, get in touch with your inner caveman.
This is some all-man stuff. Don't be afraid to start a fire and get naked and grunt while also being loving and caring. I would give Alicia lots of full-body massages. (Again, good work, if you can get it!) I tried to hold the space for calm energy and have compassion that she sometimes was nauseated. Just try to help out as much as you can to make your partner's life easier and basically try to not be annoying. Hell hath no fury like a pregnant, nauseated woman whose husband is irritating her.

—Christopher

Mama to Mama: How to Involve Your Man in Your Pregnancy

Okay, so this is basically The Mama Show because you are, after all, actively carrying and building and nourishing your baby. But make sure you're giving papa-to-be every opportunity to participate in this special process and share in its wonder and delight. Take some inspiration from these Mamas:

As a gift for my husband and myself, I bought a lovely journal that showed the week-by-week changes that were happening for our beautifully growing baby. We read it together and made notes as we shared our dreams and curiosities with each other. A prenatal yoga class for couples also helped us to connect—together—with our baby. One of the best things that we still enjoy is a project we undertook to take weekly photographs of my belly. My artist mother-in-law put all the photos together in a Photoshop file and made a gorgeous framed picture that hangs in our home as one of our family's favorite art pieces.

—Allison Rivers Samson, Nevada City, California

I got my partner involved by grabbing his hand and putting it on my belly when baby decided to dance, bringing him to appointments and birthing and baby first-aid classes, sharing birthing and baby books, watching natural birth documentaries together, and talking about the baby almost nonstop. We couldn't help it; it just seemed like such a big, exciting deal! He even listened to the HypnoBirthing CD with me at night and fell asleep to affirmations like, "My cervix opens outward and allows my baby to ease down." What a guy. If he's a mother in his next life, he'll have the easiest, most natural birth ever.

—Marisa Miller Wolfson, New York City

My husband and I frequently talked about our intentions as parents and what was important to both of us. He loved feeling her kick and hiccup inside of me, and he loved playing guitar to my belly! We talked about our birth plan so I could share what mattered most to me and he could share his concerns. Together, we wrote our plan, and he advocated for me during the birth. I wanted to involve him as much as possible because even though I was the one carrying our child, she was *ours*, and every second together as a family counted—and even more so now that's she's here!

—Kaycee Bassett, American Fork, Utah

you sneeze and have more powerful orgasms.[91] Carrying a baby and giving birth, however, are the equivalent of using a hair elastic one too many times—things just get loose. I suggest you aim to do a full set of kegels at least once or twice a day from now until after the baby's born. Knock them out in the car, sitting at the computer at work, reading a book—wherever! And by the third day postpartum, when your muscles will be up for the challenge again, you can do these exercises while you breastfeed first thing in the morning and not have to think about it again for the rest of the day.

How to kegel: Squeeze your muscles the way you would if trying to not pee. Congrats, you just kegeled! Now squeeze super slowly like your vagina muscles are a little elevator going up into your belly and back down again. Try doing that for a count of five (up and down) and work up to eight or so. My midwife recommended doing 10 of those lengthy squeezes combined with 50 little quickies.

COUNTDOWN TO BABY

Take a Class

Many people join a prenatal class to learn more about natural birth options, breathing and relaxation techniques, and birthing positions. According to Ellen Chuse, a Brooklyn-based childbirth educator who offers a lovely home birth–centered series, "A good class is where you do the emotional work and integrate the material, and that's just as important as the information." It's also a great way to connect with your partner and let him or her really be part of the pregnancy journey. A lot of midwives—mine included—recommend you take a class, if only to meet other groovy like-minded mamas. But when Christopher and I started looking around, we couldn't find a group that was for couples planning a home birth. Since we didn't think we'd get much out of learning all the things that happen during a hospital birth, we decided to rely on our own intuition plus what I was learning from a few great books and my mama tribe.

It's certainly worth investigating to see if there is a class in your community for home birthers. If there isn't, that's what I'm here for! You have this book for tons of insight and guidance, as well as other great books I've listed in Resources (page 332) and on thekindlife.com. And look to your own trusted mama tribe for their time-tested wisdom. I loved having dinner with our friends and asking them questions.

Another option to consider is HypnoBirthing. I've heard good things about this technique, which can help you let go of some of the fear and tension that can make birth more difficult and painful. If you think you may be interested in these techniques, check out the book *HypnoBirthing: The Mongan Method: A Natural Approach to a Safe, Easier, More Comfortable Birthing* by Marie F. Mongan, MEd, MHy.

Consider a Doula

Appropriately, *doula* is a Greek word meaning "one who ministers." A doula knows the drill when it comes to making the birth event as natural and beautiful as it can possibly be—regardless of whether you deliver at home or in a hospital. She is your personalized support system. While your midwife's main responsibility is safely delivering your baby, a doula's sole purpose is to bring you and your partner physical and emotional comfort. She can guide you through relaxation techniques; massage and breathe with you; administer things like hypnosis, aromatherapy, acupuncture, or pressure point therapy; suggest changing things up if she senses you're getting tired or discouraged; help the midwife facilitate birthing positions; and otherwise be a hand to hold. She can also explain to your partner what's going on at each step of labor, assure him everything is just fine, and give him the much-needed go-ahead to eat meals and take naps.

Beyond offering another pair of (very therapeutic) hands, a doula can give you the support and confidence to grab hold of the experience, look labor in the eye, and say, "I *so* have this." She empowers your partner to be there for you confidently, calmly, and completely. Like your midwife, she'll come visit you a day or two after the baby's born to make sure everyone is settling in, nursing well, and feeling good. That said, a loved one or even a friend (particularly one who's had a natural birth) can offer this kind of support. Or in my experience, my midwife provided many of these things. A doula is just another option to consider, which I might for next time! Women who employ a doula report significantly lower rates of pain, intervention, and unwanted C sections.[92]

A New Way to Nest

One of the many beautiful things that happen during pregnancy is the urge to nest, or create a snug, peaceful cocoon for your new family member. Take advantage of this time to purge your home of everything old and stale and fill it with good, fresh intentions. Like spring cleaning, a ritual that has existed for hundreds of years, deeply cleansing your living space can change its vibrational energy. When we accumulate a lot of stuff, energy stagnates. Each of our possessions carries weight, as do the dust and dirt that can settle in little nooks and crannies. This not only causes physical reactions like allergies and asthma, but also dampens our spirit and clutters the mind. Invite in a newer, lighter energy by clearing it all out. Give your house a good scrubbing (using a nontoxic cleaner). Air rugs and bedding outside in the sun, the original antibacterial purifier. Sort all your belongings and give away anything that is no longer useful or that doesn't make you happy. Open the windows and let the breeze breathe life into you and the house.

BUILDING A SAFER BABY HOUSE

By the time your baby is in your womb and the two of you are sharing a blood and nutrient smoothie, you're already passing on many toxic chemicals you may have come into contact with. These chemicals start to accumulate in baby's body. In fact, in 2004, a study by the Environmental Working Group found that on average, the newborn babies they tested had 200 industrial chemicals in their umbilical cord blood. That included things like pesticides, chemicals from consumer and home products, and by-products from industry and waste incineration, which can get into our soil, water, and food.[93] These are things that—if we're not mindful—we continue to come into contact with on an everyday basis. "Our homes should be a safe haven, a nontoxic living area that enables our bodies to use its energy for rejuvenation and healing instead of detoxifying chemicals," says green-living expert Marilee Nelson.

The great news is that adopting simple (I'm serious—so easy!) green habits now will provide enormous benefits to you and your baby's health. And by combining these preventive measures with a diet packed with plants—remember all those free radical–fighting superpowers?—you'll be giving your baby a strong defensive shield.

Hold off on large-scale changes to your home

Now is not the time to be undergoing major renovation like drywall installation, carpet removal, and painting. Demolition or the scraping up of old paint can release lead dust into your home, which can hurt your baby in utero, causing possible brain, kidney, and nervous system damage or learning and behavior problems.[94] Removing carpeting can stir up high levels of toxic chemical–laden dust and particulates.[95] The fetus is much more sensitive to chemicals and other contaminants than adults are—even if you're using green products and materials, which aren't necessarily nontoxic.

Plus, there's no need for a nursery now anyway. *What?! No need for a precious little room that's perfectly decorated and filled to the brim with toys and stuffed animals?!* Believe me, the alternative is much more fun—for you and baby. Read Chapter 10 to see all the awesome reasons for *not* building that baby suite. For now, focus on welcoming your baby into a space that is pure, calm, and clean.

Get some fresh air

It doesn't get any easier than this for reducing allergens and air pollutants in your home: Throw open those windows! As often as you can. Think of it as a reset for your entire home. Even if you keep a spotlessly clean house, things like cleaning products, synthetic fragrances, paint, carpets, furniture, mold, bacteria, mites, pollen, fireplaces, and candles release tiny irritants. In fact, the EPA has named indoor air quality as one of the top five environmental risks to public health, and it's likely a big reason why so many kids now have asthma.[96] We'll talk more about how you can reduce these gassy, dusty nuisances in the first place, but it's always a good idea to let your house breathe every now and then.

Go barefoot

According to a study conducted by the EPA, it's what we track inside from the outside that typically causes most of the lead dust in our homes. Wiping shoes off at the door—or even better, taking them off completely—can cut lead dust by 60 percent![97] It also cuts down on pesticides and any other pollutants that might be hitching a ride on your shoes.

Buy a HEPA (high-efficiency particulate air) vacuum

According to Marilee Nelson, conventional vacuums typically make the air quality *worse* after vacuuming because they release all that dust and dirt right back into the air. HEPA vacuums (not to be confused with "HEPA-type" vacuums) can suck out more than 99 percent

(continued)

of airborne bacteria and spores—including dust mite droppings, pet dander, and pollen—and even trap some of those phthalates, flame retardants, and pesticides that bind to household dust.[98] If you have carpeting in your home, it's a good idea to vacuum every other day or, at the very least, once a week. And do your sofas one or two times a month.

Chuck all pesticides and herbicides

Babies love to play in the grass and dirt outside, so you want to make sure your outdoor space is just as clean and nontoxic as the inside of your home. According to Nelson, conventional products typically used for garden and lawn care are among the most dangerous products to have in the home or garage, affecting the nervous system, respiratory system, and reproductive system. Just because you're storing them under the sink, don't think you're safe: These chemicals can still present a hazard by escaping into your home's air. Think about how you can smell chemical fragrances when you stroll down the grocery aisle—and those cleansers haven't been opened yet!

Steer clear of toxic furniture

If you decide to take this opportunity to upgrade your sofa/armchair/kitchen table, buy with your baby house in mind. If a piece is conventionally made or finished, there's a good chance that it's releasing volatile organic compounds and other unhealthy fumes into the air. The foam in the cushions may be made with polyurethane and treated with flame retardants, which have been linked to cancer, male infertility, and early puberty in girls.[99] Manufactured woods—pressed wood, plywood, particleboard, and chipboard—contain glues that give off formaldehyde, a likely carcinogen.[100] The good news, though, is that as some of these wood pieces age, they eventually release much of their noxious toxins. If you score great used pieces—the kindest way to shop!—you're not only saving a huge item from its landfill destiny but also avoiding potential nastiness. (Just make sure older items aren't finished with lead paint.) Unfortunately, items made with foam and flame retardants don't age gracefully: They degrade and create more toxic dust over time. But you can address that by restuffing and reupholstering vintage finds!

If you do buy new, invest in pieces that are clearly labeled as being made from natural or sustainable materials. Some trustworthy certifications to look for include Forest Stewardship Council (FSC), Cradle 2 Cradle, and Greenguard (which indicates low toxicity).

Reduce EMFs, or electromagnetic frequencies

Revisit the "Am I Frying My Baby?" section in Chapter 6 and keep in mind my basic rule of thumb: Would I want that cell phone/wireless router/laptop next to my baby? Most likely not. Let that be your guide as you think about adding any kind of electronic gadget—vibrating chair, DVD player, iPad dock, etc.—to your baby's space. But if you do decide to go the electronics route (a monitor, white noise machine, or humidifier), keep these things at least a few feet from where you and your baby sleep.

CLEANER CLEANING: NO MORE TOXIC CLEANING SUPPLIES

To give your nest the kindest cleansing, choose products that aren't introducing toxic agents into your living space. Today, there are more than *80,000* chemicals registered for use in the United States, and several thousand are found in our everyday environments.[101] But according to a 2010 landmark report released by the President's Cancer Panel, only a few hundred of them are tested for safety."[102] The agency also asserts that the air we breathe inside could be as much as five times as polluted as the air outside.[103] That's largely because we're swabbing down our floors, walls, and windows with freaky harmful substances that promise to get the job done better and more cheaply. Some of these ingredients are linked to cancer, blindness, asthma, hormone disruption, and damage to red blood cells and other tissues.[104] And what we're sending down our drains doesn't just magically disappear! Seventy percent of stream water contains traces of detergent, and 66 percent contains traces of disinfectant cleaners, which ends up in our water supply.

Luckily, it's so easy to find gentle, nontoxic, plant-based household cleaners that are just as effective as the nasty originals. Bon Ami, Ecover, and Seventh Generation all make beautiful alternatives to mainstream brands. Be mindful of "greenwashing," or products labeled with meaningless green-sounding promises—terms like *natural* and *nontoxic* aren't standardized or widely regulated. If you're trying to figure out whether the products you're currently using are unkind, the easiest thing to do is look for words on the label like *danger, poison, warning,* or *caution.* Look for directions that recommend wearing rubber gloves or a mask or ventilating an area after using. Check out the Environmental Working Group's Cleaners Database, especially their "Hall of Shame" for brands that aren't delivering on sneaky promises: ewg.org/cleaners/hallofshame/.

9

Third Trimester and Birth

It's crazy to think that in 1 month there will be a baby that
is mine to take care of forever. It doesn't feel real.
I love being pregnant, and I'm not in any rush for it to end,
but I'm happy and excited for you, baby. I'm ready when you are.
We love you and are so excited to meet you.

—My Journal, 8 months pregnant

WHAT YOU MIGHT BE FEELING

A Little Loopy

Pregnancy brain seems like one of those crazy myths—blanking out midsentence because you completely forgot what you were saying—but guess what? Not only is it real and normal, it's one more piece of evidence that the body is pretty genius.

There are a few reasons for that fuzzy, out-of-it feeling:

- Your brain needs extra fuel during pregnancy. DHA, the crucial omega-3 fatty acid that boosts our smarts, is at a premium because it's what's building your baby's noodle.[105] Because most of your DHA supply is being funneled into your little one, it's super-important that you protect your own neurons by getting plenty of omega-3s through your diet.

Revisit the DHA section in Chapter 5 to make sure you're getting enough foods that are rich in the stuff, like walnuts, chia seeds, tofu, and flaxseed oil.

- Your brain shrinks during pregnancy! Don't worry, you won't lose all that hard-earned knowledge, but as your metabolism changes, your brain restructures itself. Some believe it's evolution's way of preparing mothers to focus on their babies and block out other stresses. And in the week or two before birth, the brain will eventually start to grow again, this time packed with neural circuits specific to bonding with your newborn.[106]

- Toward the end of your pregnancy, you get an extra shot of the hormone progesterone, which has a tranquilizing effect and is Mother Nature's way of saying, "Just let go!"[107]

Personally, I loved feeling a bit floaty and relaxed during this period. There's something beautiful that comes with unplugging from your brain and inhabiting your body more, especially if you're type A or prone to hearing a lot of restless "mind chatter." Ironically, the more you give in to this mental pea soup, the more grounded and clear you'll feel.

WHAT YOU MIGHT BE WONDERING

Is My Baby in the Right Position for Birth?

When it comes to birth, the body's pretty much thought of everything. But sometimes, we can help the process be an even smoother and calmer one. During your third trimester, your baby is positioning herself to make her way headfirst into the birth canal. Occasionally, because of anything from the shape of your uterus to slower development of your baby's inner ears, babies prep for the big ride bottom first (breech) or back facing (posterior). Your midwife or doctor will keep you posted on where your baby's been hanging out, so you'll have plenty of time to nudge her into place if she doesn't do it on her own. Luckily, there's a variety of ways you can encourage your little one to greet the world in a manner that's easier and safer for both of you.

MAKE SURE YOU'RE IN BALANCE

Eating a clean, kind diet is more important than ever as you approach labor. If you're out of balance, it could stagnate the energy in your uterus, which holistic-minded practitioners believe can cause it to constrict. And if your baby is still bum down, that means she'll have less room to flip.

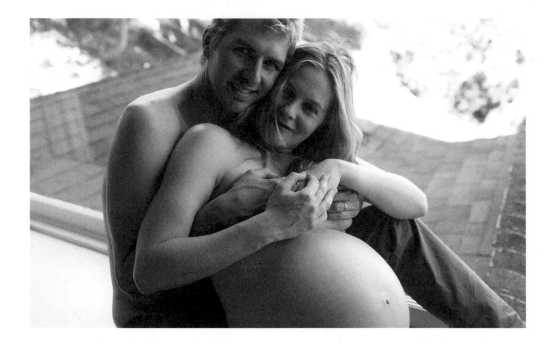

Stick with lots of healing whole foods that naturally promote circulation and ease in your body, and try to pass up things like sugar and other sweeteners, fruit, chocolate, flour-containing foods, salt, baked products, cold or raw foods, and *especially* animal foods.

DO SOME GENTLE EXERCISES

The Stretching Calf: This is a lot like the Cat-Cow posture in yoga, except it doesn't include tucking the pelvis under like a cat. On your hands and knees, breathe in, as you arch your back and tilt your pelvis while looking up to the sky. Return to a flat-back position and repeat. Try for 30 repetitions several times a day. Feel the joy as your heart bursts open to the sky.

The Lazy Calf: Lower your elbows onto the floor. Just breathe into your baby and visualize her sweet face. Sometimes the shift in gravity can help float your child out of breech position.

Handstands in a pool: This gentle inversion will encourage your baby to flip—without your having to worry about toppling over!

Sit in forward-leaning positions: This is the most commonly prescribed solution for turning a baby in the posterior position. In the car, make sure the seatback is all the way upright. When you're in a chair, shift your weight forward so you're sitting directly on your sitz bones.

Or you might find that straddling a chair, facing its back with your arms resting on the top, might be more comfortable.

CALL THE EXPERTS

Some doctors, most midwives, and even acupuncturists and chiropractors who specialize in prenatal care have techniques to turn or flip the baby.

Could It Happen to Me? Questions and Concerns about Home Birth

It's a good idea to ask your doctor or midwife about any specific concerns you have regarding labor and birth. But these are the biggies that I hear from women all the time. The answers—and reassurance—come from my midwife, Margo Kennedy.

HOW LONG DOES LABOR LAST?

"Statistically speaking, a first-time mother's labor—active labor—is 12 to 13 hours," Kennedy says. "And that's not including the first part of labor, or latent labor (when contractions are short and spread about 20 minutes apart), which alone can last up to 20 hours. So I tell my moms to plan on a 24-hour period of labor. There are so many things that go into how a body births a baby—power, passenger, pelvis, and the psyche. And all those things can contribute to how long it takes a woman to go through labor. If the mother's all right and the baby's all right, I give them all the time they need. But if mom gets tired and the uterus gets tired and stops producing strong enough contractions, then we need to reevaluate. Sometimes you just need to leave a mother by herself, just let her rest. Sometimes she needs a minute to figure it out. That's the beauty of a home birth—you don't have to follow a schedule or look at the clock. In the hospital, you feel the pressure of that clock."

WHAT IF THE BABY'S UMBILICAL CORD IS WRAPPED AROUND HIS NECK?

"In my experience, you often don't even know until the baby's born. What most frequently happens is that the head will come out, and I'll reach in and the cord will be around the neck and I just loop it over the head. I'd say that happens about 50 percent of the time—it's pretty common," Kennedy says. "It makes sense—the cord is long and the baby's been moving around.

But if the cord is pulled too tightly, that compression would cut bloodflow to the baby, and we'd be able to hear it as we monitored the heartbeat. So we'd hear the baby's heartbeat go down and then back up suddenly. Usually just changing position can fix it, which is the first course of action in a hospital, too. But if not, we would transfer to the hospital before it became an emergency. That's why we're constantly monitoring for these things. But if the mother is healthy, then her body can produce a nice, long cord and a lot of Wharton's jelly—a gelatinous substance in the umbilical cord—which makes it harder to compress."

WHAT ARE THE CHANCES OF HEMORRHAGING AFTER BIRTH?

"Hemorrhaging, or excessive blood loss, is the most frequent complication I see at home births—but even then, it's maybe 5 to 10 percent of all the births I've attended," Kennedy states. "If you're taking good care of yourself, the uterus will contract itself after birth. And midwives carry the same meds—like Pitocin, Methergine, and Cytotec as well as IVs with fluid—that they would use in a hospital in the case of hemorrhaging or just to get a mother's volume back up if she's lost too much blood."

HOW LIKELY IS IT THAT I'LL TEAR?

"During labor, the tissues have to stretch. For a woman with good nutrition, her tissues will stretch more easily. That elasticity comes from what you eat. Also, the way you push and how you allow the baby's head to sit on the perineum can make you less likely to tear. Especially waiting to push with contractions. We midwives also use methods to help relax that tissue. Warm compresses bring some relaxation, as can trying to laugh or smile or kissing your husband. Most people have no tears or just a first-degree tear, where there's just a small split in the skin," Kennedy concludes.

Should I Eat My Placenta?

Okay, so before you puke and think I've totally run off the hippie rails, let's talk placenta business. This amazing organ, which you grew completely from scratch in that magical baby house garden of yours, transfers vital nutrients from you to your baby. So some people believe that taking those nutrients back in can be a major boost to the system after delivery. But aside from being wholeheartedly supported by traditional Chinese medicine practitioners, this thinking has—until now—just been mystical lore. No longer! According to a February 2013 study done by researchers at the University of Las Vegas, the fairy tale is real! Seventy-six percent of women who participated in the study backed up what gurus, healers, and shamans have been saying for centuries: Eating the placenta helped increase lactation, boost mood, and treat all kinds of postpartum systems like blood loss, fatigue, hormone withdrawal, and the baby blues.[108]

Honoring the placenta isn't a new idea. The Aymara and Quechua people of Bolivia say it has its own spirit. Malaysians consider it to be the older sibling of the child, and ancient Egyptians believed it held the other half of a child's soul. I don't know about all that, but biologically, it's what gave your child shelter and nourishment as she grew. So it made sense, to me, to not just throw it in the trash.

I'd heard of more and more women who were eating their placentas, and I did sort of like the idea. But I was on the fence. On the one hand, I'd put all this tender care into growing the greatest, healthiest baby house, so why not process all those nutrients in a different way? I also loved that it's what many mammals naturally do and that no part of this miraculous experience would go to waste. But on the other hand, it was animal food. It was my own flesh, but it was still animal, and there was no way of knowing whether my body could tell the difference. Plus, chowing down on it like a big steak was totally unappealing. But when someone offered to encapsulate my placenta into pills as a gift, I gave it a try. I had nothing to lose.

Skipping ahead to my birth story for a second (I'll tell you much more about it later): I had a smooth and vibrant postbirth because of how well I'd taken care of my body all through pregnancy, but every once in a while, I'd have a mini-meltdown. In my sleep-deprived, emotionally wonky haze, I'd start thinking about things like how my baby was going to grow up one day, and I'd just lose it. Then I'd have my placenta pill and feel better. And I'd love when Christopher would sometimes say, "Have you taken your placenta today?" Can I be sure it was something in the pills? Maybe not. But they were my happy pills, and I wish I still had them!

Encapsulating the placenta into pills is just one way to go, and your midwife or doula can direct you to someone who will do it for you. Some women have a small piece of placenta made into a healing tincture, and some go all-in and make a series of postbirth placenta smoothies. It's difficult to say whether you'd reap different benefits from these various methods, so I say go with whatever feels true to you. And don't worry if you end up delivering in the hospital—you can still save your placenta. Some hospitals require you to sign a release waiver, but all will let you take it home so long as you bring a food-safe container. Just make sure it's refrigerated during your stay.

If you like the idea of celebrating the placenta but don't love the idea of eating it, consider burying it instead. The Navajo of the Southwest and the Maori of New Zealand bury the placenta in native soil to bind the child to its ancestral home and people. I love the idea of planting a tree in the same spot, which will grow and flourish as your baby does. And then he can point to that little sapling and say, "That's my tree!"

Cutting to the Chase: Is Circumcision Healthy?

One day, I was wondering out loud to Christopher whether we should circumcise our baby if we had a boy. My instinct was that it just didn't feel right, while Christopher was more curious about whether *not* circumcising would mean our kid would feel different. We both decided to give it some thought and maybe let the universe speak its piece. One day, Christopher was out running errands, and in a shop he came across a group of cute girls. Risking looking like a total perv, he asked if any of them had had sex with a guy who was uncut. "Yeah," one said. "And how was it?" "Best sex of my life." Score one for no circumcision.

Then we were at a pediatrician meet-and-greet, and the doctor spoke about how unhealthy he felt circumcision was—that it made the penis shorter, that it was painful, and that it was basically deemed unnecessary in the medical community. *Hmm.*

After that, I was hanging out with a friend and her son at the pool, and I noticed he wasn't circumcised. "Is that an undone penis?" I asked. "Yeah," she said. So I asked, "Has it ever been an issue that his penis was different than his dad's?" "His penis wouldn't match his dad's anyway!" she said. "His dad's is so much bigger and has hair all over it. And by the time they do look more alike, they're not going to be side-by-side comparing." Good point.

Then Bear was born. I was raised Jewish, so the second my parents found out they had a male grandchild, they wanted to know when we'd be having a *bris* (the circumcision ceremony traditionally performed 8 days after a baby boy is born). When I said we weren't having one, my dad got a bit worked up. He couldn't understand why not—I mean, it's what our people have been doing for a really long time. Then he started listing reasons for doing it, like uncircumcised penises were hard to keep clean and can get infected, and that it doesn't hurt the baby—although I'm pretty sure most babies scream and cry at their *bris*. But my thinking was: If little boys were supposed to have their penises "fixed," did that mean we were saying that God made the body imperfect? He made all this incredible stuff, and then he just happened to make the penis wrong?

When Christopher, Bear, and I were over at our friend's house hanging out in the pool, I started talking about my dad's not-so-happy reaction about Bear not being cut. And I told them about my dad's concern that Bear wouldn't fit in; that he worried about other kids giving Bear a hard time because he looked different. As if on cue, the four other moms there lifted their naked little babies out of the pool—not one was circumcised.

We're in a new world! According to a 2010 analysis from the National Center for Health Statistics, the percentage of newborn boys who are circumcised in this country dropped to 58.3 percent from 64.5 percent in 1979.[109] All those old ideas about why not to do it are totally outdated. A recent review by the American Academy of Pediatrics looked at the data from the past decades to see if there were really, truly any medical benefits to circumcision. Their conclusion? Nope![110] And according to baby doctor genius and father of eight Dr. William Sears, not only are there no medical benefits to circumcision, there are actually some pretty weighty drawbacks. The foreskin is packed with nerves (more than any other organ, actually), and removing it can diminish sexual pleasure. It helps protect the head of the penis, which, while also supersensitive, was meant to be an internal organ. When it's exposed and is constantly rubbing up against clothing, it can become desensitized, which is also bad news when your son starts getting frisky.[111]

Then there are the risks associated with what is, in truth, a minor surgery: hemorrhage, infection, septicemia, gangrene, disfigurement, or, if too much foreskin is removed, the need for skin grafting later in life.[112]

In case you're still not convinced that you wouldn't be committing your child to a life of bad Hebraic karma, consider that in Israel more and more parents are opting to celebrate the first week in their baby's life with *brit shalom* (the "covenant of peace"), a ritual alternative to circumcision.[113]

KIND ACTION

Start Winding Down Work

When I was pregnant, I vowed to give myself the 4 weeks before my delivery date as a sort of baby gift. I wanted to clear the decks of any major work projects, so all I had to do was rest and flow and stay relaxed and in harmony. I could go to the beach, play in the garden, plan fun lunch dates, make love, meditate, go to yoga, or commune with nature—anything that filled my heart and soul with whatever they craved. Sure, it was a fantasy, and this didn't exactly happen, but what was important was that I set the *intention*. Because I made it clear that this was something I valued, I managed to get far closer to the ideal than if I hadn't made the effort.

I know it can be difficult when work seems like the most important thing in the world. And even more difficult when you love what you do! Yes, it pays our bills and puts a roof over our heads and in some cases brings us soul-filling satisfaction. But you know what else is totally crucial? Being healthy and rested for labor.

Start taking more and more time for yourself so that by the 32- or 34-week mark you can, if possible, taper off completely. Do a little bit less every day until you're down to only the most critical priorities. I love how childbirth educator Ellen Chuse puts it: "Think of it as an investment in labor and birth." Going into the next phase of this journey exhausted isn't doing you or your baby any favors. In fact, spending 12 hours a day in the office right up until labor is a recipe for complications. A recent study done by researchers at UC Berkeley found that women who worked up until their due dates were nearly four times *more* likely to have a C-section.[114] That's major! "You need some time to prepare for labor," Chuse says. "It takes place in the right brain, so you have to move from the left, more analytical part of the brain into that more intuitive, dream-state brain. And it can't turn on a dime." It's so important that you do everything in your power to grab this precious time in your life. Start drawing your focus inward and fully embrace the flowering goddess that you are. For baby number two, you can bet that I'll be even better at taking my own advice.

LUNCH-BREAK GODDESS: FINDING PEACE IF LEAVING WORK ISN'T AN OPTION

If it's simply not a reality to make a clean break from work, try giving yourself small pieces of the day to be totally and utterly relaxed. If you can, set aside one whole hour for lunch: 20 minutes to serenely eat and chew, and the remaining time to rest. It doesn't have to mean taking a nap (though, curling up under your desk would probably be pretty nice!). Breathe, go for a walk or sit in the sun and close your eyes—whatever brings you fulfillment in that moment. This is what I did for myself, and it felt so luxurious. If you can't take an hour, take advantage of any time you get to find some quiet, even if it's just closing your eyes for a few moments.

Find a Mama Mantra: Empowering Words for Birth

I love some of these mantra suggestions from Marie F. Mongan's *HypnoBirthing*. Choose a couple that speak to you and stick them in your proverbial pocket. Remind yourself of these sentiments as you get closer to labor. And if you manage to think of it during labor, use them to remind yourself just how ready you are to meet any challenges.

- I trust my body, and I follow its lead.

- I fully relax and turn my birthing over to nature.

- I turn birthing over to my baby and my body.

- Each surge of my body brings my baby closer to me.

Find a Pediatrician

When my midwife suggested I do this, I didn't understand the need. They would want to see my baby so soon after being born (3 to 4 days) and then every month?! But what if nothing was wrong?? I'd managed to keep myself super-healthy with my healing, kind diet, and I knew I'd be doing the same for my baby with my top-shelf breast milk. But my midwife made a great point. She said, "If something happened to your kid and he had to go to the hospital, would you want some random doctor showing up?" Now *that* was a reasonable argument for finding a pediatrician. "You want to establish a relationship with someone for that reason, but you don't necessarily have to go regularly," she said.

After asking the other Kind Mamas in my tribe about whether they had pediatricians, I realized I was the only holdout. Granted, one of them said she walked into her doctor's office when her baby was already 2 months old and just showed him the kid. In a nutshell: He said "Fine," she said "Great," and that was that. So I knew there was some wiggle room in how much office time I'd really need. I started meeting pediatricians with the mentality that this was someone I could call in case of an emergency, not someone I'd need to visit regularly. As integrative pediatrician, founder of the Whole Child Center in New Jersey, and author of *Treatment Alternatives for Children* Dr. Lawrence Rosen puts it, "It's important for somebody—whether it's your midwife or a pediatrician and family practitioner—to check the baby during that first week of life, usually in the first 2 or 3 days. I know parents don't want to leave the home—and that's part of the reason they chose to have a home birth and ideally we'd all do home visits—but it's worth it just to say 'Hi' and let someone lay eyes on the baby."

I ended up finding an amazing (and vegan) pediatrician, Dr. Jay Gordon. I don't take Bear all the time (he's gone for about three wellness check-ups in 2½ years, and has never had to take medication), but I like knowing that I have a doctor I can call who supports my ideas about health. When finding a potential caretaker for your baby, it's crucial to find someone who supports your values and beliefs. He or she should be aware of the powerful link between your child's health and the food we eat, what we put on our skin, the products we use in our homes, and the toys our children play with. Some pediatricians are going to tell you that your child won't get enough nutrients from vegan breast milk and that cow's milk formula is a viable alternative, or that you shouldn't have your baby sleep in your bed. If you believe otherwise—and this book will give you every reason under the sun why you should—then keep looking. To me, it was important to have a relationship with a doctor who believes a plant-based diet is an essential part of well-being and who isn't too trigger-happy with vaccines and medications. If you feel the same, try to find a pediatrician or family physician who has a holistic or integrative approach to medicine.

To get a better idea of how a potential pediatrician feels about these issues, ask questions about how she raised her own children (since experience is often a huge factor in the guidance she'll give), how she might treat an ear infection (since it's the single likeliest reason for most docs to prescribe antibiotics when they are not always needed), and what kind of baby products she recommends. (Conventional sunscreens with gunk in them? Plastic bottles with no mention of BPAs? Forget it!) Also check out holisticmoms.org or join the forum at mothering.com to get referrals from parents in your area. You can also go to holisticmedicine.org, acam.org, or integrativepeds.org for further guidance.

COUNTDOWN TO BABY

Making a Birth Blueprint

Even though an "ideal" birth isn't an outcome you can control, if you are prepared, you can come close. Being healthy and rested is the first step, in addition to a few other things you can get in order now.

PICK YOUR TEAM

By now, you will have decided on a midwife or doctor and maybe a doula, too. Some women choose to have their partner support them, while others want a female friend. Some have their mothers, some include their other children, and some decide it'll be just them and their midwife. There's no right or wrong answer.

The best advice I can give is to invite people who know you so well that they'll need very little direction about how to help. People who are perfectly capable of taking care of themselves and who won't drain any energy during a time when they really need to be providing it. Because once those contractions start, it's just you, your baby, and your own little world. Seriously, there's a neural hormonal change that happens in the brain when you give birth that actually inhibits your ability to verbalize your needs.[115] A girlfriend of mine described it like being on a major drug trip—you think you're speaking up and saying things, but nothing comes out. That plus all the new, vast sensations can be overwhelming, which is why it's a good idea to surround yourself with people who can anticipate your needs.

It's also super-important to remember that this is *your* birth. You don't have to please anyone. Especially if this is your first, this is an amazing one-time deal! Don't compromise what you want just because you're worried about hurting feelings. If there's someone who's being pushy about being there, don't feel obligated to let them participate. Have your partner explain your wishes so you minimize spending precious energy. There's plenty of time to share your birth story—and baby—with loved ones.

> We go into labor as one person, but emerge as another.
> —RONI JAY, *ZEN MEDITATIONS ON BEING PREGNANT*

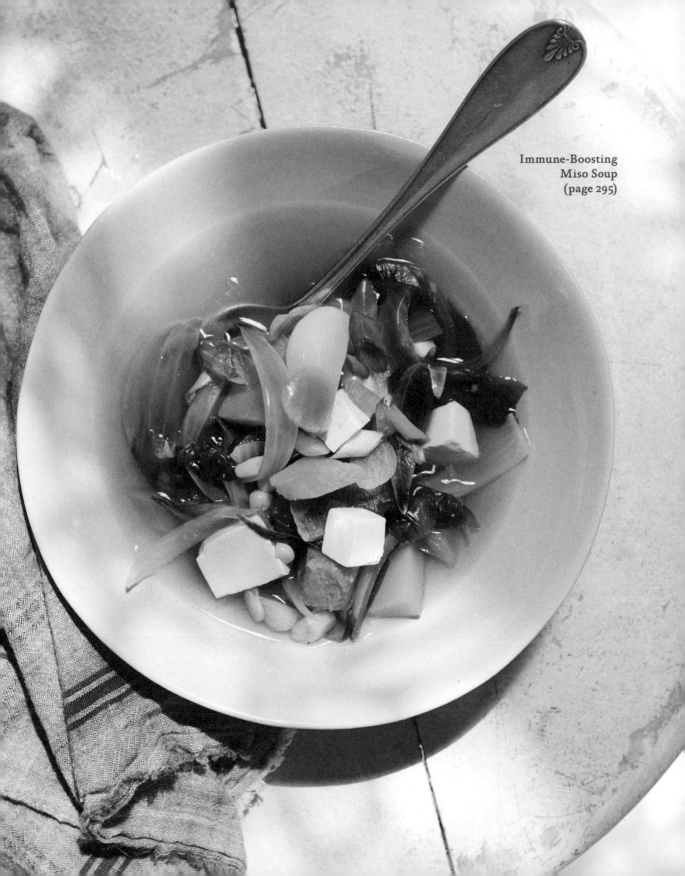

Immune-Boosting
Miso Soup
(page 295)

VISUALIZE YOUR BIRTH ENVIRONMENT

It's almost impossible to predict what exactly your needs and wants will be during labor. If this is your first child, there's no way you could have any idea how your body and mind will feel once your entire being is transported to this new and far-out place. I thought I would want someone massaging me the entire time, but whenever anyone so much as touched me, it didn't feel right. Sometimes, I just wanted to be alone in a dark place. Other times, I was comforted by my midwife and Christopher and Lalayna being right there breathing with me. There's of course no right answer, and you don't have to commit to any plan of action now, but you can try to tap into what you think your laboring self might want with a simple visualization: Set aside 15 or 20 minutes when you're not distracted by anything to close your eyes and try to imagine your birth. What feelings come up for you? What do you need to feel comfortable and secure? Think about having drapes or fabric handy for covering your windows. Consider candles or soothing music to soften the atmosphere. I loved the idea of making a playlist for birth, though when Christopher put it on, I couldn't make him turn it off quickly enough. You won't know exactly how you'll be feeling when the time comes, but give some thought to what you usually find calming.

Also think about how you normally cope with stress and discomfort. Do you usually call your partner to vent? Surround yourself with friends? Or do you like to be alone? Consider the ways you usually soothe yourself when you're not feeling your best. What is the worst thing someone could do when you're in that mind-set? What's something someone can do to make you feel a whole lot better? These are other great indicators of how you might want someone helping you—or not—as you navigate labor. Use these true desires and needs as a guide in communicating with your midwife, doula, partner, or whomever else will be with you when you give birth.

STOCK UP ON FOOD

You most likely won't want to eat past early labor, but if you feel like it, it's good to have one last good meal full of supercharged plant power. Your body is about to perform miracles and needs all the fuel it can get! Though macrobiotic counselor Warren Kramer suggests staying away from baked flour products like bread and cookies and crackers, which can make delivery more difficult. Once your labor has reached full swing, have a variety of drinks available that others can offer you. Some people will tell you to keep your energy up with crazy things like sugary sports drinks or ice pops, but those simple sugars aren't going to do you or your baby any favors—and they certainly won't give you the long-term stamina that you'll need. Coconut water, bancha or kukicha tea, sweet kuzu, water, amasake, or miso broth are the most energizing and rehydrating. Avoid anything too stimulating like sugary fruit juices, or too cold like iced or chilled beverages. They can upset the body's natural rhythms.

You'll also want to have food on hand for your support team, like a big vegan lasagna, which is what we offered. And even more important, give thought to the dishes you'll want to eat when you've finished giving birth and need to restore your strength—things that can be prepared for you so you can nest. Once you and your baby are settled and nestled, treat yourself to a hearty, nutrient-rich meal to replenish mind and body. Turn to "Your Healing Postbirth Menu" on page 179 for yummy suggestions.

Involving the Papas in Birth

When you think back to the time of tribes, the original midwives, and birth, it's pretty clear that delivering babies has traditionally been a woman thing: a time when a woman expresses her utmost womanness, surrounded by other women. We only recently started involving men in the birthing process, but that doesn't mean our male partners can't be amazing, tuned in, soothing, gentle, strong, and otherwise supportive during birth. No one knows how to love and comfort me more than Christopher does. Most of the time when he holds me, it's like he's putting me in his pocket and it's the safest place in the world. So of course he was the most important person I could imagine being at the birth of our child.

A friend up the street asked me who was going to be at my birth, and I said, "Oh, my midwife, my husband, and maybe a girlfriend." She strongly advised that my girlfriend be there, because she was concerned that my husband might be useless. I said, "No, no, no. You don't know Christopher. He's going to massage me and kiss me and be there with me. . . . " She was skeptical—from her own experience—and I was too stuck in my fantasy of an orgasmic birth with my doula-husband to hear out any of her reasoning.

When it came to seeing the woman he loves in the throes of labor, Christopher freaked. He'd never seen anything closely resembling a human trying to pass another human through her body, and he was paralyzed by fear. He was uncomfortable and anxious and scared, which in turn only made me uncomfortable. His breath, his touch, his voice—all of it broadcast just how out of sorts he felt, and so I didn't get the kind of comfort from him that I had envisioned. Later, he told me that his only thought was *My wife is wailing like she's going to die and all we have is a hot tub and some fucking candles?!* He was terrified.

During your labor, you need to be surrounded by people who are just as strong as they are intuitive. This can absolutely include your male counterpart, but know that he hasn't been conditioned to birth the same way we women have. It's another great reason why taking a class might have been helpful. Talking about labor and watching videos can sometimes alleviate a guy's discomfort. But seeing his most cherished partner in that woozy, witchy space between pain and ecstasy can be enough to short-circuit the most loving guy. Make sure your partner checks out "For Gentlemen Only: Labor and Birth Basic Training" on page 150 for lots of advice about how he can be there for you in a meaningful and reassuring way. Also, if you're on the fence about hiring a doula, this is another great reason to do it. The more experienced ones will know how to involve your partner and make sure he feels comfortable and empowered. From showing him how to physically support you to explaining what's happening to giving him the go-ahead to take a nap, her guidance can help him be there for you in a significant, confident way.

Involving Other Children

If you have kids already, consider including them in your birth experience. Here's what my midwife, Margo Kennedy, has to say about it:

I like having kids at a birth—they tend to be more accepting when they can see their new sibling come into the world. Plus, it's healthy to see and experience birth. It's a natural part of life. And when they can see the process happen and are a part of it, there's a much more natural transition in the family dynamic instead of them having to wonder, *Where do I fit in now?* That said, it depends on the mom and child. Sometimes, it's the child who's completely comfortable with birth but the mother who can't release and relax and doesn't want to make too much noise because she's afraid how it'll impact the child. But you can prepare kids for labor. There are classes that explain to little ones how the baby comes out and what it looks like. What's funny is kids are usually bored with labor, but they always show up for the birth.

I think most kids are ready by age 3, but I have seen younger children able to understand what's going on. If you want your children at your birth, make sure there's someone there to look after them since your partner's primary responsibility should be looking after you.

(continued on page 153)

For Gentlemen Only: Labor and Birth Basic Training

The fact that Bear grew inside Alicia's belly for 9 months and then came out of her was just incredible. When he popped his little head out, I just could not believe it. Alicia was so beautiful and strong during labor, even when she was exhausted. I have to say I did get a little scared seeing her in discomfort and hearing the noises she made. But you definitely feel something way bigger than you can even comprehend is happening. I was so overjoyed when I saw him breathing and my wife breathing—the caveman in me knew we were all okay. The whole thing is very primal and profound.

—Christopher

Your most special lady is about to do one of the most magical, mind-blowing things that nature has ever designed. It's seriously the most beautiful, heart-swelling, impressive, world-changing experience you could ever be a part of. And at the end of it, you get to meet your baby! But to get there, your woman has to embark on the physical and emotional equivalent of climbing Everest, except completely naked and without a Sherpa.

Even though nature has her covered, watching your partner navigate labor can be, well, a lot. My husband, whom I'd rate off-the-charts high on the loves-his-wife scale, was pretty shaken up. It was tough seeing me in so much discomfort, sometimes wailing and grunting like an animal. He said that the only thing that could have prepared him for birth would be Navy SEAL training, so consider this boot camp.

THINGS YOU CAN DO

Your midwife or doctor will be handling all the medical elements of the birth. If you've chosen to include a doula, then she administers calming solutions like massage or energy work. Hopefully, she'll put you to work, too, but I could see how it would be easy to feel like you're in the way. Just remember that only you are the father of that baby and your lady's partner for life: Your goal is to be her rock-solid foundation. Because of all the hormones surging through her brain and the all-consuming sensations of labor, she most likely won't be able to communicate to you exactly what she needs at any given moment. Remember that you know your partner better than anyone else in that room—hopefully. If not, get to that pronto! Anticipate her needs, watch her closely for cues, and give her the strength, comfort, and peace she'll need to devote her entire being to bringing your little one into this world.

Breathe with her. Try not to tell your partner to relax or breathe, or anything that can be misconstrued as asking her to change what she's doing. If you do, the politest response you might (deservedly) get is, "*You* fucking try that." Be as calming a presence as you possibly can. She'll be able to sense if you're anxious, which could make her nervous, too. But if you're strong and clear and taking charge, she'll be able to relax knowing all is well.

Keep her hydrated. Your wife should be drinking fluid from time to time (about 4 ounces an hour), but don't ask her if she's thirsty or whether she prefers tea or water. Just offer her a sip by putting a straw in or near her mouth. She might turn her head or swat at the glass—take that as a "no, thank you" and try again later.

Be the bouncer. That room or space is yours to protect. Make sure phones are turned off, voices are kept low, the door is shut, and that visitors are prohibited. Friends or family might be tempted to come by if your wife is laboring at home, but birth is not a party (unless she wants it to be!), and your wife is not a hostess.

Be quiet. You are not there to live out your football coach fantasies. If you do speak, talk slowly and softly. You don't have to take a vow of silence, but I'm pretty sure your wife isn't going to be up for chitchat (though, if she is, indulge her!). Try not to ask any questions unless you must. Limit your words to encouragements like "You are doing great," "I can't believe how amazing you are," "You are so beautiful," and "I love you."

Massage her. Women usually like to be massaged during labor. Her feet, back, and neck are particular sweet spots. Don't go full-on deep tissue, but do use a strong, firm hand that feels reassuring and present. If you can, keep your movements rhythmic with her breathing. Start practicing now by offering massages and figuring out how she loves to be rubbed. It's a double bonus because she'll feel so gooey and lovely in your hands, and you'll be a total pro on the big day. That said, if she doesn't want to be touched during labor, don't be surprised and try not to be disappointed.

(continued)

For Gentlemen Only—*continued*

WHAT TO KEEP IN MIND

If you get overwhelmed, don't hesitate to step out. Don't say anything, just leave the room, take a few breaths, and calm yourself with the thought that your partner is in the best possible professional care. You are no less a man for getting freaked out. In fact, I'd argue that your instinct to protect your significant other from any kind of discomfort is the most macho intention there is.

Don't announce when you're entering or leaving the room. She doesn't need to know your every move; just do what you have to do and try to come back as quickly as possible.

Don't bring food in. The smell of food can be sickening to a woman in labor.

If you're scared or tired, just imagine how she feels! That said, it can be a good idea for you to take a nap when you get exhausted. Labor can be long (on average 12 to 24 hours for first-time mamas), and it's ideal for at least one of you to be relatively rested. This is yet another reason why working with a doula—or having a loved one or savvy girlfriend there—can be great. She'll remind you that it's okay to take a break every now and then, and she'll take over while you get some sleep.

AND MOST IMPORTANT

Don't take anything personally—it's not about you! Your partner is in total Wonder Woman mode. Every synapse, nerve, and cell in her body is on high alert. The best thing to do is to be attentive and completely available.

How I supported Alicia during labor:
I would get in the tub with her. I would breathe with her.
I would meditate and try to bring good energy into the room.
I would leave her alone and give her space. I held her hands
and held her. I gave her lots of kisses.
—Christopher

PREPARING FOR THE UNEXPECTED

As sage and steady as the body can be, there are those times when even the most prepared, healthy, resilient mother doesn't give birth as planned. No matter how much training a midwife has or how accomplished a breather you are, labor and birth are still a part of the natural world, and anything can happen to upset its delicate balance. Even though eating well, getting rest, and enlisting the help of a professional with whom you feel comfortable will dramatically reduce the risks associated with birth, there is still a chance that things will not go as you envisioned. And in some cases, for the wellness of you and your baby, you may require medical intervention. It is overwhelming when this happens, but remember first and foremost: Labor is bigger than all of us. And if it means preserving life, then take heart in knowing that there is indeed great merit to modern medicine. Plus, birth comes in all shapes, sizes, and colors. Some of my home-birth mama friends had easy births, some had orgasmic births, and some had a crazy-intense journey—and they would all do it again.

If you have a difficult birth, processing what happened can take time. You are entitled to your experience, and no one can take those feelings away.

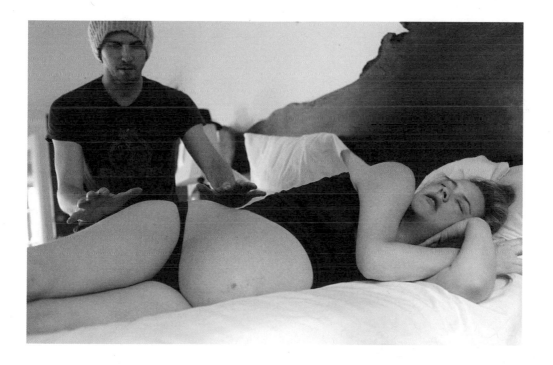

My Birth Story

I chose to give birth at home. I knew I would do it that way long before I got pregnant, since I'd seen my healthy, natural friends do it, and it made the most sense to me. My midwife was there, along with Christopher, my friend Lalayna, and another friend, Claire, who came by for a bit at the beginning.

The first 14 hours of my labor were sexy and amazing and totally blissed out.

I was on a magical mystery tour that was better than any drug in the world. With each contraction, I'd moan. It was partially from pain, but it was also coming from this deep, sensual place. My husband wondered if our neighbors would think we were having some kind of crazy-long lovemaking session! I would take little 1-minute naps between contractions and was this focused, powerful warrior. I felt like I could do anything. I also got obsessed with organizing my workspace—I wanted to clear it all away before the baby was born. Resting would have been a better choice, I'm sure, but there I was, birthing a baby, going through my papers and giving people tasks. It was funny and intense, and yeah, kinda dumb.

But the next 14 hours were more serious. I just couldn't get any relief. I labored in many different positions all over the house. We got in the tub. Margo had me walking up and down the stairs lifting my knees high (no easy feat for a very pregnant, very laboring woman!), as well as sitting backward on the toilet. When it came to pushing, Margo put me in more intense positions—lying on the bed holding one leg up with my arm while doing crunches with each push (this one sucked!), standing against the wall, squatting. It got to the point where I was so exhausted that the contractions were less uncomfortable than the resting time between. My legs, arms, abs, ribs—everything felt crazy sore. It was like I'd been working out for 14 hours straight. I found myself going from this soaring, hard-core spirit to thinking, *Get this thing out of me.*

Even though I'd been in labor for close to 26 hours and had been pushing for close to 3 (though of course I had no idea what time it was or how long it had been), it finally occurred to me to look at my midwife and ask, "How much longer?" I was expecting her to say, "Oh, 2 more hours or 5 more hours"—just *some* gauge of where I was. I didn't care how much longer; I just needed to know where I was. So I was shocked when she said, "If you don't have this baby in 20 minutes, I want to take you to the hospital."

What?! No!! But I wanted to do everything in my nature-given power to get that baby born. I pushed as much as I could for 20 minutes. Margo thought for sure the baby was going to come out hours earlier—she had even called for her time-to-deliver assistant and could see the fuzzy top of Bear's head. But for some reason, he just wasn't coming out, no matter how much I squatted. We all agreed that it was time to move. It was already 6:00 a.m., so there'd be traffic, and

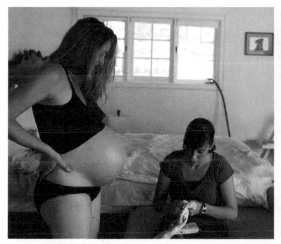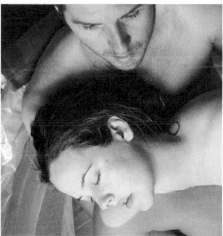

One of my midwives, Kelly, 12 or so hours into labor; in the birth tub about 16 hours into labor

the Seventh-day Adventist hospital we'd chosen in Glendale was at least 30 minutes away, without traffic. "Where's your bag?" the midwife asked. "Bag?" we said. It hadn't occurred to us to pack a bag, even though people had said I should, just in case. I was sure I wouldn't need one.

From there it was like a bad comedy of errors. Christopher scrambled around packing and then couldn't figure out what we'd done with the paperwork the midwife had us fill out, just in case I did end up needing medical intervention. He tried asking me, but I might as well have been on another planet. On the way to the hospital, he missed the exit off the freeway. The entire time, I was in survival mode, pushing like a maniac in the back of the car, where I barely fit. I was hanging off the edge of the backseat, continuing what had been 4 hours of pushing.

I asked Margo what they would do to me there, and she explained that they'd probably just use the vacuum—a suction device—but that they might have to do other things. My image of what that meant was so scary. I was too exhausted to panic, and luckily I still had all the good natural drugs that my body made pumping through me. I was calm, but I also felt sad. And there was also the shame of not being able to deliver at home. So I just kept pushing, determined to get the baby out before someone tried to cut me open.

Luckily, Christopher and I had chosen an old-school doctor who didn't believe in using surgical methods unless absolutely necessary. Back when he learned how to deliver babies properly, he told me, you didn't think twice about delivering breach babies, twins, or VBACs the good old-fashioned way.

When I got to the hospital, Dr. Wu gave me an exam and explained that my baby's head was turned to one side, making it hard to pass through. He asked what I wanted to do, and I said I wanted

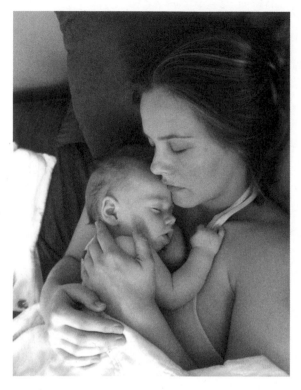

him to "get it out!" And to not do anything that wasn't absolutely necessary, because I wanted the birth to be as natural as possible. Dr. Wu attached what looked like a tiny condom that acts like a plunger to the top of the baby's head, and using what looked like nunchakus connected to it, turned his head ever so slightly and pulled him out. Even though it took him about 3 minutes to do it, that doctor was skillfully *working*. I kept thinking how if I were anywhere else, with any other doctor, I might be in surgery already.

Toward the end of labor, when I was still at home, all I could think was, *I'm never doing this again*. But just 40 minutes after being wheeled into a room in the hospital, I held on my chest my long little alien of a baby (with so much dark hair!) who was already looking for a boobie to suckle. My Bear Blu. And in that moment, I realized how I'd absolutely do this again. And I still probably wouldn't pack a hospital bag.

Emergency C-Section (ECS)

In the event that something doesn't go as planned during your birth, I want you to be prepared. Sometimes, because of fetal distress, excessive bleeding, or extremely high blood pressure during delivery, your midwife may decide to take you to the hospital. Of course, there are a number of things that your backup doctor—who you're confident understands your choices about natural birth—can do as an alternative to surgery. This might be using tools like the vacuum extractor or forceps, or maybe even a little shot of Pitocin to get the baby all the way out. But sometimes, no matter how hard you've planned or worked to have an intervention-free birth, the doctor might deem it best for mother and baby to have an emergency cesarean. And if this is what your trusted midwife, doctor, and/or backup doctor have presented to you as the best option, there is nothing wrong with this. I repeat: *There is nothing wrong with you, your values, or your resolve if your trusted backup doctor advises this course of action and you consent.*

If this does, in fact, happen, there are ways in which you can still very much cultivate a strong bond with your baby and more easily regain your strength. Your partner or doula should stay with the baby until she can be given to you in the recovery room. If you can, have someone take a digital photo of your newborn and look at her incredible tiny face as you wait. Once you are reunited, have your doula or partner guard your privacy so you can spend as much quiet time alone with your baby as possible.

Nurse the baby as soon as you can—in the recovery area, if possible—and as often as you can, ideally every 2 hours. And most important, call your support network into action. Some good company and fresh, nourishing foods will do the trick for getting you back on your feet.

Have a Postdelivery Game Plan

MAKE A BIRTH-WISH CHECKLIST

In the event you have to be transferred to a hospital during labor, the last thing you or your partner will want to worry about is fighting for the choices you've made regarding natural birth. As you've seen throughout this book, a whole bunch of medical options are handed out at the hospital door like goody bags. To keep these interventions at bay and best communicate your wishes, talk about all the decisions you might have to make with your midwife and/or doula. The beauty of working with these supporting ladies is that they can be your voice during a time when you might not be able to advocate for yourself and when your partner has more important things to do than swatting away pushy doctors and nurses. Check out the detailed checklist at earthmamaangelbaby.com/free-birth-plan and share your thoughts, questions, and concerns with your caretakers.

DECIDE ON POSTDELIVERY CARE FOR BABY

Let's talk about the alphabet soup that is the battery of tests and medicines that can be administered immediately after your baby is born: erythromyocin eye ointment, the hepatitis B vaccine, vitamin K, and newborn screening tests. Regulations vary from state to state, but the bottom line is the same: If you choose not to do any of these things, then that's your right. Full stop. However, if you give birth in a hospital, because most if not all of these things are done as standard procedure, then it's up to you to proactively say no. The doctors and nurses there don't need your consent to administer any of these things, which is why it's essential to let anyone with a pulse know what your birth plan is and, better yet, have someone there who can actively advocate for you. If you give birth at home, though, your midwife would give you all the information about these procedures and medications so you can make an informed decision before the baby is born.

To get more clarity on what these medications and tests are and whether our babies really need them, I consulted Lawrence Rosen, MD, a kick-butt integrative pediatrician, founder of the Whole Child Center in New Jersey, and author of *Treatment Alternatives for Children*. Below is what he had to say, which should be helpful when you discuss these options with your own caregiver. I also included my own point of view in cases where I made a different choice. We ultimately chose not to administer any of these tests or medications because that's what felt right in our guts. But there's no right answer, and everyone needs to decide for themselves with the help of their caregiver.

- **Erythromyocin eye ointment:** This is something I advise parents not to do in most cases. I find most hospital personnel don't even really know why they give it anymore. It goes back many, many years to when there was an unknown risk of the mom having a disease like gonorrhea, which could cause a serious eye infection in the baby when delivered through an infected birth canal. If you know you don't have these infections, then it's an unnecessary antibiotic exposure in the first minutes of life, and it can cause eye irritation and goop up the eyes. But unless you let the doctor or nurse know ahead of time, they'll administer it without asking for your consent.

- **Hepatitis B vaccine:** There's virtually no risk of hepatitis B to a newborn if mom is hepatitis B negative. Women who get prenatal care are typically screened, so you should know your status. So my advice is to not do it unless the mother has hepatitis B. In some states, it's not a mandate, but parents still feel forced into it. You have to sign a consent form either way, but sometimes with pushy nurses or doctors, parents can feel railroaded.

- **Vitamin K:** This is given to newborns in virtually all hospitals. It's usually administered as an injection in the leg within minutes of birth, and it delivers 1 milligram of vitamin K. It prevents a very rare disorder that some babies are born with in which their blood can't clot normally unless they get that 1 milligram of vitamin K. Even though it's a rare disease, it can be severely life threatening, causing things like internal bleeding and bleeding in the brain. The problem is, there's no test to do ahead of time to know which babies have it and which don't. So while we're giving it to a lot of babies who probably don't need it, in my opinion the alternative is far worse.

    In the United Kingdom, there was concern about a link between leukemia and vitamin K injections—that's when the oral version became popular in Europe and is still offered as a choice there. But here in the United States, most pediatricians, myself included, believe that studies show injectable vitamin K is more effective than oral vitamin K and that there's no link between the injection and cancer. While I don't advocate for oral vitamin K, it's still an option some parents will choose. This is definitely a case where you need to let the hospital know that you're choosing to not do the injection, because they don't need your consent to do it. If you'd prefer they didn't, they'll have you sign a consent waiver.

My take: I felt that Bear could get the vitamin K he needed from my diet, having learned that consuming vitamin K–rich foods like Brussels sprouts, broccoli, cauliflower, leafy greens, and chickpeas can be sufficient on its own.[116]

- **Newborn screening test:** This is also known as a metabolic screening test or the heel-prick test. Every state has one, though it varies from state to state what exactly they're looking for. Usually it's a whole battery of things—congenital thyroid disease, PKU, cystic fibrosis—and it gives us good information that we can act on. I don't see any downside to doing this. If you're giving birth at home, your midwife will sometimes come back to the house to do it, or a trained doula can do it. Or you can go to your pediatrician or primary caregiver's office and he or she will do it. It should be done in the first 24 to 48 hours, ideally after 24 hours of feeding. There are private labs that do extra testing on top of this, but check with your OB or midwife to see if that's worthwhile. It's typically not.

  My take: I opted to not do this test because I felt in my heart and my gut that Bear would be shielded from these diseases by my diet and health practices. And my midwife said that these conditions were so rare, and the tests can yield false positives. I also didn't want my baby being pricked in the first moments of life. Or anytime, for that matter!

- **Newborn hearing test:** This is an easy, noninvasive screening test that is required by law in some states. It rules out hearing problems at birth and only takes a few minutes.

  My take: I didn't like the idea of funky waves near my newborn's head. Plus, I'd heard from a friend that her pediatrician said there's all kinds of false positives in the early days (turns out at a rate of more than 30 percent![117]). I felt comfortable gauging my son's hearing using my own observation.

Cord Blood Banking

You will probably hear about this from your caregiver, who will ask whether you want to save the blood from your baby's umbilical cord so that the cells can be used one day to treat various diseases. But here's the deal: There's still a lot of controversy about the practice's benefits. And most important, in order to collect the necessary amount of blood, your midwife or doctor would have to clamp the umbilical cord almost immediately after birth, before it's done pulsating. This means your baby might not receive every last drop of oxygen and nutrients from your placenta, which according to Margo Kennedy, can help him better transition to his new surroundings. Not to mention that it's also expensive—there's a $1,500 to $2,000 collection fee, plus an annual $100 to $200 fee just for keeping the stuff frozen. Just some things to consider.

Prepare to Start Bonding at Birth

Skin-to-skin contact with your newborn is one of the most delicious sensations this world has to offer. When you can finally hold your baby in your arms, gaze at his face, and feel his teeny tiny heartbeat next to yours, it's hard to imagine life being more right than that. What's even more beautiful is that you're helping each other's bodies cope with the enormous feat they just accomplished. Your warmth keeps your newborn snug since he can't yet regulate his own temperature, and your newborn—who will instinctively start wriggling toward your breasts—will jump-start your body's oxytocin production when he begins suckling. Oxytocin, or the "love hormone," will seal your bond forever, help the uterus contract so that the placenta can detach and be delivered, and seal off any blood vessels it was attached to. Isn't that amazing?! It's nature's special way of getting you all sorted out.

Within minutes of birth, most babies enter a still, calm state. Researchers have found that this "quiet alertness" happens for about an hour after babies are born and is when they are best able to take in their new environment.[118] There's no question that you'll realize exactly how to let your baby know that she is safe, secure, and the most precious thing in the world. But just for inspiration's sake, here are some tips for how to have a beautiful first meeting with your little one.

HOLD YOUR BABY SKIN-TO-SKIN AS SOON AS POSSIBLE

Holding your baby tummy to tummy or cheek to breast is one of the most intimate ways you can wordlessly tell your baby that you're here for her in this strange new place. Aside from it being the gooiest, most blissed-out feeling ever, skin-to-skin contact has been linked to teaching babies to deal with stress, stimulating nerves in the brain that help with food absorption, improving immune function, and helping them sleep more easily. Some research shows that touch is crucial to neurological development.[119] This little ritual definitely isn't just for the first moments after baby's born—you'll want to do it for months to come. And it's a nice way for dad to share the love, too.

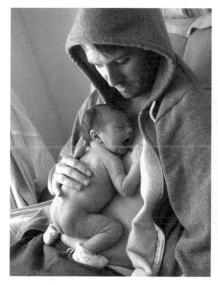
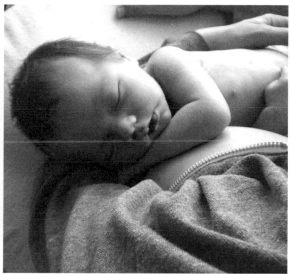

CARESS YOUR BABY

You won't be able to keep your hands off your tiny nugget of joy, but it's helpful to know that you're doing so much more than just giving her a gentle and therapeutic hello. Stroking your baby's whole body, whether with the palm of your hand or the tips of your fingers, stimulates the nerve-dense skin, which as the largest organ in our bodies, can actually help your baby breathe more rhythmically.[120]

GAZE AT YOUR BABY

Newborns can see best at a distance of 10 inches, which, pretty magically, is the distance from your nipples to your eyes.[121] During the first hour after birth, a baby's eyes are usually open (all the more important to have low, soft lighting), so it's the perfect time to make deep, meaningful eye contact as your baby nurses.

SAY "HELLO"

Studies have shown that newborns can distinguish their mother's voice from everyone else's very early in life.[122] It's not surprising—you were roommates for a pretty long time—but it bodes well for keeping your baby soothed during her first days. And don't let papa worry, baby will learn his voice soon enough and find solace in having him close by.

GETTING THE SHOW STARTED: INITIATING LABOR NATURALLY

If there's one thing nature doesn't do, it's absolutes. Even though some doctors like to pin down an exact day for your due date, most women don't give birth on their assigned day. In fact, only *3 percent* do. And if it's your first baby, then there's an even smaller chance you'll give birth on your given day. It's much more natural and realistic to have a 4-week window for your baby's birthday, with 2 weeks on either side of your due date. Think of overshooting your due date as a really beautiful thing. According to the Kushi Institute's Diane Avoli, a little extra baking time means baby will be more developed. That said, your midwife will want to frequently monitor both you and baby for any signs of distress. If there's none, then there's no reason to worry that your baby's birth date is later than you originally thought. Your baby will let you know when it's time!

Some doctors and more conservative midwives may want to induce labor if you've significantly overshot your due date. Before you consider this route (which typically involves the use of Pitocin[123] or stripping the membranes), and assuming there's been no distress detected in you or the baby, try advocating for more natural alternatives. Before exploring any of these options, though, be sure to run it by your doctor or midwife first.

For the Planner

There are effective preemptive measures you can take to prep the body for labor:

Raspberry leaf tea: This tea's natural properties can be a uterine and pelvic tonic and relaxant, which preps both for labor and for more effective contractions. Have a glass a day for the month leading up to your due date.

Evening primrose oil: Though I didn't use this (maybe next time!), my midwife recommended it. Taking evening primrose oil in gelcap form can help "ripen" the cervix. At 32 weeks, take 500 milligrams or one or two gelcaps a day. At 34 weeks, increase to two to four gelcaps, and by 36 weeks, if your membranes are still intact, you can additionally insert three caps vaginally at night. Just prick the capsules with a pin first.

Relax: Some healers—like the very wise Diane Avoli—believe that a big reason for delayed labor is that a woman's constitution is too yang, or tight and not relaxed. Bodywork like light massage or acupuncture can help loosen up the mama flow, as can drinking relaxing natural teas like chamomile and avoiding "tightening" foods with a lot of strong spices. Listen to calming music, scent your pillow with yummy essential oils like lavender or geranium, go for a gentle walk or swim, surround yourself with the positive energy and let come what may.

For Faster Results

Lovemaking (if your water hasn't broken—and you feel like it): Semen carries the hormone prostaglandin, which can help soften the cervix. And sometimes, just getting a little frisky without doing the deed can do the trick because it can trigger oxytocin production, which in turn triggers contractions.[124]

Pump: If you're approaching the 2-week-postbirth date mark, then using a breast pump to stimulate your breasts is an effective way to get oxytocin flowing and, as a result, trigger labor. This is not recommended for jump-starting labor any old time you feel like delivering the baby.

Walking and gentle yoga: I say go for a long walk every day until that baby pops out!

Acupressure, acupuncture, reflexology, or massage: I'm always hearing the most unbelievable stories about how just one session with a skilled healer can speed things up.

Castor or borage oil: Taking ½ tablespoon of either every half hour for up to three doses can create a pulsating action in the bowel, which can stimulate labor. This is best done under the supervision of your caretaker, since it can be pretty gnarly and can make you feel not so hot.

YOU'VE PLANNED, NOW LET IT ALL GO

You've gazed at your belly and dreamed. You've been buzzing with anticipation. Maybe you've even been a little afraid. But let me tell you something: No matter what, there's nothing you can do to truly prepare for birth. I don't mean this in a scary way. It's the opposite: Because there is nothing you can possibly do to know what to expect, the only thing you can do is just let go. Submit. Your birth will still unfold exactly as it will, and no matter what, it will be exactly how it was meant to be.

Remember the long line of women who have done this before you. Think about how wise and knowing your body is. Imagine the divine plan that has been unfolding in your belly and all the millions of miracles of biology that have already happened to bring you this far. Just as your body will tell you when it's time to labor, trust that it will see you through this adventure as a faithful guide. Because birth is just that—an adventure!

IO

The Kind Nursery

I think one of the biggest misconceptions about having a baby is that suddenly you're going to need all this *stuff*. When I was close to giving birth to Bear, people would share their roundup of "the essentials" . . . then send me six-page lists with everything that you *absolutely* needed to keep this baby happy, healthy, and developing. According to these well-meaning advisors, if you didn't at least have a bouncy seat ("one for every floor of the house!"), play center, activity mat, swing, bassinet, Diaper Genie, monitors ("with video!"), and changing table and matching crib, then you were not properly equipped.

Pretty overwhelming, right? Not to mention expensive! If you've been on the receiving end of one of those megalists, no doubt you've started wondering if maybe having this stuff would make raising a baby a little easier. But I promise you that that's not the case. Do you need some things when you have a baby? Yes. Do they require batteries or fancy linens or a decorating scheme? Nope. It might feel as if not having the right things will make more work for yourself. But take a step back and think about how you've chosen to raise your baby so far.

First, you cleaned out your baby house. You got rid of the junk that you and your body didn't need in order to create the brightest, purest space for baby to grow. So why not keep building this big, beautiful house for him? You can create that space by *not* cluttering up what you have in the first place. To my mind, the kindest nursery is no nursery.

When you choose the kind parenting path—which we'll talk more about over the next few chapters—you're naturally doing away with excess. Because *you are* your baby's food, solace, entertainment, transportation, and education, your need for things diminishes dramatically. Introducing too much stuff, on the other hand, can distance the connection we have with our babies. When you distract her with toys or leave her to entertain herself in a playpen, you're replacing yourself with things. And that could mean the difference between a baby with an innate sense of contentment and belonging in the universe and one who is always searching for happiness in that next candy bar/cigarette/pair of shoes.

YOUR NEW "ESSENTIALS"

As we'll talk about in upcoming chapters, babies thrive when they're a part of our lives. They both want and need to be held and carried and nursed, and at night it's much more natural for them to continue to be with you than alone in a separate room. That's really what it boils down to: The more you fight nature, the more stuff you need. Because the less you embrace your baby's innate sense of what's good and right in the world, the more work you need to do to convince her that everything's okay.

At the most basic level, all you need when you have a baby is something for her to eat, somewhere for her to poop, and a place to sleep. That really just means having your boobs handy, in addition to some cloth or eco-friendly diapers and wipes (or a bowl and some shrubs, if need be!) and making your own bed into a baby-friendly nest (which we'll talk all about in the next chapter). If you wear her in a sling or carrier, then you don't need swings and play mats to keep her happy when she wants to be held. And all those toys that you see taking over the homes of all your friends? You won't need them because they're not nearly as interested as seeing the world with you.

But I will concede there's a bit more to it than that. Of course, you'll need things for diapering, breastfeeding, and carrying baby, which you'll learn about in upcoming chapters. As for the rest, here's my version of the "essentials":

Organic, natural fiber blanket for swaddling: You'll get more of these as gifts than you'll know what to do with, which is great because they're handy for so many things—swaddle, burp cloth, sun shield, boob cover. It's nice to have at least three or four because they'll inevitably get covered in pee, milk, and spit-up.

A few items of clothing: Your baby doesn't need a closet full of clothes. You don't need very much for the first 6 months, and babies grow like little weeds, so 12 outfits (like onesies or kimono-style snap shirts and pants) will do the trick. A combination of short- and long-sleeved is perfect, though consider the weather in your area. The rule of thumb is to dress your baby with the same number of layers as you're wearing plus one. (FYI—skin-on-skin counts as a layer!)

Soft surface for putting baby down: Something like an organic cotton throw rug or blanket, or even something as simple as your bedspread or a yoga mat. (Ideally an old one; a new one will need to off-gas in the sun for a few days first.)

Car seat: This is a total necessity if you plan on driving anywhere with baby, but unfortunately, there aren't a lot of 100 percent clean green versions out there. Many car seats are made with polyvinyl chloride (PVC), which is widely used in plastic baby gear.[125] It contains phthalates, which you already know are nasty for you and even more so for your little one. Restrictions or bans have been placed on phthalates in PVC toys and baby gear in the entire European Union, Japan, Iceland, Mexico, and Norway due to their risk to children's health.[126]

But until our lawmakers wise up, there are a few brands that are making a cleaner car seat. Orbit Baby (which we have and has been great for us), Graco, and Britax are phasing out the use of flame retardants and PVCs. This is one instance where buying used isn't such a great idea. Many states have laws against selling and/or using secondhand car seats because the safety standards change so frequently. Also, once a car seat has been in an accident, it's not considered a safe

---

Baby Entertainment Centers, Bouncers, and Walkers

WHAT THE HEALER SAYS The Kushi Institute's Diane Avoli

Babies need a combination of lots of hugs and love and touching and then quiet time without constant stimulus. You don't need flashing lights and all those new things out there. It's overstimulating, and it actually keeps them from developing their own imaginations. I think of kids as their own home entertainment centers—you can just sit and watch them, and in reverse, they can sit and watch, too.

WHAT THE PEDIATRICIAN SAYS Lawrence Rosen, MD

Toys that "assist" motor skills like bouncers and walkers can actually be detrimental to baby's development. Both have been associated with head and neck injuries. In fact, babies who use walkers actually walk later, not earlier. I never recommend these and in general advise against expensive, probably toxic "baby furniture/toys."

product anymore. And while hand-me-downs may have off-gassed, they could actually have higher levels of contaminated dust from cushion degradation.

Stroller: You won't need this for a little while and may rarely use one—particularly if you use a sling or carrier—but see my tips below for how to find the most healthy, eco-friendly options. And while there are a ton of different models out there, keep in mind that research suggests that rear-facing versions are better for baby's brain development.[127] Instead of getting overwhelmed with street noise, the elements, etc., she can more easily see and hear you.

GETTING THE THINGS YOU DO NEED

Clothes and apparel: Try to find hand-me-downs whenever possible. Ask friends, family, and neighbors; join a local parenting network; shop at the local thrift shop; and check out sites like thredUP, StorkBrokers, Rascal's Resale, and BabyOutfitter. If you buy new, look for items made with organic cotton or other natural fibers and without things like bleach, chemical softeners, and harsh toxic dyes. Some favorite brands: Under the Nile, The Little Seed, and Adooka.

If you receive more than you need—or things you have no use for—pay it forward and donate it or pass it on to someone who really needs it.

The rest: Although there are plenty of great brands making eco-friendly baby gear—from strollers to carriers—again finding gently used items is ideal. You won't have to worry about nasty parts leaching chemicals, and you definitely can have the peace of mind that you won't be contributing one more piece of plastic to the landfill. See if anyone in your tribe is looking to lend or sell their hand-me-downs, or check out super-handy sites like the Freecycle Network, eBay, RockaBuyGear, Swap Baby Goods, or Craigslist. Try to source things as locally as possible.

A KINDER BABY SHOWER

If a loved one offers to host a baby shower in your honor, gently suggest that your guests either bring something that they've already used and loved and want to contribute to your baby treasure chest or consult a green registry stocked with things you need. Use a site like BabyList (babyli.st/index) that allows you to register for gift cards for postpartum doula services and groceries, baby-and-me yoga classes, or even donations to charities that mean a lot to you and your partner.

WHAT ABOUT EDUCATIONAL TOYS?

There's a secret to raising little geniuses, and it's not subjecting them to hours of Baby Einstein CDs or classical concertos. It's totally free, and it's a lot more fun that dragging baby around town to all kinds of classes. Want to know what it is? Play! For the first several years of a child's life, one of the most significant ways for her to learn, boost her brainpower, and tap into her creative prowess is not doing flash cards or memorizing her ABC's. It's banging pots and pans, waving around that spoon, and—Bear's favorite—rearranging all the food storage containers in your cabinets. Being able to explore and touch and move coupled with getting to see the world by your side means she's learning neat things like sequencing, cause and effect, color, communication, and language.[128]

After 3 months, the age babies typically start playing, you'll see that when your baby does what you do all day, he wants to play with the things you're playing with. He wants to hold the sponge while you do the dishes, take things off shelves and then put them away again, check out the nifty gadgets in the garden, bop around the colorful bottles in the bath—all the things he sees you doing when you're just living. And frankly, your baby's criterion is pretty basic: Can I put it in my mouth?

The same goes for books. I read to Bear when he wanted me to, but I found it more worthwhile to simply let him live and breathe the world around him. I never saw the point in drilling him on things he'd eventually learn naturally. I love that he's using the world around him as his teacher, not a bunch of books. Yes, reading with your child makes for cuddly, beautiful, quiet time together. But is it the most important thing for making sure your baby grows up *smart*? Nope. Babies learn language by being repeatedly exposed to words, which in turn builds lots of neural pathways to process that information. The more language they hear, the more they learn.[129] Evidence is now showing that the key to early learning isn't having an iPad or watching television— it's talking! Even something as simple as pointing out how beautiful the trees or clouds are or saying hello to a doggie that goes by. And researchers are beginning to understand that the more exposure our babies get to people talking to them from birth to age 3, the better.[130] So while books are one way to achieve this, you can do just as much good by carrying your baby as frequently as possible. That way, she's not only hearing all the sweet things you say to her throughout the day, but she's also learning about how to interact with other people.

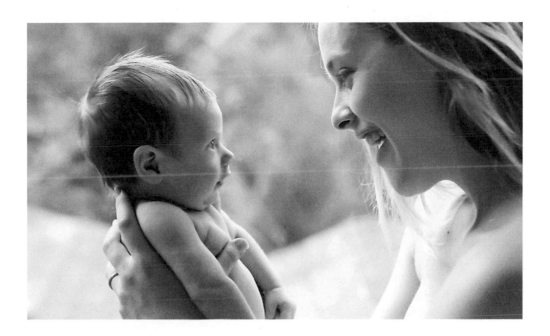

A SAFER TOY BIN

You're going to end up with more toys than you want. If you decide to keep them, make sure that they're not made with any of the nasty chemicals that manufacturers are, sadly, including even in our babies' playthings (particularly those manufactured in China, India, and other Asian countries, where regulations are looser). In the United States, toys may be made using BPA (which has been linked to everything from hindered brain development to neurological problems[131]) and PVC (which can contain toxic phthalates and heavy metals)—all of which have been identified by regulatory agencies as problematic because they have been linked to long-term health impacts.[132] And while I love giving old items new life, when it comes to antique toys, an exception should be made. The paint on vintage trucks and dolls is likely to contain lead, since lead safety regulations were put in effect only in 1978.[133] Similarly, the US Consumer Product Safety Commission changed the laws regarding phthalates and lead in toys back in 2009 to lower the allowable levels, so anything made prior could have significantly higher levels.

Here are some tips for how to make sure your little one is having good, clean fun.

Scrap the Soft Plastic Toys

These are the biggest BPA and PVC offenders. Instead, stick with playthings made with natural materials like solid wood (either unfinished, with a nontoxic finish, or painted with no-VOC

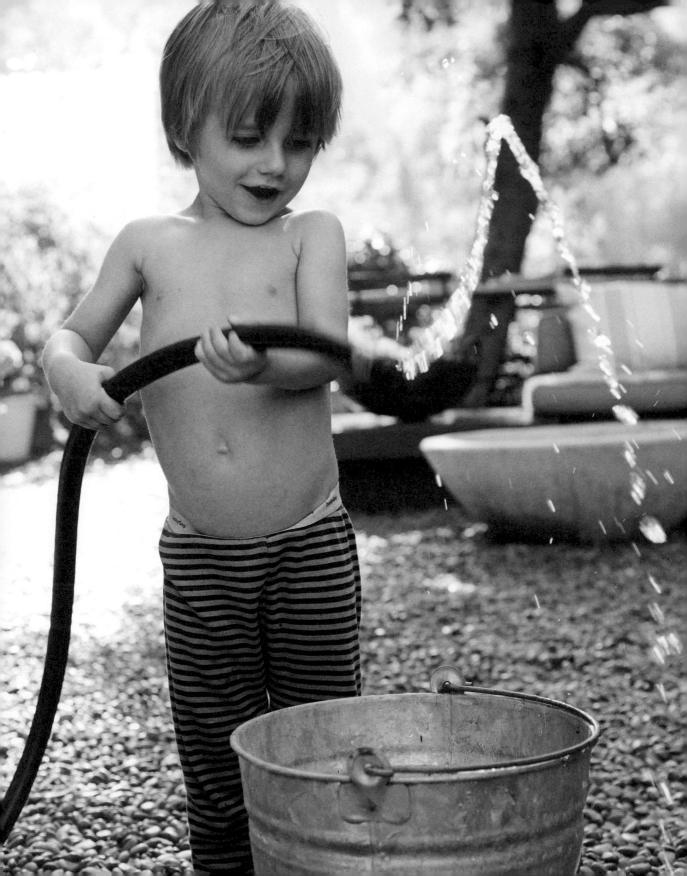

paint), natural rubber, or organic cloth like cotton and hemp. Some hard plastic toys can be safer options. Just make sure you double-check with one of the Web sites listed below.

Be Wary of Plush and Fuzzy

Since some stuffed toys are treated with flame retardants and most are made with petroleum-based foam filling, try to make sure baby's favorite lovey is made out of organic, untreated fibers like cotton or hemp.

Check a Database

Instead of trying to memorize all these crazy-making details, go to HealthyStuff.org, where you can search their database of more than 5,000 products that they've tested. Or go to MomsRising. org and check out the text-messaging system they developed with the HealthyStuff.org toys database. You can text "healthy toys" and the name of a particular toy, manufacturer, or retailer to 41411 to find out whether a toy was made using any toxic chemicals. While the database isn't comprehensive, it's a great starting point for anything you truly need.

Buy New but Kind

If you want to splurge on something new for baby, some of my favorite healthy and responsible toy brands include Apple Park, Under the Nile, Kid O, Plan Toys, and Palumba. And keep checking out thekindlife.com, where I post my newest discoveries.

BUYING LESS STUFF SAVES THE PLANET, TOO!

The more we set our minds and hearts to not consuming quite so much—and in turn creating less waste—the greater the gift we give our children in years to come. Any parent who watches TV knows we're told that if we just buy the latest, greatest, coolest things for our babies, our lives will be easier and our children will be happier. And in turn, we're sending all the packaging, disposable goods, and perfectly fine old items to the trash. In 2006, Americans generated 250 million tons of garbage, more than half of it from our homes. Of that, 3.6 million tons alone were disposable diapers, and a third of it was a toxic mishmash of packaging from all the "convenience" items that save us from having to cook, clean, and take care of objects for more than one use.[134] We can't just bury it and forget about it, because that's turning our landfills into toxic waste sites,[135] and incinerating it all would mean creating dangerous emissions that are linked to nasty things like cancer, birth defects, and autism.[136] It's dangerous for our babies *and* our planet.

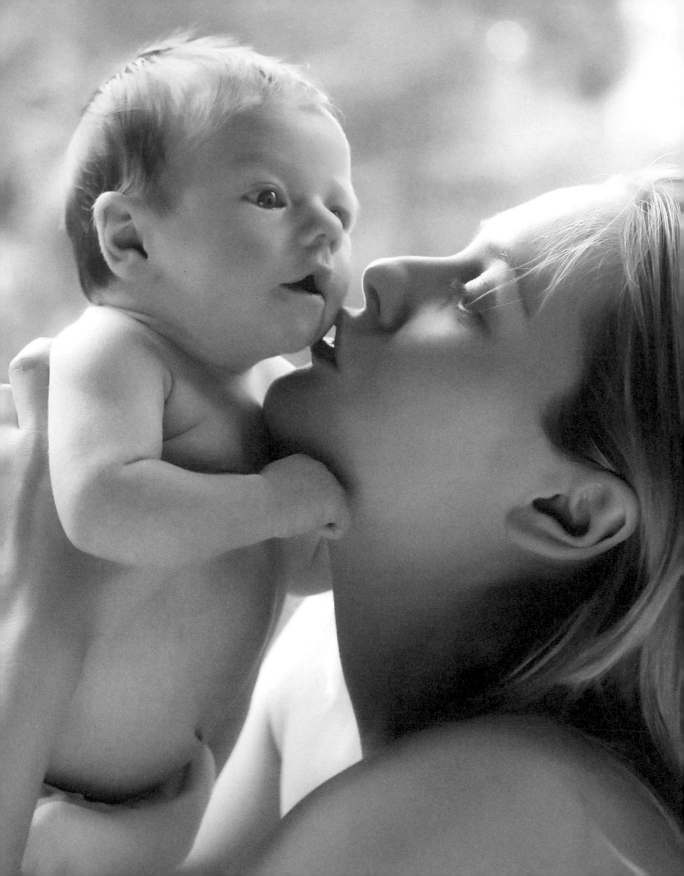

PART III:

welcoming baby

Lying-In and Creating a Space to Heal

II

Lying-In,
aka Your Most Amazing
Baby Vacation

Everyone tells you how you're going to love this
baby so much that you won't even believe it. And you're like,
"Duh, of course!"...But you don't know. You can't know! It's simply
the greatest thing in the world. There's nothing more soothing than
Bear's little face and his little mouth on my boobie and his smile—
everything he does is all so delicious. I love smelling his feet and
kissing his little butt. Now Christopher and I lie in bed and
instead of staring into one another's eyes, we stare at the baby.
It's not that we don't love each other anymore, it's just that now
there's this Martian love ball that you can't help looking at
and being with and just inhaling.

—My Journal, Postpartum

The world is a different place after you give birth. It feels brighter and even more full of possibility, and you are filled with the most unparalleled love you could ever feel for another living creature. It is, simply, magical. That's why you should do everything in your power to savor the bliss.

Think back to a time when you went on the most relaxing, soul-nourishing vacation. Do you remember how you wanted to bring that feeling back with you and hold on to it for as long as possible? But little by little, the real world creeps back in. This is no different. That's why for my post-baby experience I looked to cultures around the world that observe a ritual called lying-in, which honors a new mother with all the peace, rest, and nurturing she needs in the first 40 days after birth. It's a time when mama and baby retire from the world and focus solely on healing and bonding, not worrying about how quickly she can get back to the office or lose all the baby weight.

In our culture, people actually admire moms who can get back to "normal" as quickly as possible after giving birth, but that mind-set seems backward. On a very basic level, your body needs this time to mend. Lying horizontally encourages the uterus to return to its normal condition and helps prevent too much postbirth bleeding. A well-rested mama produces richer, more nourishing milk for her baby. And nursing is like a full-body healing salve for you and for your newborn.[1] The deeper significance is that this time is for bonding with your baby because she, too, is healing. She's getting used to this crazy new world, some of her systems are still developing, and her bones need to settle back in place. All she needs is your warmth and nourishment, not to be passed around like a doll. Too many visitors or too much chaos can make your baby fussy and cranky. Instead, embrace this time as the tender transition that it is and make yourself a therapeutic little nest. And research backs up the importance of this period: According to a 2009 study done by UC Berkeley researchers, women who took fewer than 6 weeks of maternity leave were four times less likely to breastfeed.[2] You're setting yourself up for a rich, profound connection with your baby instead of hurrying on to the next thing.

Lying-in can look different for everyone. I took 10 days to do nothing but tend to my baby. I stayed in bed and saw as few people as possible. I'd eat my meals there and nap as much as I could. After those 10 days, I would do a few light chores a day, but I always put rest and baby first. Because I'd planned ahead, I didn't need to worry about things like cleaning the house or keeping the fridge stocked with lots of yummy, healing foods. I burrowed into my baby nest and completely gave myself over to my baby. What I got in return was this magical experience in which I had the freedom of doing absolutely nothing but spend time with my new little family.

I know what you're thinking: Who am I to tell you that you should consider taking time away from work? But I assure you that it's not something that only the super-privileged and trust-fund endowed can afford. A friend of mine, who is a teacher married to another teacher, decided to take a year off to take care of her son. They saw spending more time with their baby as being more valuable than the income, even if it meant living more simply. They knew things would be tight, so they took the opportunity to leave New York City for that time and get some fresh air out in the country. Even if that scenario isn't realistic for your family, there are ways you can protect the time you do have to spend with your little one, and I strongly urge you to explore them. After all, this is a once-in-a-lifetime opportunity: to be with your brand-new family, or newest addition to it, and revel in the fact that you have no idea what you're doing and yet it doesn't matter because you actually know exactly what to do.

PREPARING TO LIE-IN

Lying-in isn't a one-size-fits-all prescription. Some women take 10 days of complete bed rest and then spend 40 days doing little aside from resting and nursing and bonding and nurturing around the clock. I'd maybe do a load of laundry here and there or take a quick shower, but I tried my best to stay in my blissed-out baby bubble. Try not to spend a lot of time on your feet, avoid stairs for as long as possible, and certainly don't lift anything too heavy. At some point during your lying-in, you can go outside for walks—my midwife recommended 3 weeks—but keep them short. I loved spending time in our yard, and I eventually strolled around our neighborhood, which provided just enough fresh air.

If you were part of a tribe, the other men and women would be making food and tending to all your needs. That way, you could devote all your time and attention to your baby and, no less important, yourself. Think of all the people in your community—family, friends, anyone you can count on—who can swathe you in much-needed support after your baby is born. Now is the time to call upon these cherished individuals.

Consider tapping one of your friends to take the lead and have her coordinate your mini-tribe. Make a list of all the things you know you'll want help with—walking the dog, preparing or gathering food, cleaning the house, running the washer and dryer, holding the baby while you nap or shower—and have her put together a rotating schedule where people can drop by and lend a hand. Once the baby's born, you can keep a chore list on your fridge, so anytime people ask, "Is there anything I can do?" you can direct them to the list. You'd be surprised how many folks get pumped about things like helping with the laundry and scrubbing down a bathtub! It makes people feel good to be truly helping.

If you don't feel comfortable asking for that kind of assistance or don't have a lot of backup living nearby, consider hiring a cleaning service. And it can be beyond valuable to bring in some-one to prepare meals. It doesn't have to be a super-fancy private chef, just someone who maybe likes to cook for fun and will follow recipes from this book and *The Kind Diet* for a low hourly fee (which will be way less than you'd spend on takeout, since you'll have days' worth of food in the fridge). Ask around at your farmers' market or touch base with a local culinary school. You'd be surprised what people are willing to contribute in exchange for experience and good karma. Or engage a postpartum doula, who can help with light housework in addition to supporting you in other ways, like help with breastfeeding.

I know it can seem extravagant to bring in "help." But this special treatment is what you automatically would have gotten had you given birth in tribal times, because the tribe knew just how essential it was for new mamas to make some sacred space for baby. Paying someone to clean, make healing food, or otherwise lend a hand is not being lazy or diva-like. Think of it instead as an investment in getting the healthiest, most vibrant start with your baby. That said, it's worth noting that a baby nurse is a very different kind of help from a postpartum doula. While a postpartum doula is there to help you with the baby, her first and foremost role is to help the mama. Because if you're rested and healing and healthy, then you'll be a better mama for it. A doula's job is to make the space—whether it's doing laundry, preparing light meals, tucking you in with a foot rub, or sharing wisdom about anything from breastfeeding to first baths. Most postpartum doulas will assure you that they are not there to tell you how to parent, they're there to help you tap into your own wisdom. It's important that you let your gut speak about what you feel is best for your newborn. Baby nurses, on the other hand, are there only for the baby. The idea is that you can leave the baby with her while you go about your day and she'll bring him over whenever he needs a feeding. But then you're missing out on all that crucial, heavenly mama-and-me time that these first weeks are for.

Even though I didn't have anyone come in to help me with the baby (no doula, no baby nurse)—for which I'm so grateful because it gave me and Christopher the opportunity to really tune in to our parenting intuition—I did have someone cook and someone clean every once in a while. Don't, under any circumstances, be tempted to tackle this all yourself. Sometimes, after birth, a new mama might feel a rush of vitality because of all the gooey hormones surging through her body. It can be completely euphoric. You've just accomplished this amazing feat of Amazonian strength and now you're caring for this tiny creature with your very own body. It's

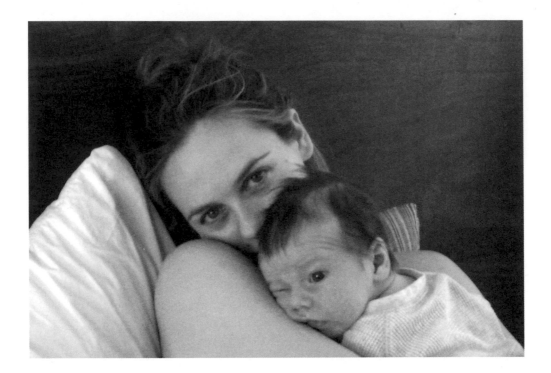

such a high! But don't waste all that energy on things that truly aren't as important, such as getting your "body back" or paying bills or making phone calls. Those tasks can distract you from the precious charge of learning every nuance of your baby's existence. Sleep, dream, nurse, gaze into your little one's eyes, and let nature take its course. If you have a tiny bit of energy to spare, channel it into inspiring activities like meditating and journaling. If you need to scratch the e-mail itch while you're up nursing at 3:00 a.m., or if you feel like picking up a book every now and then, go for it. But try to remember that you'll be back in the swing of things soon enough, so cherish this precious and all-too-fleeting period.

You can turn this time into an even more beautiful ritual by taking cues from women around the world. In Indonesia and Malaysia, a new mother is given weekly massages with special herbs and oils to encourage her body to return to its natural condition.[3] Indigenous Mexican and Native American cultures emphasize warmth for a new mama by making sure her room is comfortably heated so she can nurse more easily while also helping her baby feel snug and secure. And in India, mama and baby are given a ritual bath after their lying-in and are then presented at a special party to celebrate them both.[4] Consider planning similar "coming out" festivities so that you can cherish your alone time even as you look forward to a gathering of loved ones. You could have people come and visit with you while you're tucked in bed, or you could greet people in your living room and keep your bedroom off-limits so you and your baby have a sacred space to nurse or seek quietude.

MAKE A BABY HIDEOUT

Sometimes well-meaning loved ones who come to see the baby end up taking more than they bring. Of course, people are visiting to share your joy and celebrate and shower you with well wishes and love, and that's beautiful and welcome. But occasionally, no matter how pure the intentions, people can sap a lot of your energy. That's when you need to do whatever it takes to preserve that precious resource so you devote every ounce to your baby. Even just sitting and talking may feel like too much effort. That's okay. Give yourself permission to step out of the room if you need to recharge, or invent a signal so your partner can be the one to say in the most loving manner possible, "We love you, but get the hell out now . . . and come back soon!" Another way to deal with eager well-wishers is to send an e-mail blast with a sweet birth announcement sharing the news of baby's arrival, that mama and papa are in love and resting, and the heads-up that you won't be returning calls or e-mails for a few weeks. Read more about this and other tips for how to preserve this sacred space in "For Gentlemen Only: Protecting the Nest" on page 186. The reason I put the advice there is so your man (or woman) can spearhead those measures instead of your having to worry about them.

I can't stress enough that the secret to healing after birth—and to keeping healthy forever after—is to remember the most important things you need right now: food, sleep, and (eventually) exercise. If what you're eating isn't giving you all the nutrients you need, then you can't sleep well. If you don't get rest, you won't have the energy to do much of anything. If you focus only on resting and not on what you're giving your body to rebuild and sustain its peak condition, then you still won't feel completely well. Being a mom takes every single morsel of your being, so you want to have as much energy as possible. Food is your ally. Eat well and you will rest well, heal well, and live well.

YOUR HEALING POSTBIRTH MENU

How smoothly you heal after birth is hugely affected by the foods you nourish yourself with. Loading up on kind whole grains, legumes, and veggies just like you did before having your baby is the best way to ensure a quick recovery,[5] but there are also some special foods and dishes that are really restorative—and that help you produce more luscious, nutrient-rich breast milk.

- Your best first food is Immune-Boosting Miso Soup (page 295).

- Next would come Kinpira Soup, which is wonderful nourishment. Have a bowl or two daily for 5 to 7 days and then two or three times a week for at least 6 weeks. You can find a recipe for Kinpira Soup in *The Kind Diet* or on thekindlife.com.

- Try to have nishime (a Japanese vegetable stew) four times a week. Using squash in this dish is particularly tasty (page 299).

- The best proteins during this time are tofu, tempeh, and seitan. All of these can be stir-fried, deep-fried, or added to soups, barley stew, or nishime.

- Vegetable tempura is nice a couple of times a week and is great with noodles and broth.

- Work in plenty of grains like amaranth, barley, quinoa, and brown rice.

- *Mochi*—pan-fried, deep-fried, or eaten as a snack—is very nourishing for mama.

- Have healthy oils daily, even twice a day. This will prevent you from getting depleted, especially as you're nursing. Your food shouldn't be greasy but should simply have some oil in it—dishes like stir-fried noodles or pan-fried *mochi*. Treat yourself in moderation to richer, good-fat foods like avocados, nut butters, and creamy dressings.

- Other excellent dishes include lightly steamed or sautéed vegetables; root vegetables and their tops, especially turnips; dried daikon cooked with carrots and fried tofu or tempeh; sweet, creamy pureed soups; fried rice and fried noodles with vegetables; sweet rice and brown rice cooked with kombu; and lightly steamed bread with tahini.

- For something sweet, refer to "Conquer Your Cravings" (page 114) to see what's on the kind menu. My top picks for this important time are a bowl of cooked pear or apple (just a little; not every day), warmed carrot juice, Sweet Calming Kuzu (page 297), and Tangerine Kanten (page 319).

Just as kind food can help you, the wrong foods—especially animal products and sugar—can hinder. These nasty foods can weaken your uterus and slow its return to normal size, and that recovery can be more painful. Nasty foods can cause the normal bleeding after delivery to last longer and be heavier[6] and at the same time make your milk thin and watery.[7] Also, steer clear of raw fruits and vegetables or anything that's iced or chilled. You're aiming to nurture your body as much as possible, so treat it to warm foods and drinks, which are soothing to the system.

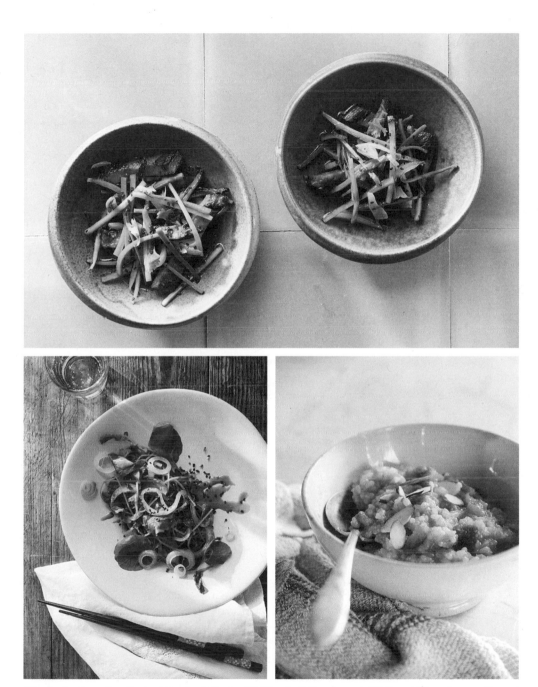

Clockwise from top: Braised Burdock Root with Hearty Seitan (page 306); Sweet Rice, Amaranth, and Apricot Breakfast Porridge (page 301); and Watercress with Creamy Tahini Dressing (page 298)

If you crave sweets, instead of eating processed sugar that will only upset your body and most likely your baby, try scratching the itch with a little barley malt or brown rice syrup in your tea (barley or kukicha) or oatmeal or even some of the Goody-Goodies treats listed in Chapter 8. But if that's not going to do it for you, try something kinder than a Snickers first—like some So Delicious frozen dessert or any of the other Naughty-but-Nice sweet treats listed in Chapter 8.

Cooking During Your Lying-In

Eating clean, nourishing food during this crucial time will be your lifeline. Make it a priority. Not planning ahead will most likely mean that you'll end up ordering in or grabbing something less than ideal, and it's only going to make you feel lousy. That's why I highly recommend you find someone else to prepare food for you, so you don't even have to think twice about it. But if your partner, friends, or family will be doing the cooking after your baby is born, keep things simple to get the most mileage out of their time in the kitchen. By making bigger batches, 1 to 2 hours of cooking can feed you for up to 4 days, with just the quick addition of freshly prepared vegetables each day. Bean dishes and soups are good for 3 to 4 days in the fridge, and grains can last 2 to 3 days. Then once you're all healed and back on your feet, wrap your baby up in a sling, bounce around the kitchen, and commit to giving yourself the gift of pure healing food.

GET YOUR BUTT IN BED

After eating well, sleep is one of *the* most important practices you will have as a new parent. Being rested makes everything so much sweeter—it will seriously save you. Plus, if you get too exhausted or depleted, your milk supply could be affected. This makes eating well that much more crucial. Giving your body clean food that delivers energy and nutrients and that your digestive system doesn't have to wrestle with all night means that you can get deeper, more effective sleep. And don't be like me and try to tackle everything in life while your poor husband begs you to get some rest! Here are some other tips for slipping in as much shut-eye as you can:

- Especially in the first 6 weeks, whenever baby is sleeping, get your behind into bed.
- Ignore the temptation to get stuff done while baby is napping. Sleep is more important.
- When you wake up in the night to nurse or soothe baby, try not to look at the clock. Sometimes, meditating can help ease the mind back to rest.
- Try breastfeeding while lying on your side—you and your baby can doze off together.

- Do whatever you have to do to get the sleep you need. Decide how much it takes for you to be a functional human being and then stay in bed until you've gotten that amount. Think of it as banking hours and not going anywhere until you've hit your goal. Even if it takes 12 hours of effort to get 8 hours of sleep, try to respect that. In our case, Christopher got great sleep while I nursed all night, so once he woke up he'd take Bear and walk him for hours so I could catch up on some of what I'd missed. You're going to be exhausted no matter what, but doing this makes it way better.

THE ICKY STUFF THAT NOBODY TELLS YOU ABOUT

When you're pregnant, it seems like everyone is quick to tell you every single detail about giving birth. But what can you expect *after* the baby's born? It's odd that no one warns you about those issues. I was in utter heaven in my lying-in baby cocoon, but there was no denying the fact that my body had just been to the top of Everest and back. Yet there's no way you can dominate an achievement like that without a few bumps and bruises along the way.

I mean, let's get real—you just carried around a Tofurky loaf in your body for 9 months and then pushed it through your lady parts. Things are going to need a little loving care! For me, sitting on the toilet was zero fun, and my chichi was on fire. Even though I tore only a teeny bit when the baby came out, I was swollen and sore.

But your body is genius, and it can pretty much get back to fighting shape on its own if you give it nourishing foods and lots of rest. Here's a heads-up about some things you can expect in the first few weeks after birth, plus ways to give yourself a little extra TLC:

Your Bottom/Chichi/Vajayjay/Vagina Is Going to Be a Hot Mess

It'll be sore, it won't like it when you sit on the toilet, and it may burn. Luckily, you can get relief:

- **Calendula tincture or bottom spray:** My midwife recommended that I buy a bottle of calendula tincture, and every time I hobbled to the bathroom to pee, I'd mix a dropperful with some warm water in a squirt bottle and spray it all over my poor little chichi. It felt so, so good! And doing it every time I went to the bathroom meant my tender bits were constantly getting some love. Calendula is a natural remedy for speeding up healing after childbirth and can prevent infections. Make sure you're buying the tincture in the dropper bottle and not the essential oil. Using oil on the area right after birth can trap bacteria and cause infection instead of letting the area breathe and heal. I also recommend Earth Mama Angel Baby's New Mama Bottom Spray, especially in the first week. It's a *lifesaver*.

- **Bottom cream:** After about a week, when things down below had calmed down a bit, I couldn't get enough of Earth Mama Angel Baby's Mama Bottom Balm. The olive oil base soothed the stinging and burning. And it smells delicious!

- **Cold pack:** Cold is good at bringing down inflammation and offering respite, especially in the first 2 or 3 days after birth. Store your sanitary pads (which we'll talk about in a minute) in the freezer, or keep your bottom cream in the fridge.

- **Aloe vera poultice:** Aloe is a natural healing remedy, and it's particularly good for mending a tender or torn perineum and providing comfort. My midwife told me to spread a good-size blob on my chilled sanitary pads or directly on my skin. Keep an aloe plant in your house so all you have to do is break off a tip and scrape out the flesh. Or buy pure aloe in bottled form, which you can find in most natural food shops, and store in the fridge. Chilled witch hazel will also do the trick.

- **Sitz bath:** This is a small bowl that fits into your toilet. Use it to soak your bottom without having to get into the tub. A lot of midwives recommend this remedy, and it's true that the warm water is good for getting fresh, healing blood circulating to your tender bottom. But I don't advocate going out and buying a piece of plastic just for this one temporary task. Putting a couple of inches of warm water in the tub can offer amazing relief to a sore perineum, and you can add some Soothing Ginger Tea (page 296) to the water, which is miraculous in helping with itching and soreness.

- **Fresh air:** Above all, get your butt in the air! Nothing breeds bacteria better than dark and damp. Sunlight and fresh air, on the other hand, have natural antibacterial properties. If there's somewhere private you can be outside, great; otherwise just have some nice naked time in bed. Either way, getting a little breeze up there can feel so good.

You'll Feel Kinda Like You Have Your Period

For about 3 to 6 weeks after birth, you'll experience some bleeding from where the placenta was attached to the uterus. For the first few days, the flow will be similar to the beginning of your cycle, though it could be heavier. The bleeding will taper off and stop altogether after the site heals completely.[8]

A Note on Homeopathic Remedies

Your caregiver might recommend healing boosters other than what you see here, which is great! But be mindful that most commercial homeopathic remedies in pill form are made with lactose, a sugar found in animal milk. Even though very little of this remains in the actual remedy, consider this a heads up that it's technically not vegan. This isn't a free pass to use them, but then again, no one's going to call the Kind Police. So double-check the label before bringing the remedies home. If you're having trouble finding a version that's completely kind, see if there's a homeopath in your area who can make you a special lactose-free formula. Apply the same mindfulness to liquid and topical remedies, too.

Even though you wear a pad only for a relatively short time, pick one that's made out of organic fiber. (See "Why Your Tampon Sucks" on page 59). Otherwise, you'll be making your poor lady bits—which have already been through enough!—keep close company with the nasty chemicals that we talked about in Chapter 5.

You May Still Have Contractions

As your body works to shrink your uterus back to its original size and shape, you'll very likely experience afterpains, or what feel like menstrual cramps or labor pains. If it's not your first baby, these might be more intense, because additional pregnancies make the uterus more relaxed and stretchy, which means your body has to put in more effort to get it back to where it was.[9] Lying on your stomach can sometimes help, as can drinking some calming kukicha or Soothing Ginger Tea (page 296).

You Might Get Backed Up

Your entire body needs to recalibrate after giving birth, and that includes your bowel movements. The foods and dishes recommended in "The Food Remedy: Your Healing Postbirth Menu" (page 179) will help your system return to its regular self.

(continued on page 188)

For Gentlemen Only: Protecting the Nest

By the time your baby is born, your lady will have been on one of the trippiest rides she could ever have imagined. Her body, her brain, her hormones, her spirit, her emotions—just about every particle of her being has been taken out, shaken up, and rearranged. She'll need to physically heal and she may need to emotionally recalibrate, too.

That's where you come in. You are the protector of the mama-baby cocoon. Any actions you can take to ensure your partner is nourished, comfortable, content, and free to do nothing but bond with baby is helping your little family put down strong roots. But remember to take time for yourself, too. This incredible baby vacation is yours to enjoy just as much as it is your partner's. By making it your job to soak up every bit of this incredible time, it'll be so much sweeter for everyone.

Here are a few tips for navigating this new territory:

Run interference. Of course, your friends and family will want to see the new baby. But visitors are not always beneficial in the first few weeks after birth. If "zero visitation" is how your lady chooses to proceed after the baby comes, let people know that she and the baby are happily nesting and that you'll gladly open your home to visitors when the time comes. If you do have guests over, let them know what kind of foods to bring, whether there are any errands they might be able to run on their way over, or if there's something around the house they might be able to handle on your new family's behalf.

When guests are there, pay close attention to your partner and her body language. If she's looking a little droopy or is giving you the wide-eyed "Get them out of here!" look, it's time for you to escort everyone out the door. No one will think you're being a jerk for asking them to leave. You're simply practicing an important part of being a parent: preserving your energy so baby can have the best of you.

Keep the nest neat. There's nothing more irritating to a new mom—or most women, really—than clutter. Every morning, take the time to walk around the house and straighten up anything that might be distracting.

Anticipate her needs. Healing and nursing mamas need plenty of nourishing snacks and fluids. Take a peek at the special healing foods listed earlier in this chapter and surprise your partner by making sure the house is well stocked with healthy provisions. Offer them to her from time to time without her having to ask, and she'll melt with gratitude.

Assert yourself. While the most important thing a new mama can do right after birth is spend all day touching and nuzzling and nursing baby, it is just as essential for you to form your own father-infant attachment. Snuggle into that healing cocoon with your partner and baby, and relish the warmth and joy of your family. And give mama a break by taking a walk with baby in the sling around the house or the neighborhood. She can try to get a little sleep, and you and the little one can talk about your big plans for the future. Your whole mission as a new father is to dote—and the more you love on the baby, the better the daddy you are and the sexier we ladies think it is.

Be there. The more time you can spend bonding with your baby, taking care of his needs, and supporting your lady as she heals, the better. I know you don't always have a choice about how much time off you can take from work without being penalized, but be honest with yourself. Will you truly get fired if you rally for another week at home? Will your income seriously suffer if you take unpaid time off? Being there to share this incredibly special, unparalleled, once-in-a-lifetime space with your new family is often far more valuable than a paycheck.

Be a superparent. By shouldering the weight of running the household—making dinner, getting everyone dressed for school, making sure teeth are brushed—you'll be giving her the essential space to complete her recovery.

There would usually come a point where Alicia had been feeding Bear on and off through the whole night, and she would be delirious. She would ask me to take him for a while so she could sleep. Fellas, this is no time to dilly-dally. Don't rub your eyes or stretch or any of that stuff. Treat it like officer training school and your general just came in with the bugle. Don't just tell your wife how appreciative you are of her, show her. Get her to drink water and make sure she's nourished. Change diapers and get your baby in some clothes so your wife doesn't have to do as much.

—*Christopher*

BABY BLUES AND POSTPARTUM DEPRESSION

It's hard to imagine, but sometimes the afterglow of birth isn't so rosy. Though it's less common among kind mamas, some women experience the blues after giving birth.

Keeping a clean, balanced diet is crucial. Even though there hasn't been a big push to identify a definitive link between certain deficiencies and postpartum depression specifically, we do know that eating plenty of foods rich in things like zinc (nuts, beans, greens), selenium (whole wheat), and magnesium (red foods like berries, beets, and purple-top turnips) has been shown to reduce feelings of depression, increase emotional stability, aid sleep, and fend off irritability.[10] Definitely steer clear of processed sugar, which makes us feel unbalanced. To help recalibrate the major hormonal shift that happens postpartum, look to foods like burdock root, tofu, and tempeh. Burdock root supports liver function, which helps break down excess hormones. And the phytoestrogens in tofu and tempeh work to rebalance estrogen. Consuming plenty of magic foods like leafy greens, whole grains, legumes, and foods rich in omega-3 fatty acids (flaxseed oil, walnuts, soybeans/tofu) also supports brain and emotional health. These foods can give your body the nourishment it needs, promote much-needed restorative sleep (another potent cure for feeling low), and bring you back toward balance.

That said, if you're experiencing anxiety, crying spells, appetite loss, or any of the afore-mentioned symptoms and have "scary thoughts" like thinking you might harm your baby, then you should call your caregiver. Sharing your honest and true experience and getting the help you need are steps toward becoming the bravest, strongest, most loving mama you can possibly be.

SELF-HEALING TECHNIQUES

Okay, even after all that, I assure you from the bottom of my heart that giving birth is still the most enchanting, intensely satisfying experience that exists in this universe. And there are some other ways, besides eating super-clean, that you can help yourself strengthen and recover.

Starting on your third day postpartum, get back to your kegels to help tone back up your lady bits and boost circulation. Also, keep up with your journaling. Keep a notebook by your bed and write down anything that comes to mind before you go to sleep, which can help clear your head before you drift off. This practice can also help give shape to what your new needs, hopes, and wishes look like now that you're a mama.

Let Your Birth Story Heal You

Spend some of this precious quiet time writing your birth story—you've been to the moon and back! How could you not want to recount every single detail?! Try to do it as soon after birth as possible, while the events are fresh. You seriously won't regret it. One day, your story will be an amazing thing to share with your little one or maybe just to revisit yourself. I read my mom's labor reports as I went into labor, which was so incredibly neat.

Let Your Baby Heal You

If you're ever overwhelmed or anxious about how your transition into mamahood is going, take a cue from your baby and bring it back to the boob. As your baby nurses, look into his eyes and just be there, in that moment. Breathe as he breathes. Feel the magnetism that will forever weave the two of you together in this world. Know that you are giving your tiny baby everything he needs, and, in return, he'll completely nourish you if you let him.

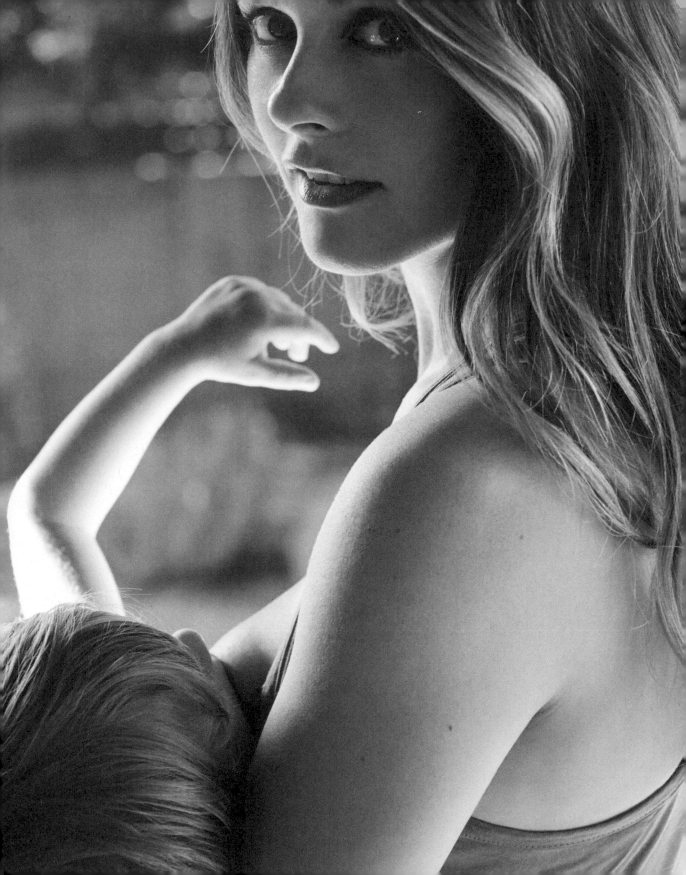

12

Breastfeeding

*I love to smell your little hand while you're feeding; the way you
put it up to my nose and just stare at me is so delectable.*
—My Journal, Postpartum

Breast milk is the purest expression of a mama's love for her baby. It's no wonder that the American Academy of Pediatrics says breastfeeding is the healthiest choice you can make for at least the first 6 months.[11] It has the unmatched ability to nurture, fortify, cure, and soothe. It is, to my mind, the ultimate act of kindness. It's sensual, adorable, satisfying, empowering, and, at times, insanely funny. I can't imagine life without it. And I suppose, in a way, God or Mother Nature or the Supreme Being or Zeus couldn't either, because he and/or she created us with breasts and the milk that was designed to give our babies life.

Breastfeeding is primal. As mammals, we're designed to nourish our young this way. We have our boobies for a reason—it's to feed our children! Within minutes of being born and placed on my chest, Bear was nuzzling his way toward the breast. He intuitively knew to go there. When I breastfeed, I feel more deeply sensual and connected to my most powerful woman self than I have ever felt in my life. And then there are the faces babies make—watching your little one on the breast is like the best film you've ever seen. When Bear first started breastfeeding, he'd get this look like he was a little squirrel that fell out of a tree. Sometimes he gives me these soft, flirty eyes. And sometimes he just looks bored. It's all so priceless.

BREAST MILK: THE MOST PERFECT FOOD

From the beginning of our human form, mothers—like their mammalian sisters in the wild—nursed their children. For good reason, too: It's nature's most perfect food. It's always available, just the right temperature, sterile, and completely free, and it keeps babies thriving and healthy.

By the turn of the 19th century, though, women across America had begun to embrace artificial infant food or formula. A 1910 Boston study found that 90 percent of poor mothers breastfed, while only 17 percent of wealthy mothers did.[12] In response to the growing number of women who either couldn't nurse or, more likely, didn't want to because it was seen as dreadfully lower class, cows were proclaimed the new "wet nurse for the human race."[13] Unfortunately, many of the babies fed modified cow's milk died, but that only prompted scientists to step up their laboratory-made-formula game. Meanwhile, more and more women started giving birth in hospitals, and so with doctors promising new mothers that these marvels of modernity could ensure their babies were getting the best possible nutrition, boobs didn't stand a chance. By the time World War II and the baby boom rolled around and women were being liberated from their aprons, portable, science-backed, doctor-approved formula was the new "perfect" food.[14]

Today, formula companies still stand by that claim, even though the World Health Organization says that infants should be breastfed exclusively until 6 months to "achieve optimal growth, development, and health,"[15] and the American Academy of Pediatrics suggests that women breastfeed for at least 12 months to give their children the full health benefits.[16] You would think the government could maybe step in and let Americans know what's what, right? Well, the WHO certainly agreed, stating that promoting formula—especially in hospitals—caused unnecessary confusion among new moms. In 1981, a code to restrict the promotion of infant formula products was drafted and put to a vote. The final tally: 118 to 1. Care to guess who the lone naysayer was? (Hint: It rhymes with "Shamerica.")[17]

So we have to take matters into our own hands. Just as natural birth is still an unpaved road, so is breastfeeding. They're both the oldest, most nature-made, God-given roads there are, but we need to pick up some of the downed trees that have been blocking the path for some time. Like any other journey worth taking or brave decision worth fighting for, the secret is to get your knowledge on, understand your rights, and let your boobies reach their full, glorious potential! Here are a few more reasons why boob food is perfect in every way:

Breast Milk Is Nature's Magical Elixir

The breast milk you produce is perfectly designed to meet all the needs of your baby's developing brain and body. Your body knows exactly how to calibrate the calories, fat, protein, and vitamins delivered to your baby based on how often and how long she feeds.[18] In fact, your milk changes as your baby grows.[19] When your baby is first born, she needs more fat to build her brain and help her body insulate itself.[20] As she gets older, her needs change, so a 6-week-old will get a different protein, fat, and nutrient shake than a 6-month-old. And if your baby is born prematurely, your body will automatically provide her with its own superboost brew that's easier to digest than formula.[21] Milk also changes throughout a single feeding. "Hind milk," or the milk that is highest in baby-fortifying fat, is delivered only in the second half of a nursing session, as if it's some kind of sweet reward for baby finishing everything on her plate.

Breastfeeding Makes Healthier Babies

Breast milk is nature's bodyguard. Unlike any formula, breast milk delivers a complete immune system to your baby. Our little ones aren't born with all the bacteria- and disease-fighting antibodies that they need to defend themselves, so they have to get the antibodies through our milk.[22] By breastfeeding, you're passing on the antibodies to every virus you're exposed to, which protects your baby from getting sick or at least helps him get better faster.[23] Breast milk seals off your baby's intestines, kick-starts his digestive tract, and populates his gut with all kinds of good bacteria, which fend off intestinal issues.[24] That also helps your baby absorb food more quickly, so that he can grow, resist contaminants and infections, and even avoid lifelong digestive diseases like Crohn's.[25] Breastfeeding has been shown to reduce a baby's risk of obesity, asthma, diabetes, leukemia, lymphoma, and sudden infant death syndrome (SIDS).[26] Breastfed babies have a reduced chance of developing allergies,[27] and because they're also getting a good workout of the jaw muscles, tongue, and lips to get every last drop from your boobies, they have a lower risk of TMJ disease later in life[28] and a reduced chance of needing braces.[29] And amazingly, nursing your little girl reduces her lifetime risk of breast cancer by as much as 25 percent![30]

Breastfeeding Makes Happier Babies

Breastfeeding isn't just for mealtimes. It's also a magical antidote for a baby's fear, anxiety, loneliness, pain, and overstimulation.[31] Breast milk has chemicals that induce sleep,[32] which is sometimes all an infant needs to make the world right again. And being close to mama forms a powerful calming balm for a fretting baby. Breastfeeding is cuddling, caressing, nuzzling, and warm, decadent skin-on-skin nesting. You're telling your baby in the most powerful way that he's safe and cared for. And when you do that, you create a path for him to feel emotionally and psychologically secure for the rest of his life.

Breastfeeding Makes Happier, Healthier Mamas

Your baby's not the only one who benefits from breastfeeding. When your newborn settles in for a meal, your body releases a groovy hormone cocktail. I think it's nature's ultimate thank-you for doing it. There's almost no describing how delicious and lovely it feels to breastfeed. It's like you're so high with joy and love and yet so deep with mama-goddess purpose. The act itself is unbelievably delicious—a full-body tingling. Sometimes I'll cradle Bear's feet or he'll hold my

---

Breast Milk Is Your New Pharmacy

Aside from giving your baby every single health advantage there is at mealtime, breast milk is also the ultimate cure-all for almost every ailment that might come up in baby's early days. It's a natural antibiotic and has almost otherworldly power to both soothe and heal. Try it:

- Dabbed as a salve on cracked or tender nipples, baby acne, heat rash, or other skin irritations like diaper rash. (Though breastfed babies get *way* less diaper rash, and babies in cloth diapers get almost none. And no diapers equals zero rash! But more on that in a bit.)

- Squirted in baby's nose on an airplane or other germy places to protect the nasal membranes. It also triggers the sneeze reflex, which can help force out any nasty germs that might have snuck in. Another bonus is that nursing during takeoff and landing helps keep baby's little ears from popping.

- For red, irritated eyes—though you should check with your pediatrician to make sure the irritation is nothing more serious than a plugged duct or a minor infection.

- Dropped in the ears, it can potentially reduce the discomfort of an ear infection (though in my experience, kind babies are less likely to get these).

- Applied to relieve and heal cuts and scrapes.

hand, and it's so romantic. I say the universe wouldn't have made it that way if it wasn't completely normal, and it just feels *right*. I'm providing for my baby in this incredibly physical, animal way, and it's exactly what my body wants to be doing in that moment. Every time I feel a little grumpy and Bear latches on to my boob, I'm instantly the most contented woman on earth.

Breastfeeding is a powerful emotional and physical tonic. When our babies latch, we get a boost of oxytocin for bonding, shrinking the uterus back to its normal size, preventing the baby blues, and chilling us out;[33] plus prolactin for energizing mother's intuition,[34] stimulating even more milk production, and giving you the warmest, fuzziest feeling.[35] Breastfeeding moms sleep more (according to a 2007 study, an average of 45 minutes a night more than mothers who were formula feeding; nursing moms also reported feeling less tired!).[36] And nursing helps mamas burn about 500 calories a day (making it easier to return to prepregnancy weight),[37] protects against breast and ovarian cancers,[38] lowers blood pressure, and decreases the risk of osteoporosis.[39]

Breastfeeding Is Kind to the Planet (and So Much Easier)

The boobie is the original green food! Breastfeeding creates very little waste—none of those icky plastic bottles and liners. My mother-in-law, who was part of the culture of women who were told that formula was better for working moms, couldn't believe how much less there was to clean and how much less "stuff" there was to deal with.

Breastfeeding Is Kind to the Wallet

Breast milk is free! A year's worth of formula—not including all the equipment you need for bottling, sanitizing, storing, and transporting it—can run around $900.[40]

GETTING STARTED: SET YOURSELF UP FOR SUCCESS

So now that you know what an incredible, powerful, and downright scrumptious miracle breastfeeding is, let's talk about how to do it. I'm going to keep it brief because, guess what? You already know how! And so does your baby. But because most of us didn't grow up watching our moms, sisters, aunts, friends, or tribe mates, I know you may have a lot of questions and concerns. Here are the basics for sweet breastfeeding success the first time.

Keep It Kind

The first and most important factor in successful nursing is your diet. Restorative, nourishing, strengthening food is key when it comes to boosting the chances that you'll produce milk quickly and also enough of it. Just as you built the most luxurious baby house by eating clean, kind foods, you can make sure you're making the most magical breast milk tincture by continuing to fortify yourself. Plus, the better you feed your body, the better it can rest and heal and ward off stress, all of which add up to ultimate breastfeeding prowess. I'll talk more about this and which foods can give you a superboost in the section "Your Breastfeeding Menu" (page 199).

Master the Latch

Babies are born understanding the power of the boobie, but sometimes they need a little nudge to get the hang of the right latch. Without a good latch, a baby needs to do a lot of work to get just a little bit of milk, which can tire her out and mean she's not getting everything she needs in a feeding. It can also affect how much milk you're able to produce, since your body takes cues from nursing sessions to figure out how much to make.[41] Milk left in the breast signals to your body that it doesn't need to make as much for next time, and it can lead to not-so-pleasant maladies like engorgement and plugged ducts (more on that in a second). And last, an unsuccessful latch can be a real zinger on the nipples, which will make nursing more uncomfortable than it should be and lead to cracked, bleeding bits. Make sure your baby is opening nice and wide and taking in your areola, not just your nipple. It's called *breast*feeding for a reason!

Nurse Like It's Your Destiny

During your baby vacation, you'll have all the time in the world for your new job as mama and letting those boobies reach their full potential. Feeding frequently around the clock will help prevent jaundice in your baby; boost your milk supply; ward off engorgement, plugged ducts, and mastitis; and make that milk as nutritious as possible. The more frequently you feed your baby, the higher the fat content will be in future feedings, which is exactly what your baby needs to grow.[42]

Sometimes babies nurse when they're just thirsty or looking for comfort. Those little snacks also support good milk supply and weight gain.[43] If that's happening frequently, though, make sure he's getting in some good, long, slow swallows at his mealtimes. Otherwise, his wanting to snack might indicate that he's not getting enough milk.

At first, it might feel like you're doing a whole lot of nursing—and you will be!—but that just means you're setting you and your baby up for a long and vibrant breastfeeding relationship. And as for those super-sleepy late-night sessions, my friend Lalanya put it in such a beautiful way: "It was actually pretty amazing to think of all the other mamas up feeding their babies at the very same time. It's almost like a whole network of women are connected by the nighttime nursing." Plus remember that as tired as you are, this time in your life is fleeting. Cherish these tender sessions with your little one while they last.

Go for the Breast Defense: Have an Expert On Call

If you run into a hitch, call in an expert. There are so many easily remedied things that can become bigger obstacles if not addressed, and they usually only take tiny tweaks. Consider enlisting the help of a lactation consultant. The $100 or $200 you spend to help you establish a fruitful, long-term nursing relationship will ultimately save you money, whether on formula or medical costs down the road. Plus, many health insurance plans will reimburse you for these services. If paying for a consultant isn't an option, you can get free guidance from the La Leche League International (llli.org) advice line or by attending one of their meetings in your area. Also check out kellymom.com, an amazing site that even lactation consultants sometimes visit.

THE BREASTFEEDING BASICS

Make Way for Colostrum

Before your milk-milk comes in, your breasts will start expressing something called colostrum. This creamy, golden miracle food is packed with proteins, vitamins, minerals,[44] and special properties that help your baby's intestines finish developing,[45] fend off disease and allergies,[46] and offer a turbocharge of antibodies and natural immunity.[47] It acts as a gentle, natural laxative to flush out meconium, or waste built up in utero, and gives your baby strong protection from illness.[48]

Your colostrum is plenty of food for baby until your milk comes in, which usually happens 2 to 5 days after birth.[49] It's normal for your baby to lose a small amount of weight in that time,[50] so don't feel pressured to supplement with formula. Even though it's now completely medically acceptable to stick with a colostrum-only diet, nurses and doctors used to be trained to think that babies needed a lot of milk in their early days. Give a kind but firm "no thanks" to anyone who still thinks this is the case and tries to convince you as much.[51]

Making Kind Milk

The happiest, healthiest babies are the ones who get the happiest, healthiest breast milk, and if you're a Kind Mama, then you're already on the case! Kind milk has fewer—or no—chemical pollutants[52] and the perfect amount of protein,[53] essential fatty acids, and vital nutrients like iron and zinc.[54] Kind milk helps babies sleep better at night, is effective at warding off disease and allergies, and comes with an insurance policy from your body that you'll most likely produce enough.[55]

If you're splurging on cranky-making sugar—or worse, hormone-laced, toxin-filled meat, fish, and dairy—that all gets passed on to your little one. Susan Levin, MS, RD, explains, "Tox-

ins and hormones like to store and accumulate in animal fat. Because breast milk production is dependent on mother's fat supply, the mom's toxin buildup will inevitably be a part of the milk." And baby doesn't yet have the defenses in her tiny body to ward off things that might harm her. Because these foods keep your own body from balance and harmony, there's a chance they can

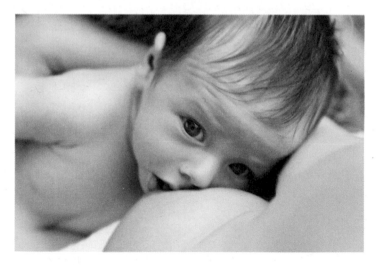

prevent you from making enough milk, which means baby won't be able to get all the amazing, lifesaving miracles your breast milk would otherwise be able to offer.

And these foods aren't only harmful for your baby, they're disruptive. The same culprits that are at the root of pregnancy discomfort can make your baby aggravated and cranky. They can also mess with a baby's sleep,[56] which any new parent will tell you is the *last* thing you want.

To keep your milk as fresh and clean as possible, stick with whole, plant-based foods that make you feel good. At least for the first 6 months, strive to make clean eating an art form. Remember that you're *building* milk for your baby, and that your only job is to feed your baby (and to sleep!) and to be totally present for the pure joy available to you through your little love ball. If you focus on that, you'll make the best milk in the world. This isn't a special diet; it's very simply eating balanced, nutrient-dense food. This not only ensures your baby is getting everything she needs but also gives you the energy to adjust to your life's new rhythm.

YOUR BREASTFEEDING MENU

The foods on this list should be familiar friends by now. They're the exact same ones we need to boost when we're growing and nurturing a baby! We're still doing exactly that, so the same wisdom applies. Eating a kind diet across the board will address these needs, but here's a cheat sheet so you can see which nutrients and minerals are in especially high demand, and those that are particularly potent milk-makers.

As for eating three square meals a day, don't get too stressed out. If you're feeling peckish all the time, feel free to indulge in lots of mini-meals. After all, you're giving out a lot! Complement this boosted intake with dishes like pressed salads, nishime, and greens (all of which are very nourishing, balancing, and medicinal), in addition to all the other sautéed, steamed, baked, or blanched veggies you love to keep your body happy and harmonized.

Sweet brown rice: This has more protein and fat than regular brown rice, which is ideal for nursing mamas. I always mix it with other grains like regular brown rice or some rye if I am eating it like a grain, or with some amaranth if I'm making more of a porridge. See page 294 for how to make tasty and balanced grain medleys. You can also eat it in its compressed form, mochi, which puffs up like a scrumptious waffle for breakfast or as a crouton that's great in soups.

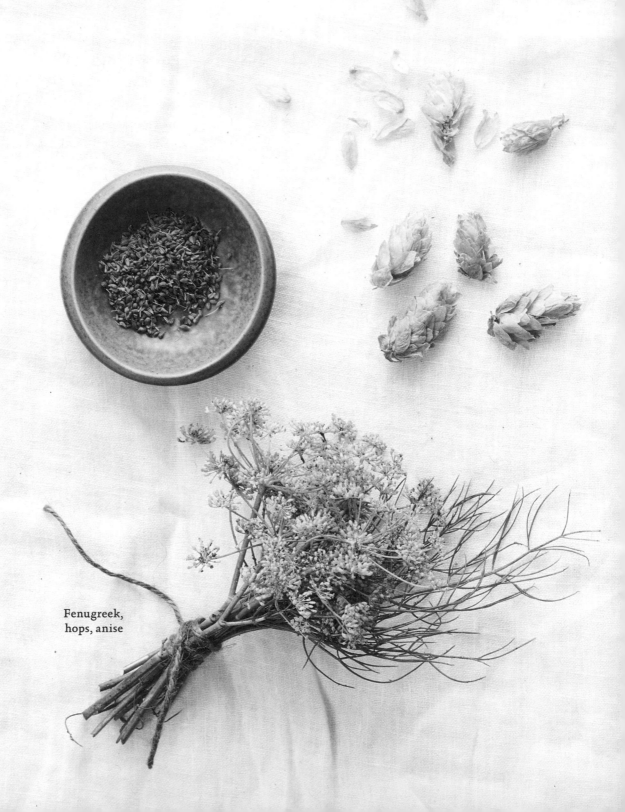

Fenugreek,
hops, anise

Beans, tofu, tempeh, and seitan: Because milk production is a full-body workout, try to get as much energy-rich fuel as you did during the second and third trimesters of pregnancy.[57] Each meal should have some protein.

Good fats: You need enough of these to help build your baby's developing brain and eyes,[58] and they also happen to prevent mild depression like the baby blues.[59] Sprinkle some flaxseed oil on your oatmeal and some olive oil on a light sauté a couple times a week, or treat yourself to some fried mochi three or four times a week, which is a good source of fat and so great for your milk. Other fortifying options are richer foods like seeds, stir-fries, nuts, and nut butters (just don't go crazy on the nuts and nut butters!).

Iron-rich foods: Just like during your last trimester, iron is still in high demand.[60] Continue loading up on things like seaweed, quinoa, greens, sesame seeds, tofu, pumpkin seeds, raisins, beets, and molasses (in moderation).

Something sweet: Enjoy treats like gently cooked fruit. Things like applesauce, steamed pears, and fruit stews are all yummy and simple options, or sweet and creamy amasake, a thick fermented drink made out of rice, which is nice diluted with a little water and heated up. Or make a batch of Tangerine Kanten (page 319) or Baked Peaches with Gooey Nut Crumble (page 320).

Water: Drink as much as you need and want. Don't drown your organs, but listen to your thirst.

Vitamin D: Revisit page 51 for a vitamin D refresher, since your baby will get her vitamin D through your milk.

Oats: Like the rest of the foods below, these guys are called galactogogues, or foods with a special active ingredient that stimulates milk production. To get the full effect, use whole or steel-cut oats instead of instant or rolled varieties.

Dark leafy green vegetables: Just one more reason to love these veggie superheroes!

Borage: This herb grows like crazy and sprouts beautiful purple-blue flowers. Pull off the little flowers and sprinkle them on your salad, or take a small dose of borage seed oil, if needed.

Fenugreek, blessed thistle, fennel, anise, hops, and alfalfa: These herbs can get things moving in high gear and can be taken in capsule, tincture, or tea form.

High-quality dark beer: According to Christina Pirello, dark stout beer like Guinness makes for great breast milk! Having a tiny bit of a stout—and I mean tiny: 12 ounces or less—a couple times a week is an age-old remedy. Dark beer is high in iron, and the malted barley gives your milk a boost.[61] Have your brew right after you've fed baby so the alcohol is out of your system by the next feeding. Samuel Smith makes a nice organic stout. If you're buying Guinness, make sure you get their extra-stout, because their other brews aren't vegan.

Soothing Ginger Tea: This restorative drink not only helps produce milk but also strengthens the nervous system! See the recipe on page 296.

FOODS TO AVOID OR REDUCE WHILE NURSING

Despite their kind label, some foods can be less than ideal for you and baby in the very beginning. These normally good-for-you provisions can be hard for your baby to digest and make him gassy, bloated, or fussy. Avoid them for the first few weeks, then slowly introduce them one at a time to see how your baby reacts.

- **Cruciferous vegetables** like broccoli, Brussels sprouts, cauliflower and cabbage.

- **High-acid fruits and vegetables** like oranges, grapefruit, and tomatoes.

- **The onion family** (including scallions).

- **Dried fruits** (especially prunes): Babies can sometimes be sensitive to these foods.

- **Beans:** Since they can be hard on baby's digestive system, hold off on adding these back into the rotation for 3 to 4 weeks.[62] It's okay to have a small amount every once in a while if you mix adzuki beans or chickpeas with rice and cook them together in a pressure cooker. For now, eat more tempeh, seitan, and tofu for your protein needs.

- **Certain herbs:** Sage, parsley, and peppermint can slow down your milk production. Steer clear of these herbs in your food, teas, or supplements.[63] Peppermint in particular is too stimulating for an infant and can upset her digestion.

- **Nasty foods:** By now, it's pretty obvious, but it bears repeating: Animal foods, high-sugar foods, and stimulating drinks like coffee do nothing to help your body and all its parts work the way they should—including making milk that's plentiful and not full of nasty toxins. They only add stress to your body, and if there's one thing that stands in the way between you and letting down your most luscious boobie offerings, it's stress.

IF YOU'RE FEELING NAUGHTY

When I first started nursing, no matter how stocked my fridge was with the cleanest, yummiest foods, all I wanted was to be bad. I craved toast, pasta, sweets—you name it. It didn't help that suddenly food tasted so good after being so uninteresting during pregnancy. It was like I discovered eating all over again! I asked Christina Pirello why I was being such a maniac. Her answer: "When you're nursing, you lose a lot of nutrients. Your body's instinct is to get those nutrients back in the easiest form to digest—carbohydrates." She suggested eating four or five small meals throughout the day. And she recommended foods like light, protein-loaded, easy-to-digest quinoa plus lots and lots of veggies (especially steamed, boiled, and sautéed greens). She reassured me that there's no law saying that life has to be reduced to beans and rice. So long as I was loading up on the good stuff and feeling okay, I didn't need to beat myself up over a little indulgence every now and then, as long as my treats were naughty but not nasty.

Rest!

I've said it once and I'll say it again, so listen up: Rest is what's going to make the difference between a baby adventure that's soulful and delicious and magical and one that feels strenuous.

Lactation consultant Beverly Solow, IBCLC, sums it up well: "Taking naps is not a luxury; they're an *essential*." Not getting enough rest is one of the most common causes of a dip in milk supply. Consider these small stretches of sleep as vital, baby-nourishing must-haves. It's why leaving the laundry, cooking, phone calls, bills, etc., to someone else is so important. You have more crucial duties to attend to, and taking care of yourself is taking better care of baby.

GEARING UP: HANDY STUFF FOR BREASTFEEDING

One of the most beautiful things about breastfeeding is that pretty much everything you need is attached to your body. But it's super-helpful to have a few thoughtful tools.

For Baby

BOTTLES

We got by with eight glass bottles until Bear was 8 months old. I thought we had a great system—it was enough for feedings and for storing milk from my pumping, and at the end of every day, we'd clean them. But then Christopher went to a friend's house and saw they had, like, a *thousand* bottles. He came home that night and said, "Baby, could we maybe get a few more?" It definitely would have made life easier to have that many, but I felt it was so wasteful to have more than we needed. So we took the cue and added a few bottles to the rotation.

I recommend having somewhere between 10 and 12 bottles if someone else will be giving baby your milk sometimes. That way there's a little wiggle room for the nights when doing dishes just isn't in the cards. When you do need to wash a batch, a great tip I got was to throw all the bottles, caps, and nipples into a mesh laundry bag and then place the whole thing in the dishwasher or a large pot of boiling water. No more searching for missing pieces!

We'll talk more about when and how to introduce bottles into the mix in the next section.

As for nipples, green-living expert Mary Cordaro recommends Natursutten's natural rubber version as a first choice. Unlike silicone nipples, which are manufactured with chemicals that over time can leach into their surrounding environment, natural rubber nipples are made without chemicals or artificial ingredients. The next best option is nitrosamine-free latex.

A PILLOW OR TWO

In the very beginning, when you're nursing around the clock, it can help to have extra padding to prop up both you and your babe. It makes the affair so much yummier when both of you are comfy and secure. Try stuffing one pillow behind your lower back and using a second to support your arm while you hold baby. Friends have told me that another great option is to repurpose your body pillow, if you bought one. Wrap it behind your waist and bring the ends together toward your front. You can sneak in a little extra rest, and you'll be saving your back and neck from crazy nursing contortions.

There are pillows made especially for breastfeeding, but they aren't the kindest option. Even though you can buy organic covers for most versions, the stuffing or foam is usually synthetic and not ideal for what your fragile little one should be breathing. A February 2012 report on toxic flame retardants used in baby products tested 20 popular items, including nursing pillows. *Seventeen* of the items tested positive for noxious chemicals that have been linked to cancer and hormone disruption! If you still like the idea of a nursing pillow, though, there are more planet- and baby-friendly versions by brands like Blessed Nest and Organic Caboose.

For You

MILK SAVER

When I first had Bear, I noticed while I was nursing him that he was soaking wet. It was on his chest, so I knew it couldn't be pee . . . then I realized that my other boob was leaking on him! We're not talking just a few drips, either. It was like full-blast boobie lasers. I e-mailed my friend Heather, asking, "What's the deal?" She said, "Stuff your bra with a big sock." That worked for the first 8 weeks when I didn't leave the house, but once I was out, I needed a better solution.

Then when I was in New York, I discovered something I wish I'd known about it since day 1: The milk saver was the answer! When you feed your baby, this handy-dandy gadget collects milk from your other boob. Instead of soaking up all my extra milk with a sock, I could save it. Sometimes, it would be as much as an ounce or more, and all those ounces add up! We mamas work so hard for every little drop of milk we pump, and this way every bit gets put to good use.

Even though the best model out there is plastic (Boo! Hiss!), Milkies Milk-Saver is BPA and phthalate free. Otherwise, it's completely perfect in every way and so low fuss. You don't even need to use a plastic storage bag like the company recommends—just use it upside down (which I discovered by accident). Put the cup inside your bra, then put your nipple in the hole. Voilà—it will collect your milk. If you're a total klutz like me, remember to take it off when you're done nursing. Once you bend over with it still on your boob, there goes all your fabulous milk!

Choosing a Bottle

For the deepest green: Go for traditional glass bottles. They're sturdy, heat resistant, and don't leach chemicals. Companies like Lifefactory, Evenflo, Born Free, and Dr. Brown's make great versions. Or you can try one of the newer stainless steel options made by Kleen Kanteen and organicKidz, which offer the same benefits as glass without the breakage factor when your baby starts to launch them across the room. OrganicKidz offers one that converts into a sippy cup *and* a lunch box–friendly water bottle, so less waste and less to buy down the road!

A lighter green option: Choose a plastic version. This isn't my favorite path because (a) it's plastic, and (b) although all bottles are now BPA free, you still have to be careful not to expose them to hot water (even though most manufacturers say theirs are dishwasher safe) or any hot liquids.[64] According to a 2011 study that tested 20 top-brand plastic baby bottles, virtually all leached chemicals that acted like the hormone estrogen, even though many were BPA free. The researchers ultimately concluded that there are thousands of possible chemicals in plastic that can act just like BPA, especially when heated.[65]

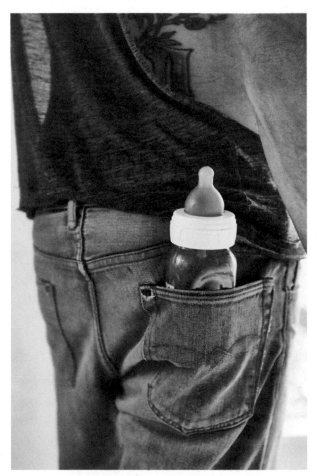

Two of the cleanest options in this category are bottles made by thinkbaby and Born Free. Their offerings are free of BPA, phthalates, nitrosamines, lead, PVC, PET, melamine, and biologically harmful chemicals. You can also buy a conversion kit, which means your bottles can double as sippy cups.

NURSING TANKS

At first, I didn't want to wear a bra because they weren't comfortable, but with my boobie sprinklers being so feisty—and the inevitability that I would one day have to leave the house—I wanted a solution that was comfortable and that kept the rest of my torso warm while I nursed. Because really, who wants to sit around in just a bra all the time? I went back to my friend Heather, and by the next morning, I had her nursing tanks in my mailbox.

I pretty much didn't take those things off for 7 months. They were lifesavers! All I had to do was snap off one of the little bra straps for instant boob access. On top of being comfy and functional, they looked good layered under shirts and jackets. I still wear them if I'm going out on a date with Bear, so he gets easy access without showing the world my belly or getting drafty.

The best way to score a nice stash of these is by asking your mama friends or mamas in the neighborhood for their hand-me-downs. Otherwise, try to find an organic version.

NIPPLE PADS

Thanks to these little pads, I could ditch the sock. Try looking for a reusable version in earth-gentle materials like those from Bamboobies or Heavenly Hold. Or better yet, you can make your own personalized pairs by cutting up an old sweatshirt or cotton washcloth. You won't need them as much if you use the milk saver, but they do come in handy from time to time—especially when you're out in the world. Nipple leakage at a meeting or nice dinner isn't so cute.

What You Don't Need

HOOTER HIDER

I fully believe that breastfeeding is natural and beautiful and should be honored and celebrated instead of hidden away—especially under a big, crazy-patterned apron. That said, I understand there are times when breastfeeding in public calls for a little discretion. One trick is to wear a light cardigan on days when you'll be out, and you can simply pull it over your boob while you nurse. Or position your sling—more on these miracle contraptions in a bit!—so that your baby and boobie both have a little privacy. Throw one of your baby's light blankets in your bag for such an occasion.

BOTTLE WARMER

Instead of wasting money, electricity, and space on one of these gadgets, heat your baby's bottle the old-fashioned way by leaving it in a bowl of warm water until it's the perfect temperature. Or better yet, don't bother! If you're going to be using your milk within 10 hours of pumping, you can leave it at room temperature.[66] And you might even find that your baby doesn't care what temp his meal is so long as it's in his belly!

A NURSING APP

I have heard so many women raving about these handy apps that tell them when to feed and which breast to start with at their next nursing session. I think it's too easy to overrely on a little device that tells you how to connect with your baby. Instead, tune in to his hunger cues and pay attention to what his needs and rhythms are. When it comes time to figuring out which breast to start with, just give them both a little squeeze. You'll be able to feel which is more full! I'm pretty sure all of our ancestors figured out this nursing thing just fine without an iPhone.

INTRODUCING A BOTTLE

As smart as your baby is, he might get a little mixed up if you introduce other nipples besides your own too soon. Some studies have shown that introducing a bottle prematurely could negatively affect breastfeeding.[67] It might be because each nipple calls for a different kind of sucking, which can confuse your baby, or if a bottle replaces too many feedings, it could lead to a decrease in your milk production.

It is recommended that you wait at least 6 to 8 weeks before introducing a bottle. Make sure you're in a steady nursing rhythm, which means that at every nursing session, your baby can latch, get a full meal, and is gaining weight.[68]

Don't try pulling a boobie-bottle switch up on the actual first day of your absence. Allow your baby a couple of weeks to adjust to the change by giving him a bottle instead of the boob every now and then. It can be a meaningful way for dad to get in on the feeding action and to let baby know that everything's going to be okay even if the boobies sometimes can't be there.

Packing It Up to Go

When you do decide to introduce a bottle, you'll need to start storing milk, so pick one or two feedings a day when you can pump afterward. (Your supply is highest in the morning.[69])

If you're going to be using the milk within 8 days, store it in the fridge—freezing destroys some of milk's immune-strengthening properties.[70] That's why I suggest storing your milk in glass containers in the fridge, which Dr. Lawrence Rosen agrees is ideal (versus plastic storage containers or bags). You can even keep adding cooled, just-pumped milk to already-stored milk.

If you happen to make a lot of milk or need to build a bigger backup stash, freeze your milk in itty-bitty 1- or 2-ounce amounts. That way, you only have to defrost what you need, since defrosting, refreezing, then defrosting again can further obliterate the good stuff. And if you

The Formula of Formula

Manufacturing baby formula looks a little like this: First, companies start with either nonfat or whole milk from cows and then strip it of the fat that infants can have trouble digesting. Next, it's diluted with water to reduce the level of protein, pumped full of lactose—or milk sugar—plus some synthetic vitamins and minerals, and topped off with a blend of vegetable oils to stand in as a more digestible form of fat.[71] But remember all the icky stuff that dairy does to our bodies? All that inflammation-causing, hormone-introducing, mucus-making, allergy-promoting gnarliness? Add that to a yummy cocktail of synthetics and voila! Breakfast, lunch, and dinner.

Gerald Gaull, MD, a pediatrics professor at Mount Sinai School of Medicine in New York, said it best: "For us to think that in 40 years we can duplicate what has happened in 4 million years of human development is very arrogant."[72] Amen! Innately, there's no way that formula can be a biochemical match to our own milk. And because we're not built to digest other species' milk in the first place (as adults or babies), there are harmful effects—especially to infants. The proteins in formula have been shown to cause allergic reactions such as diarrhea, vomiting, abdominal pains, and skin rashes.[73] And that's not to mention all the diseases and chronic conditions that dairy is linked to down the road, like obesity, diabetes, cancer, joint pain, fatigue, depression, headaches, immune deficiencies, stroke, osteoporosis, blindness, kidney disease, multiple sclerosis, rheumatoid arthritis, and hyperthyroidism.[74] Plus, formula lacks 100 of the identified components that make breast milk so awesome.[75] Most notable is taurine, which may be involved in early brain development.[76]

find yourself with more milk than you know what to do with, donate it! There are a lot of mamas in need of your superior kind goods. Go to thekindlife.com and look up the Kind Mama Milk Share to connect with women in your area.

MILK EMERGENCY RX

There's going to come a time when the idea of a late-night pumping session so you have something for baby the next day while you're out is the last thing on earth you have energy for. In a perfect world, would you give your baby your beautiful breast milk for every single feeding? Absolutely. But is it the most calming peace of mind to know that every once in a while you have a little safety net? Sweet Jesus, yes. Enter made-with-love Grain Milk.

This golden little recipe (see page 321) is a rich, nourishing breast milk alternative that the macros swear by and babies love. I'm not recommending it as a substitute—though healers in this community don't discourage that if absolutely necessary—but keep this tucked away in your back pocket for a time when your baby is older than 4 months and you need a quick milk-sub fix. It's very kind, unlike formula, and can be adjusted in consistency and flavored with yummy things like rice syrup or toasted sesame seeds. You'll be able to read much more about this when you get to Chapter 17.

BREASTFEEDING CONCERNS AND CONUNDRUMS

Getting on Track after Medical Intervention

In the event that you have to be separated from your baby at birth because doctors are tending to one or both of you, then make certain that hospital personnel know your wishes to breastfeed as soon as possible. If you've had a C-section and required anesthesia, it's still safe to feed right away.[77] Your baby might be a little groggy—as will you!—but it's a good opportunity to get in a relaxed and pain-free feeding before your incision site begins to hurt. If it's going to be more than a couple hours, ask for a breast pump so you can start stimulating your milk ducts and save up precious colostrum. As soon as your baby is returned to you, ask that she room in—sleep in the room with you—so you can nurse as frequently as possible. If your midwife or doula isn't still with you, ask for a lactation consultant to help you figure out which nursing positions put the least amount of pressure on your incisions.

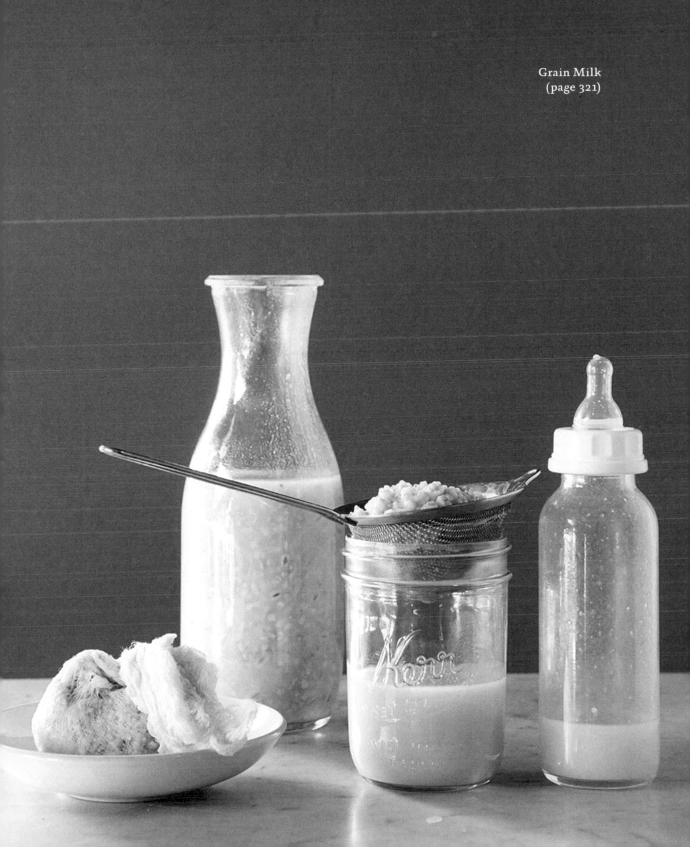

Grain Milk
(page 321)

Talk to your doctor about how to best manage your pain while you recover. It's not ideal to be on unnecessary medications while you're nursing, but it's more important that you can manage any discomfort so you can still breastfeed. There are several safe options that your health care provider should be able to offer.

Ouch, That's My Boob! Doing Damage Control

Although breastfeeding is not supposed to hurt in the long run, for some, having a small person attached to your chest might take some getting used to. It's normal to feel a bit of tenderness or even occasional pain in the early weeks while your nipples are more sensitive and adjusting to the sensation, but if baby is doing things right, the discomfort, if any, should ease over the first month. If there's no excruciating pain, cracking, or bleeding—which are signs you should call your lactation consultant (more on that in the next section)—then your sore nipples are normal. Below are some ways you can pamper your mama parts.

- Skip the soap when you're washing your breasts. It can dry out your nipples and cause soreness. And according to Dr. Mehmet Oz, babies prefer to nurse on a mother's unwashed breast.[78] So stick to just rinsing with water.

- Moisturize your nipples with a little olive oil or, my favorite, the very yummy chocolate-scented shea butter nipple cream from Earth Mama Angel Baby. Whatever you do, skip the lanolin, which is very unkind.

- Express a little milk after you feed and dab it on your nipples—it's nature's magic balm!

- After nursing, let your nipples get some fresh air. A little sunshine and a breeze are the best healers in the world.

What about All the Yucky Things My Friends Say Will Happen?

I'm sure by now you've heard the horror stories: "My nipples were bloody!" "My boobs were on fire!" It's really bad news that so many mamas have such dreadful breastfeeding experiences while there are yahoos like me saying it all should be fluffy clouds and butterflies. But guess what? It can be! Sure, it might take a little getting used to, and there may be small bumps in the road, but that's all the discomfort you should experience. With a little know-how—and maybe a visit from or a call to a lactation guru like your midwife, doula, or IBCLC or a trip to your local La Leche League meeting—you can sidestep these all-too-common maladies.

Boobies, Babies, and Booze

According to the National Institutes of Health, less than 2 percent of alcohol reaches the mother's blood or milk. It also peaks in the milk and bloodstream about 30 to 60 minutes after consumption. Most experts agree with current research that finds that any alcohol transferred from a drink or two will not harm a baby.[79] La Leche League's *The Womanly Art of Breastfeeding* backs this up by saying that when a breastfeeding mother drinks occasionally, or has a drink a day, that amount of alcohol hasn't been proven harmful.[80] So no need to worry that your boobies have become little beer taps!

That all said, I feel the same consideration should apply to drinking while nursing as it did to drinking while pregnant (page 72). It might be deemed "okay" by the medical community—and I completely value that having the occasional glass is how some women unwind and feel a little better about life—but it's still putting something in our bodies that isn't completely supporting how we nourish ourselves or our little ones. And when you consider that a newborn's liver is still developing,[81] it makes that somewhat unnecessary indulgence seem a little less appealing. But I am, after all, human, and a glass of wine would sometimes sound so deliciously decadent. If I wanted to have one well-deserved libation, I'd have it right after I fed Bear so that it was out of my system by the time he needed to eat again. I also tried whenever possible to opt for sake and high-quality beer, which contain minimal sugar and were less likely to make Bear fussy.

CRACKED AND BLEEDING NIPPLES

If your baby latches correctly, your nipples should not crack or bleed. So if they start to look even remotely irritated, mention it immediately to your lactation support person. Most likely, you can make little tweaks now before things turn sour. According to Beverly Solow, most nipple damage happens at night when mama's too tired to correct her baby. If your nipples do crack, she recommends applying a warm saltwater compress. Dissolve about ½ teaspoon of salt in ½ cup of hot water, soak it up with a cloth, then leave it on your tender bits until it cools.

ENGORGEMENT

Solow advises that the best prevention is to not skip feedings and to drain the breast well at each nursing session. If you still get engorged, continue to regularly breastfeed or pump to bring things back down. She says if you're not freely leaking milk, then apply a cold compress to the breasts; if you are leaking, apply a warm one. The best remedy is getting the milk out.

Another reason for engorgement, according to healing experts, is that your diet may be too rich. Make sure that you're not having too much oil, salt, flour products, and baked foods and that you're eating enough veggies. Go super-simple for a few days to bring things back into balance—take in lots of grains and beans and leafy greens, and definitely revisit the magical daikon, which can help flush out your system.

PLUGGED DUCTS

Sometimes, when the breast doesn't get drained well or your nursing routine is thrown off because of a hectic day or your baby is sick, your milk ducts can get stopped up. This usually appears as a hard lump or wedge-shaped area of engorgement that may feel tender, hot, or swollen or look reddened.[82] Continue nursing and/or pumping to keep the milk flowing in addition to applying warm and cold compresses and massaging your poor boobies from the top of the breast down along the blocked duct to the nipple (especially while nursing, which can coax the plug out). If for some reason that doesn't clear things up and a lump of backed-up milk forms, or you develop chills and a fever, then you need to talk to a doctor or midwife.[83]

MASTITIS

This is an inflammation of the breast often caused by obstruction, infection, and/or an allergy. Symptoms are the same as for a plugged duct, but the pain/heat/swelling/redness is usually more intense and typically includes a fever, chills, or flulike achiness. Not draining your breast well is the most common culprit.[84] According to Solow, the first treatment is frequent breastfeeding and pumping. And macrobiotic expert Warren Kramer suggests avoiding sweets, flour, and oil to help your body fight off infection. But you should absolutely call your midwife or lactation consultant if you experience these systems, especially a fever.

Is It a Bad Idea to Nurse If I'm Sick?

Nope—the opposite! Your milk will be chock-full of antibodies as a result of fighting off the illness, which are the best protection for your baby against that same bug. Wash your hands frequently and, hard as it might be, try not to cough on your baby, but keep up the nursing.[85]

What If Baby's Sick?

When your baby's sick, breast milk is the best thing you could possibly give him.

What If My Doctor Says My Baby Is Too Fat or Too Skinny?

It's important to know that your doctor's size chart is not the final word on the health of your baby—it's just the culmination of a lot of data. So your little one, who is unique and special in every way, is being compared to an *average*. And that includes babies who are fed formula.

Remember that so long as your baby is eating frequently and effectively, seems satisfied with the food she's getting, is gaining weight, isn't abnormally fussy, is peeing and pooping plenty, and doesn't seem weak or sick to your eye, there's no real reason to worry. Find a doctor who won't get all judgy about your veggie-grown baby being a little on the lean side. According to the Physicians Committee for Responsible Medicine, breastfed babies tend to grow more slowly than bottle-fed babies. And less rapid growth during the early years is thought to decrease the risk of disease later in life.[86] Or maybe baby's a little on the chunky side—then know that babies fed on demand cannot be obese, and they have a higher chance of having a healthy body weight as they grow into adults.[87] Seriously! According to Dr. Rosen, it's a total myth that giving babies all the breast milk they want can lead to a weight issue.

How Long Should I Breastfeed?

The American Academy of Pediatrics recommends that babies nurse exclusively—no solids, formula, or water—for at least 6 months.[88] The academy also asserts that continuing to breastfeed, in addition to introducing solid foods, until 12 months can be super-beneficial[89] because our milk becomes even more concentrated with disease-fighting antibodies the older our child gets.[90] Then there are WHO and UNICEF, who recommend that we breastfeed for at least *2 years*.[91] Additionally, there are researchers who suggest that to get all the amazing benefits of breast milk and breastfeeding—nutrition, security, health—our little ones are designed to breastfeed for a minimum of 2½ years![92]

Our boobies are so much more than breakfast, lunch, and dinner. They're also comfort and closeness and security and love. So deciding when to stop placing them on the menu isn't something any book or timeline or pediatrician or other parent can dictate. There's no one magical answer, no one-size-fits-all solution, no breastfeeding law. But what all these really smart people are saying—and what women in most cultures around the world are already doing—is that we should breastfeed as long as our children still want to do it.[93] It's called "natural weaning" or "child-led" weaning, and it's a personal decision that you and your baby should make together.

When we let our babies (and by "babies," I mean toddlers, little people, children, etc.) tell us when they're ready to move beyond the boob, they reap more miraculous benefits than breastfeeding alone. Despite what so many mamas are being told by scaredy-cat naysayers, breastfeeding for longer doesn't lead to needy, whiny, wimpy kids. Just the opposite! Research has shown that kids who are part of a weaning team—and not kicked off the boob too early—are more independent and more confident and easier to reason with.[94] All the time you spend breastfeeding, even after your little one is eating solids like a champ, is so gooey and delicious and heavenly for both you and them. So why put an end to that just because someone else says you should?

Here's what Dr. Rosen has to say on the matter:

> In my experience, 99 percent of the time there's a tacit agreement between mother and child about when to wean. It's about accepting the fact that you're going to look to your baby for cues, and if you're at peace and they're at peace and everybody's happy, then it's all fine. As to when that is, most women who are breastfeeding, they'll know when it's time. And their babies will know. It could be at a year or 2 years or 3 years; it'll vary. If you're getting pressure from other people, you need to ignore that. Trust your intuition and what feels right to you. That will guide you the vast majority of the time.

Try to relish this all-too-brief time we have to care for our babies in such a deep, meaningful way. So many moms have come over to me while I'm nursing and said, "Oh, I miss when mine was that size" or "I wish I had breastfed for longer because I miss it so much." But there's no rush to stop! And you can fine-tune it along the way.

My plan was to figure it out as I went along. I expected that one day Bear would say, "You know what, Mommy? I want some *amasake* instead." And that would be that, because I trust him. He has this divine knowledge about his needs. Or maybe—even though I can't imagine it right now—I'll be the one to kick him off the boob. The lactation consultant at my pediatrician's

(continued on page 218)

What's the Deal with Colic?

We've all heard about those poor inconsolable babies screaming nonstop, driving even the most well-intentioned parents to a dark, frustrated, and completely exhausted place. The cause, most often, is colic, or a digestion condition that causes babies to cry more than 3 hours a day more than 3 days a week. Don't worry—it's not some mean spell sent from the heavens to make life difficult. There's a solution. It starts with what we mamas eat.

If you notice your baby is fussiest between 6:00 and 10:00 p.m.—when colic usually makes its presence known—and occasionally pulls up or stiffens her legs in an attempt to let out the gas that's causing sharp pains in her intestines, then she might have colic. In most cases, it's caused by baby's digestion difficulties. Luckily, because you're the gatekeeper of all that is good and milky, you have a lot of control over what might be irritating baby's little belly.

First, make sure you're avoiding nasty foods, especially dairy, which is one of the most common causes of colic.[95] Then there's caffeine and sugar—which, while not directly connected to colic, will do nothing to soothe your baby to sleep. Think about how cranky you are after your buzz wears off! On the kinder end of the spectrum, there are some foods that can contribute to colic. First, make sure you're avoiding the gassy-making foods listed in "Making Kind Milk" (page 198). And if you're already a clean, mean, nursing machine, then look to other, more subtle changes like chewing better, eating more slowly, not eating while standing up, and cutting back on natural sources of sugar like fruit along with carbonated beverages and oily or flour-based foods.[96] You'll notice in about 2 weeks whether these changes are helping.

As for short-term "what will make this poor baby stop crying?!" remedies, midwife Margo Kennedy put it this way: If something doesn't work, move on to the next trick. Start with the boob to see if it will offer some comfort. If he won't take it, try the sling or a soothing bath to calm him. Offer a few drops of Sweet Calming Kuzu tea (recipe on page 297), which, according to Christina Pirello, can help alkalize baby's intestines and moderate digestive stress. Or try chamomile tea; according to Dr. Rosen, it contains natural chemicals that relax a baby's intestinal tract and nervous system.[97] One ounce of very strong tea (let it brew for 5 minutes and then cool to room temperature) three times a day will sometimes do the trick. Gentle touch is also worth a shot for colicky babies. According to Kennedy, craniosacral therapy has been known to work wonders, and my friend Laura recommends gently rubbing baby's belly in a clockwise motion to see if you can coax out any gas from there.

Do Pacifiers Suck?

Pacifiers offer comfort, but if you're just shoving one in your kid's mouth every time he cries, then you're overlooking an important interaction between the two of you (especially if the pacifier is taking the place of nursing sessions!). Instead, Solow recommends you consider what else may be bothering him—"Are you hungry, little guy? Cold? Just want to gaze into my eyes?" And if nothing seems to be working, then she agrees that it's fine to try introducing a pacifier. For us, my boobs were the main event, then whenever possible, we'd use our fingers for Bear to suck on. But there were times when a pacifier came in handy, like during car or plane rides. The best option out there is the all-natural rubber ones made by Natursutten. Just keep in mind that rubber versions tend to wear out more quickly because they're not being held together by toxic polymers, so skip the dishwasher.

PACIFIER FUN FACT

When a pacifier falls on the floor, you gotta do what you gotta do. As any parent can probably tell you, there's a good number of times when that means popping that thing into your own mouth to clean it off. But before you call social services, consider this: A recent study published in the journal *Pediatrics* reported that infants whose parents sucked on their pacifiers to clean them developed fewer allergies than children whose parents rinsed and boiled them. They also had lower rates of eczema and fewer signs of asthma. Researchers chalk this up to "immune stimulation" through exposure to new microbes.[98]

office, who advocates letting babies nurse whenever they need to for as long as they want, said she was once watching a sheep with her lamb. The lamb went to nurse and the mama kicked her away, as if to say, "That's enough." And that, too, is a completely natural decision. Ultimately, the one that makes everyone happy is best.

Bear is 2½ years old and he still loves breastfeeding. But he also loves his food so much and seeing the world so much and he has big ideas and places to go, so sometimes he just forgets to nurse. He still wants his boobies first thing in the morning, before and after naps, when we take a bath together, or when he's getting sleepy. And as of late maybe I don't always love having such a boob-crazed little animal who's groping me all day, but every time we share these moments, I'm blown away all over again about just how exquisite it is. I could eat him up! And then suddenly, he'll hop off and go about his business.

You and your baby will find your rhythm—whether it's his showing readiness or you asserting yours— and take those steps together. But in the meantime, treasure the journey while it lasts!

IF BREASTFEEDING IS NOT AN OPTION

Sometimes, no matter how strong your resolve, breastfeeding is not a possibility. Maybe you've had breast surgery or maybe you're a beautiful soul who's chosen to adopt instead (in which case, major karma props to you!). Either way, know that you have options and that your baby will not lack from love or health or happiness. Let me say that again: Your baby will feel cared for and nourished even if you can't breastfeed. Is breastfeeding an optimal choice? Of course. But are there also amazing benefits to being a calm mama who is at peace with the world and present for her baby? Without a doubt. As weird as it sounds, there is more than one way to breastfeed. Let's think of it in terms other than just milk and boobs. Breastfeeding is an act of bonding, too. So regardless of how you ultimately have to feed your child, know that it is absolutely in your power to give that baby everything nature intended. It may just look different from the next mama. And as for those thoughts of "What does it mean if I can't do the one thing I was supposed to as a mom?" To that I say: You grew this baby! You made the cleanest, most immaculate house for him to live in for 9 months, then brought him into this world with the ultimate strength and intention. Or if you adopted, you made it your mission to give your gifts to a child who needed them most. And with conviction and grace and love, you will help him navigate his way. *That* is being a mom. As for what your baby eats, here are some options to consider:

Find a Macrobiotic Counselor

These experts are specifically knowledgeable in how to use food for healing. Either they can work with you to see if it's your diet that's preventing you from breastfeeding successfully, or they can help you create a breast milk alternative that's going to give baby everything she needs.

Seek Out Donor Milk

This formula alternative—one backed by Dr. Rosen and many other doctors, midwives, lactation consultants, and mamas in the know—is an amazing way to get your baby some of earth's finest food. You can go through a milk bank, but those goods are oftentimes expensive and

Mama to Mama on . . . Their Nursing Journey

My son, Kai, nursed until he was 1 month shy of his third birthday. He was the kind of kid who loved nursing; it was how he self-soothed and how he fell asleep. I didn't want to just take that away from him. However, much to our surprise, he was very involved in his weaning process. I was 5 months pregnant at the time, and as I got further into my pregnancy, every nursing experience was painful for me. My son is very intuitive, and I believe he could sense my pain. His nursing sessions got shorter and less frequent. Sometimes, he would even go a day or two without nursing, or he would have a few suckles and be done. I can't even pinpoint his last breastfeeding because of how easy the transition was. It was bittersweet—on the one hand, I was relieved to be rid of the pain, but on the other hand, I was sad to say good-bye to my firstborn's babyhood. But my son immediately found a new way to soothe himself—elbow rubbing! He literally started doing this within days of weaning, both to my husband and me. When he's sleepy, sad, or hurt, he calms himself by rubbing our elbows. It's so sweet and touching. I love that, even without nursing, he has found his own way to remain physically connected to me.

    —Rachel Chiartas, Cranston, Rhode Island

I nursed until my boy was almost 2. I had been wondering when it would happen, why it would happen, and would I know? Would he know? But it became clear that we were feeding less and that we both were ready to begin to separate. He was looking for other ways to connect with me and wasn't asking for the boob as much, so I followed his cues. I wanted this process to be largely driven by his wants and needs. I started dropping feeds and noticed that he didn't ask for them again. It was shocking. I was dreading giving up the night feed, but he never even missed it. I was sad and cuddled him with his favorite lovey and was cautious not to show him too much of that sadness. He needed the space to be okay and to move on—and so did I. I was relieved and happy and anxious all at the same time, but eventually I was thrilled. He was growing so nicely and we got to nurse together for nearly 2 years. The best thing I ever did was nurse my boy.

    —Lora Appleton, New York City

Both of my sons weaned themselves just after turning 4 years old. One time, 8 months pregnant with my second, I said to my first, "There's not much milk, is there?" He unlatched for a moment and said, "No, but I don't mind." It dawned on me that more than nutrition was happening when we nurse. Sometimes, being pregnant and sore, I would ask my son to wait and be still for 1 minute before nursing. And he would often fall asleep before the minute was up. That began our weaning process. I was the only sad one when the nursing was done for good.

    —Nina Vought, Salt Lake City

reserved for babies who are ill, and you have no way of knowing anything about the mama who donated it. The milk is screened, but they're not asking questions like whether the donor eats a lot of meat or dairy or processed food. That's why I posted the Kind Mama Milk Share on my Web site. It's a place for like-minded women to connect and share this most precious resource. I also recommend reaching out to mom groups in your neighborhood, asking your lactation consultant and midwife to tap into their networks, putting the word out among friends and relatives, or checking out other mom-to-mom milk-share sites like Eats on Feets (eatsonfeets.org) and Human Milk 4 Human Babies (hm4hb.net). Your midwife can help you figure out what questions to ask a potential donor (you want to rule out certain illnesses and medications), but women enlightened enough to share their milk are oftentimes so proud of their hard-earned goods that they'll brag about just how pristine it is!

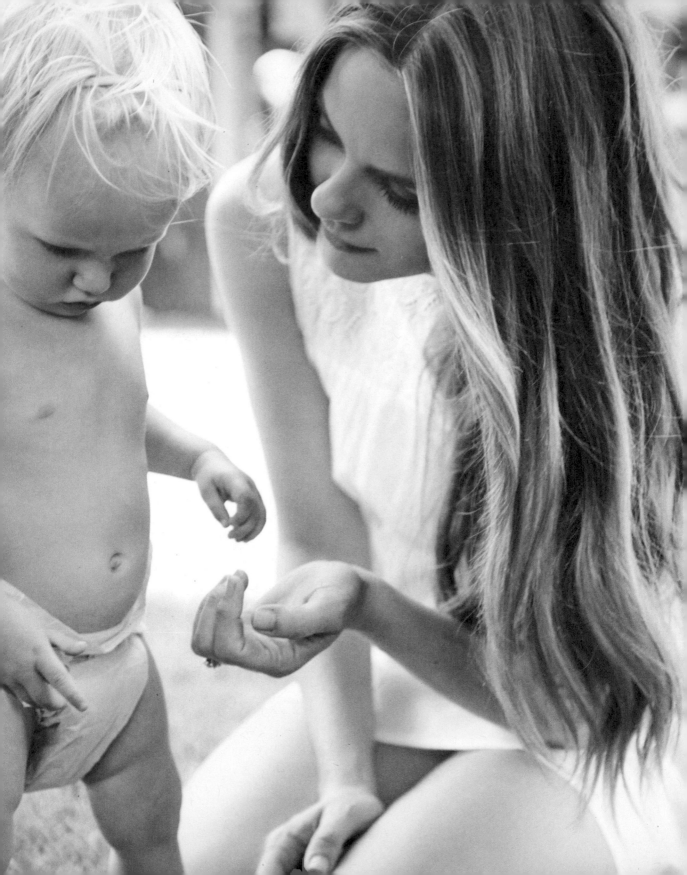

13

Mastering Doodie Duty:
The Diaper Solution

We've talked about input (breastfeeding), so now let's talk about your baby's output. We all know that babies are little pee and poop machines. But the amazing secret I learned is that your baby's need to go is just one more opportunity for us moms and dads to tune in. It's just as essential as being carried, held, and nursed. And better yet—when you do start paying close attention to this need, the less stuff you have to buy, the less waste you make, the fewer messes you have, and the more you get to know your little one. But before I introduce you to the kindest path, let's first take a look at the alternative.

THE POOP ON DISPOSABLE DIAPERS

When it comes to these landfill-clogging, nasty chemical-laden butt bags, it's all about business. Disposable diapering is a multibillion-dollar industry, and it's one that's fueled by corporate-backed pseudoscience. Since 1962, companies like Pampers have enlisted pediatricians to tell mothers that their children are not "toilet ready" until they're verbal.[99] That means more diapers for baby and more dollars for them. And it's worked! More than 90 percent of American baby bottoms are covered in disposable diapers. They're even made for 4-year-olds! But while that's great news for companies like Procter & Gamble, it's bad news for your baby and for our planet.

Although ingredients vary by brand, most disposable diapers include a variety of plastics and elastic materials, wood pulp, and a freaky-sounding substance called superabsorbent polymer, or SAP, which can ooze out of diapers and crystallize on baby's bum if he's left in his own pee for too long.[100] These materials certainly aren't biodegradable, so when you do the diaper arithmetic that a baby averages eight diapers a day in her first year, and so uses between 3,000 and 7,000 before she's "potty trained," that means that about 3.7 million tons of waste every year is sitting in landfills and isn't going anywhere.[101] What those diapers are doing, however, is leaching all kinds of junk into the land, air, and waterways. Typical diapers are bleached with chlorine, dioxins—persistent chemicals—that seep into the surrounding environment. And the poop from all those dirty nappies soaking into the earth is a real concern for human health.[102] As if that's not enough harm to the planet, consider that disposables require up to 3.5 billion gallons of petroleum—a nonrenewable resource—a year to manufacture[103] and that we cut down 250,000 trees each year to provide all that wood pulp.[104]

Plus, all the junk that goes into these diapers—and I'm not talking about poop—is potentially dangerous for your baby. While there are few studies on how chemicals in diapers might affect a baby's health,[105] here's what we do know: Disposables emit gases like toluene, xylene, and styrene—all of which have been identified by the CDC as VOCs, or volatile organic compounds[106]—and your baby is inhaling them. Because babies inhale more air per pound of body weight than adults do and are typically more affected by the toxicity of air pollutants, that's pretty nasty.[107] Some disposable diaper manufacturers also add synthetic fragrance to mask odors, dyes to add decoration, and lotions to allegedly prevent diaper rash. But these additions aren't as helpful as they sound and may actually be harmful. In fact, researchers from the University of Massachusetts Medical School found that up to 20 percent of diaper rash cases could be caused by exposure to the petroleum-based dyes used in diapers.[108] Also consider that for boys, disposables may even impact sperm development because of all the heat they trap.[109]

We'll talk about a kinder way to use disposables if absolutely necessary, but let's first explore some even kinder alternatives.

WHAT ABOUT CLOTH?

The cloth diaper has come a long way from the days of giant safety pins. There's a huge range of styles now, and each is, in its own way, easy to clean, affordable, and, most important, effective. Plus, cloth is hands-down less expensive than disposable, and these diapers generate 100 percent less landfill waste, carry no risk of toxic off-gassing that can irritate baby's lungs and skin, and cause far less diaper rash.[110] Embrace your inner earth mama and hang a clothesline and run washer loads on cold to save energy. (FYI—90 percent of the energy used to wash clothes is spent heating the water, so switching from hot to warm can cut your energy

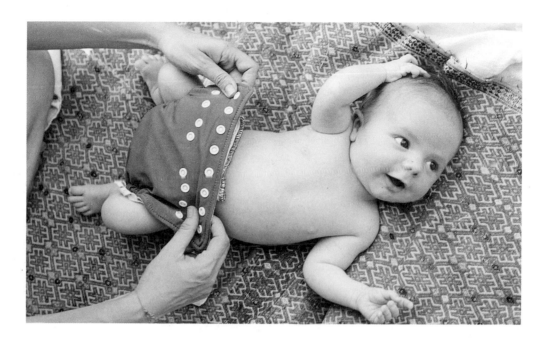

expenditure by *half*![111]) As my mother-in-law (who's a clean freak, in the best possible way) taught me, "Heat shmeat"—there's no need for hot water for clothes. All those loads of dirty diapers do use energy and water, but they're still far better than their disposable counterparts.[112]

HYBRID DIAPERS

These have a reusable cover like a cloth diaper and disposable inserts that can be biodegradable. They're often touted as the best of both worlds, but here's the catch: Most of today's landfills lack the sunlight, air, and moisture for items to actually biodegrade. Are you producing less waste if you go this route? Yes. Is it better than nothing? Yes. But the best possible scenario is not throwing anything away. A slightly better option is choosing a hybrid that's flushable, like gDiapers, which have inserts made out of chlorine-free, tree-farmed wood pulp. They meet the Water Environment Research Foundation's criteria for bowl and trap clearance and have also received the Cradle to Cradle certification. But I still think there's an even *better* way to diaper.

What is this magical arrangement that means spending less, using less, and feeling much, much more of a connection with our babies? It's what I like to call potty whispering.

Alicia loved changing Bear. It would take her like half an hour every time. She would talk to him and dance—they would have this whole little love affair.

—Christopher

BECOMING A POTTY WHISPERER: ELIMINATION COMMUNICATION

Infants aren't born with the instinct to eliminate in their diapers—we teach them that! In nature, they'd be much more content leaving their business in the grass than having to sleep and eat accompanied by their own pee and poo. But because of convenience parenting and the multibillion-dollar disposable diaper industry fueling it, we've convinced ourselves that the good and natural thing to do is to train our babies to embrace their shrink-wrapped tushes, and then *retrain* them to go in a toilet 2 or more years later.

The only problem is, it's not what baby instinctively wants to do. Babies are born with an innate sense of their body rhythms. They know exactly when they'll have to go to the bathroom, and within just days of birth, they're equipped to let you know, too. But infants who are left in their diapers all day get out of tune with their bodies. When you don't acknowledge their cues that they have to go to the bathroom, they *learn* to go without communicating their needs. And because they get used to walking around in a toilet, by the time you want to take that diaper away, it can be pretty difficult for a small child to relearn how to pay attention to this need and do something about it.

By tuning in to your baby's elimination needs, however, you're not only mastering potty training by the time your baby is as young as 9 months old, but you're also reinforcing that you're there for baby's every natural need, creating more opportunities to be loving, stay completely present, and save our planet from landfills full of poopy diapers. You're telling your baby that she's seen and heard, which leads to emotional security, a sense of inner "rightness," self-reliance, and joy.[113] Plus, there's nothing better than being able to squeeze that little naked baby butt all the time—I mean, come on!

Elimination Communication? Say What?

I swear this isn't half as kooky as this sounds, so step away from the Pampers! Even my husband was like, *What is this hippie up to now?!* But after he saw me and Bear do it together, he was a believer. And I promise you'll be a believer, too.

First of all, elimination communication, or EC, has been practiced by families all over the globe since the beginning of time. In traditional cultures, this tuning-in is the norm. Take China, for instance. Women wear their babies, and when they feel their babies' legs clench, they take them off and pee them. Or in India, women hop off the bus to pee their babies. When you tune in, you'll see that from the moment your baby wakes up in the morning, he is sending you cues about his need to pee and poop. His whole body could tighten up or he might start getting restless or he'll stare into space or he'll give you flirty eyes or make a little puckered face or maybe something else entirely. Luckily, it's not all guesswork. Most of baby's potty needs coincide with specific moments in the day, like waking up, after nursing, or getting up from a nap. (If you've housebroken a doggie, you know exactly what I'm talking about!) You'll start to notice patterns in your baby's cues. And when *that* happens, you're already a potty whisperer in training.

All you have to do is practice. When you think baby has to go, take him to the potty/bucket/ bowl/shrubs and let the call of nature take its course. At first, you might barely notice his cues, but once you get the hang of the timing and use your mama instincts, you'll get the hang of it. I would take Bear to the potty every 20 to 30 minutes and make our cue sound—we used *pssss* for pee and grunting or *caca* for poo. If he truly wanted nothing to do with it, it meant he didn't need to go. Giving baby some time without a diaper, is an even *more* delicious practice. Babies with fresh air–kissed bottoms get way less diaper rash (as in none, usually), and they also get all kinds of scrumptious naked time.

With elimination communication, you'll have many fewer soiled diapers, which means less to wash or throw away, less of an expense, and definitely less of a mess. (Seriously—have you seen a baby's bottom after rolling around in his own poo?!) And it's also crazy fun! I can't tell you how satisfying it is that my kid goes poo on the toilet and has been doing it since 6 months. When we were just starting out, I began to notice that when Bear looked like he was flirting with me, smiling sweetly, or looking deep into my eyes, he'd be peeing. Or he'd stare off into space for a second and then pee would come. (These are common cues, actually.) I'd take him to the potty, and if he went, we had a little celebration. He made the cue, I saw the cue, and then we did it! One time, we had all just gotten in the car, and Bear reached for his little toilet. I put him on it, and he went. How cool is that? He was 10 months old! The way Bear smiled at us when he was done—like he was having a ball communicating with this newfound secret language that we shared with one another—it made us all feel so proud and empowered.

The Potty Whispering Basics

There are all kinds of ways you can incorporate EC so that it realistically fits into your life. Take inspiration from mamas in India and South Africa, who start with just the first cue of the morning. After a few weeks, they'll add in other times of the day. Our method is a mash-up that we've adjusted as Bear's gotten older and his needs have changed. Now he's diaper free by day, but we use cloth diapers for naps and nighttime. If we're away for a few days and not wanting to do laundry, he'll get an eco disposable. When he was little, I would take his diaper off when I was feeding him to let him get a little fresh air and also tune in to when he'd need to pee or poop. Or he'd wear pants and no diaper. Because when I was with him—most of the time—he had my undivided attention. And the more time he spent without a diaper, the more he could tune in to his need to go and the stronger his cues were to me. I'm thrilled because we used so few diapers, and I never had to "train" him to go to the bathroom. And it's never something else to do—it's just always been another part of the time that I spend with Bear that makes it more fun and special. Of course, there were accidents—like when I'd sometimes forget to put him on the pot and we'd have a little pee slip—but it wasn't a big deal. What outweighs it by far is how fun it is to have a diaperless kid and to see that cute butt running around.

Since these are just the basics, I highly recommend a great book called *Diaper Free: The Gentle Wisdom of Natural Infant Hygiene* by Ingrid Bauer, a guide about what's possible when you get in sync with your baby's potty needs. Even though I didn't discover the EC technique until Bear was 6 months old, you can totally start from day 1. It's my plan for baby number two!

The Whisperer's Arsenal: This Is All You Need!

CHOOSE A DIAPER

For those times when you need a little insurance:

Cloth diapers: Some cloth diaper covers have snaps, some have Velcro, some have cloth inserts that make it an all-in-one system, and so goes the list. Try a few styles until you find something that works for you. We liked the kind that snap and grow with the baby. These covers are mostly made out of polyurethane laminate, or PUL, which, while a type of plastic, is kinder than its other synthetic compatriots and definitely kinder than wool.

If you're concerned about how much laundry you'll have to do with cloth diapers, look into local services that will pick up your dirty diapers and deliver clean ones each week. It's usually not that expensive, and services are still cheaper than buying disposables. Check out super-informative sites like jilliansdrawers.com and kellyscloset.com.

Hybrid diapers: These certainly produce less trash than disposables, but be mindful of what's still ending up in the waste stream. Companies like gDiapers and GroVia make versions that you can flush and/or compost.

Disposable diapers: The good news is that you can find versions that are chlorine and fragrance free, but the bad news is that they'll still end up in a landfill. Brands to consider are Nature Babycare (which contains no oil-based plastics, and the wood pulp core comes from sustainable forests), Seventh Generation (which uses less SAP than the standard national brand diapers), or Earth's Best and Honest Baby Company.

EVERYTHING ELSE

Wipes: Choose cloth wipes (organic cotton, hemp, or flannel) or repurposed T-shirts. For easy tush wipe-downs, you can keep a spritz bottle filled with water by the toilet, and after 3 months, you can add in a few drops of essential oils like lavender and chamomile. If you're tempted to think disposable wipes might be the way to go, consider this: If every mama in the United States used one fewer wipe today, we'd keep more than four million of them out of landfills![114]

If you decide to use disposable wipes when traveling or on the go, make sure you steer clear of the conventional kind that are frequently soaked with a not-bum-friendly blend of alcohol, fragrances, and other skin irritants.[115] Look for brands that are unbleached and free of dyes and chemicals. Honest Company, Earth's Best, and Seventh Generation all make nice versions.

Changing pads: Since I hadn't yet become the champion potty whisperer that I am today when Bear was first born, there was a lot of pee in my life. Everywhere. If you're not practicing EC, there's going to be some wet and wild times. Which means that you could go through a rotation of three or four changing pads in a day. I highly recommend avoiding the more expensive variety in favor of old cloths or towels, which you can throw in the wash. Or go with the Keekaroo Peanut Diaper Changer, which is latex, PVC, BPA, phthalate, and formaldehyde free; doesn't require a cover; comes in super-fun colors; and just wipes clean.

Bottom creams and powders: Even though cloth diapers cause far less diaper rash than disposable, sometimes baby's bottom needs a little TLC. Breast milk works like a charm for diaper rash, as can a dab of olive oil, balms made by miniOrganics and Earth Mama Angel Baby. (For more of my favorites, check out thekindlife.com.) All these remedies are much gentler alternatives to talc or talcum powder, which have traditionally been used to keep small bums dry but can irritate baby's lungs.[116]

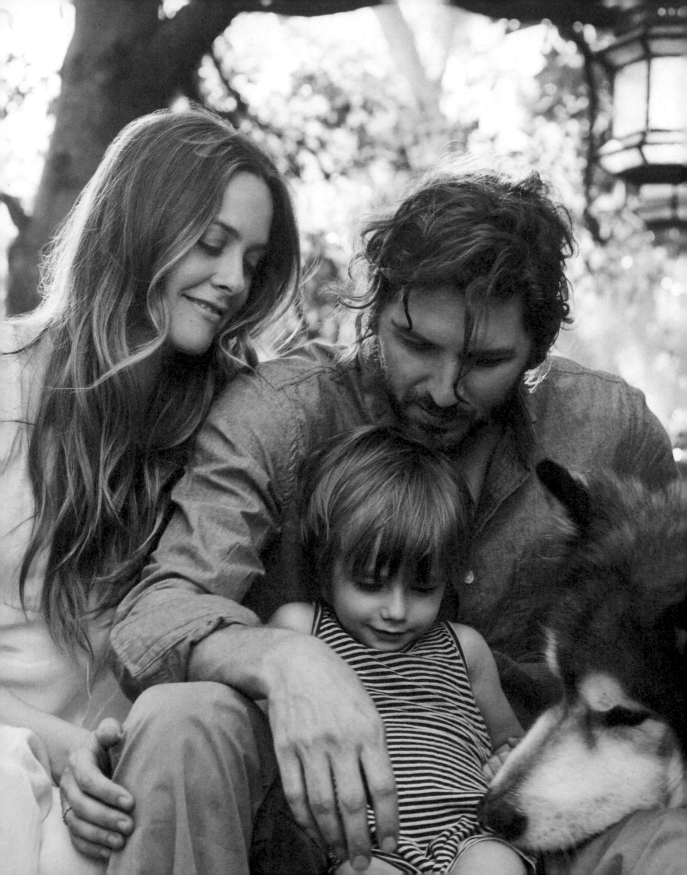

PART IV:

raising
baby

The First 6 Months and Beyond

14

Kind Parenting:
The Healthy,
Happy Baby Plan

May 8—You're puckering your lips as if you are thinking;
I can't stop kissing them.

May 11—You love sucking daddy's fingers.

May 14—You sleep between us at night, so sweet.

May 16—Dad says he can see your features
more—you're turning into a little man.

—My Journal, Postpartum

I know everyone says that babies don't come with an instruction manual. But what if I told you they kind of do? The truth is, there's a formula to raising happy babies: When a baby's needs are met, they're content—not only because they're warm, dry, and fed, but also because they trust they're being valued and heard. And a baby who feels right, acts right. Everyone tells us we have the happiest baby. They're right—Bear is a completely edible ball of sweetness. Sure, it could be his unique God-given spirit, but I don't think it's simply a lucky draw that my baby is so alert and present.

Kind parenting is all about tapping in and asking, "What does my baby need at this moment?" It's using every comforting resource Mother Nature gave to us—our boobies, our skin, our touch, and our instincts—to create a haven where baby can grow confident and secure because he knows his needs really matter. It's the physical and emotional ease that a baby gets from being held, cuddled, caressed, cooed to, breastfed on cue, comforted when fussy, and not left alone to calm himself. It's the ultimate in building trust and in turn molding a blissful, smart, healthy, child.

Think about how babies used to be raised. They'd be swaddled into a little papoose on mama's back or burrowed into carriers under mama's clothing and taken into the fields or the woods or the tundra to do the day's work. They could nestle into their mother's warmth and sleep, or they could watch the world go by in all its wonder and color. The gentle rocking and closeness to mama soothed them, and if they grew hungry, the boobie was right around the corner. And because mama spent all day with her baby from the moment the little one was born, she knew exactly what baby's needs would be. Why did women do it that way? Was it because they all read some kind of sacred scripture on child rearing? Or because Oprah said it was better? Of course not! It was completely out of necessity: Babies needed their mamas!

The beautiful thing that happened is that babies were woven into the fabric of everyday life. These women didn't worry that their tiny, defenseless babies were taking advantage of them or were going to need years of therapy because they weren't "given enough space." These mamas were guided by their natural intuition and what they saw everyone else doing. And it just made good sense—innately, babies could be comforted, rocked to sleep, nursed, and educated about the world simply by tagging along. And did all those kids grow up to be whiny, spoiled, needy brats? No way! The exact opposite: They grew up understanding where their place in the tribe was and how to be a part of a larger working community.

In our culture, everyone is in a race to figure out how to have their kids not need them. They get passed from the nurses at the hospital to a baby nurse to replace mommy's attention, fed from a can to replace mommy's milk, and left with vibrating electronics that are supposed to replace mommy's comforting hold. Somehow, parenting became an inconvenience. The problem with being the convenient parent, though—aside from possibly stunting your baby's development (which we'll get to in a bit)—is that you're missing out on so much joy! Sure, you're maybe sleeping more or able to go out with your girlfriends more often, but how much satisfaction are you getting from that? Think about why you had a baby in the first place. Didn't you want a deeper, more special relationship in this world? Aren't we all just looking for more love? Everything our babies do is for such a short time—nursing, crawling, cooing—why miss that because you're too busy worrying about how to make your child more independent? Guess what—no matter what you do, independence is going to happen. So why not spend this precious time savoring every moment you can be there for your baby in the most significant way possible?

This is how women have been successfully raising their babies pretty much since the beginning of time. It's written about beautifully in the book *The Continuum Concept,* by Jean Liedloff, and it's also completely backed by research:

Kind Parenting Makes Sweeter Babies

Babies whose needs are met cry less, get sick less often, can usually sleep better at night,[1] and are rarely bored, colicky, fussy, whiny, and clingy.[2] Instead, because they know how to trust and love, they're more prepared to form close emotional bonds as older children and adults.[3] Basically, every single study done on child development and behavior shows that the more physically and emotionally attached an infant is in his first year of life, the more emotionally healthy he'll be later.[4] And because every day he's learning about our world by how we treat him and respond to his needs, it means he's likely to be more sensitive, optimistic, empathetic, easier to reason with, and more bonded to people than to things.[5]

Kind Parenting Makes Smarter Babies

Many studies now show that the most powerful contributor to brain development is the quality of the parent-infant bond and an environment where all the baby's needs are met on cue.[6] And because content babies don't cry as much (usually only when they need something), they spend more time growing and learning. In fact, these babies have higher IQs than "playpen babies," or those little ones who are left to play alone and comfort themselves.[7] The "quiet alertness" of a calm, happy baby allows her to fully experience everything in her environment, which leads to not only getting smarter but also to a neat kind of "inner organization" that allows even the physiological systems of her body to work better.[8] I can't say enough about how true this is. Every time I'm out and about with Bear, I *see* him learning: *Ah!* There are the trees. *Ah!* There are the birds. He's taking in everything. None of it comes from my showing him or teaching him. He discovers and learns on his own. And by being there to support him—not to drill him on his ABC's or colors—I'm allowing his knowledge and experience of the world to be much deeper.

Kind Parenting Makes More Independent Babies

I can tell you firsthand that practicing kind parenting leads to kids who feel confident and safe in the world. From the time Bear was born, people were always telling me how amazing it was that he never cried whenever I handed him to someone else to hold. It was like he felt so sure of who he was and where he belonged that he wasn't the least bit afraid of the world or other people. By 8 months, he was crawling around like a maniac. At first, he'd go a little ways away from me or Christopher, testing his boundaries, then scramble right back. But at one point, he scooted around the corner, and Christopher and I looked at each other and realized, *He's not coming back.* We went into the next room, and there he was, perfectly content playing by himself. Then back he came. Now when I maul him with too many kisses, he looks at me like, "I've got other things to do, lady. I don't want to kiss you. I want to see the world!" Then *he* pushes me away, and while I'm always a little sad to let him go toddle around, I love that he has so much confidence.

One of the biggest myths about attending to your baby's needs on cue is that your baby will be spoiled and needy. But both experience—mine *and* the experts—and research show that kind parenting fosters independence. Bear and the kids of so many of my mama-tribe friends are living proof. They're not clingy or shy at all. They're incredibly social and happy and free.

It turns out that the spoiling theory was just a fad in the 1920s. So-called baby experts were trying their hand at commercializing baby rearing and telling parents that holding a baby a lot, feeding on cue, and responding to cries would make for clingy babies. But there was not one drop of scientific research to back up their claims.[9] On the other hand, those experts who do have the goods to back up their claims are confident that it's a completely natural instinct to want to be attached or intimately bonded to our parents. In fact, the more secure a baby feels with his "home base," the more likely he'll be confident enough to explore his environment.[10]

Kind Parenting Gives You Wisdom

One of the most important lessons I've learned in my life is one I learned from being Bear's mom. If Bear is crying or upset or scared, I don't make him process those feelings on his own and I

Does My Baby Need a Schedule?

I know you've heard the moms who rave about how they have their baby's day mapped out to a T. But it turns out scheduling your baby isn't the coolest thing since sliced bread. Every single baby is different. Not only that—every single *day* for every single baby is different. So how can we stuff them into one preset mold?

For young babies, it's much more of a comfort to know their needs are being met when they need them to be met most. That means feeding baby when he's hungry and letting baby sleep when he's sleepy, no matter when he's feeling those vibes. It's also great for mama and papa because it means living less rigidly and going with the flow more. But don't just take it from me that having an around-the-clock baby love fest is the easiest, simplest, most satisfying way to go; listen to Dr. Lawrence Rosen.

"During the first 4 months of life, babies typically don't understand schedules—they do things on demand. If they're hungry, they eat. If they're tired, they sleep. If they're awake, they're awake. You're not going to spoil your baby by holding them, feeding them, or letting them sleep. You just have to be mindful of what they need. It's something I try to teach parents early on. If you can learn to be in the moment, surrender to being in the now, and not worry about anything a minute from now or a minute before, then life becomes a lot less stressful. Babies will teach you how to live in the present more than anything in your life."

don't tell him to stop having those feelings. I honor them. I hold him or sit with him and say, "I see you're feeling sad" or "I see you're really frustrated," and after a moment or two, it passes.

Through doing this for him, I'm finally learning that everything passes. If I'm scared or anxious or sad or mad, it will all pass. You have to allow these feelings and ride that wave. It's kind of like yoga, where at first you feel discomfort, but if you breathe into the discomfort, the sensations can fade. Growing up, I never internalized that it was okay to sit with feelings and let them move through me. Instead, I would become scared by how upset I could get by something or anxious that I should be doing something to fix it or stop it from happening in the first place. But by being an attuned parent for Bear, I'm teaching both of us that these feelings pass and everything will be fine. I'm not perfect at it yet, but I'm thrilled to help him have a head start.

HONORING BABY'S INSTINCTS: YOUR BABY NEEDS YOU FOR A REASON!

There's a very good reason for your own instinct to scoop up your baby and protect her: Human babies are among the most helpless of newborns. Aside from knowing how to root and suckle, they're not equipped with many survival skills at birth. Being alone, flat on her back, and left on a cool, firm surface with no noise surrounding her is not a natural environment, and separation is not an option if she wants to survive.[11] Crying is her way of expressing herself. That's why it's important to point out that kind parenting isn't about never, ever letting your baby cry. Rather, it's about tapping into *why* your baby is crying and trying to meet her needs. In your baby's earliest days, keeping her close and snug is the most meaningful way of expressing your deepest love.

Wearing Baby

Wearing your baby in a carrier or sling is one of the most natural ways to care for your baby from the moment he's born. Mamas around the globe have been doing this forever! In ancient times (and in many of today's traditional cultures), babies were wrapped up and wiggled and jiggled all over the mountainsides and deserts. What these wise mamas knew was that good things happen to babies who get to come along for the ride. It's not just human mamas who have figured this out, either. Ever wonder why those lion cubs look so blissed out when they're being carted around in mama's mouth? A recent study done by neurobiologists found that when babies—and

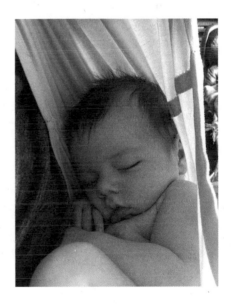

other mammals—are picked up and carried, their heart rates slow almost immediately.[12] Before we credit mamas for monopolizing this effect, let's note that the researchers saw similar reactions to nuzzle time with papas.[13]

Carrying baby kangaroo-style has been shown to benefit all elements of neurological and emotional development. Babies sheltered on your body can smell you, listen to your heart and lungs, and feel the warmth of your body.[14] According to researchers at Stanford University, carried babies cry less because little ones are most settled when they're rocked in all directions, not just side to side.[15] All that soothing and holding leads to daytime calmness and helps baby mellow into better sleep at night.[16] Cultures that carry their babies rarely see incidences of colic, and they also report that their babies gain weight more reliably. That could be because boob-on-demand is a lot easier when baby is just inches away. And because carried babies get to eavesdrop on all your conversations, it enhances their speech development and teaches them how to communicate better.[17] Bear was talking long before he had words. Even at 3 months, he was a clear communicator—he had so much to say with his noises! And now he's the chattiest little man. He loves stopping to talk to people and is constantly asking us questions because he's curious and excited and wants to know everything there is to know. When a baby gets to see and hear and touch the world as you're doing it, too, he's getting inspired by it all and he's learning.

I still love toting Bear in the Ergobaby carrier, and Christopher loved his sling. I adored that Bear could be a part of so much of my day, and that even when I wasn't gazing at his face and cooing at him, I was still giving him the nurturing he needed. I loved that as he got bigger, I got stronger. Because he was nestled into my front, I could nurse easily and discreetly, which meant he never had to fuss out of hunger or overtiredness. His naps were deep and sweet, and when he was awake, he was my little travel buddy. And because he cooked with me and gardened with me and cleaned the house with me, everything became a toy.

CHOOSING A CARRIER

There are many styles to choose from: soft cloth pouch slings that you can just throw over one shoulder and need no adjusting, and "ring slings" that are similar in style but can be adjusted as your baby grows. Wrap carriers can be tied in different ways for the most comfortable position. Some carriers, like Ergos, look like little backpacks you wear on your front. Even if you have special considerations, such as a bad back, there are ways of wearing baby that can work. And don't feel like you need to commit to just one type, either. Depending on your preference and comfort, you'll find that a certain style is better for, say, long walks and another for getting chores done around the house.

That's why getting hand-me-downs can be such a lifesaver—you can learn what works and what doesn't without having to buy a whole bunch. If you do buy new, be sure you're opting for natural and organic materials. You definitely want to go with a model where baby is facing you, at least for the better part of her first year. Your baby will still get to see the world, but without too much overwhelming, cranky-making stimulation.[18] Plus, it's so much more fun when you get to gaze at your partner in crime all day long!

TRANSITIONING INTO A CARRIER

Most carried babies dive into a burbling blissed-out trance right away, but if yours doesn't seem to be having any of it, it's not because he doesn't like his new ride. Babies sometimes resist a carrier if they are too hungry or too tired, want the boobie, or need to go to the bathroom. Or sometimes, if they sense your own apprehension with the whole arrangement, they, too, can become anxious.[19] Make sure your baby is as comfortable as possible before loading him up, then take just a few laps around the house. You'll both get a feel for how safe and secure the new carrier is, and you'll share that peace of mind.

One of my tricks was to put on my Ergo, then pick up Bear and give him a cozy snuggle. Then I'd start walking while putting on the arms of the carrier, which felt like a nice big hug. He'd fuss for a second at first, but then he'd be in heaven.

Naked Time

The most heavenly, delicious thing in the world is to hold your naked baby against your skin. There are so many benefits, especially when they're first born—it helps babies deal with stress, stimulates nerves in the brain that aid in food absorption, improves immune function, and helps them sleep more easily.[20] Babies feel so content and secure and at peace when they're attached to you. Not that we're naked all the time, but the more Bear can go naked, the better. Sometimes, I would quietly cradle Bear after I'd nursed or set him up tummy to tummy in a Moby Wrap carrier or wildly kiss him all over his edible little body while he laughs hysterically (which I still do!). Or Christopher might lie with him on his bare chest, and Bear can feel in that moment that his world is a beautiful and special one.

Bath Bonding

Taking a bath with your baby is an adorable, precious, lovely thing that's not to be missed. It's seriously one of the greatest joys and is relaxing for mama and baby. A rubdown in the sink, while cute, is not as much fun! Seriously, there's no need for those plastic baby tubs. They cost money and take up space and detract from some of the most pleasurable moments you could be spending with baby.

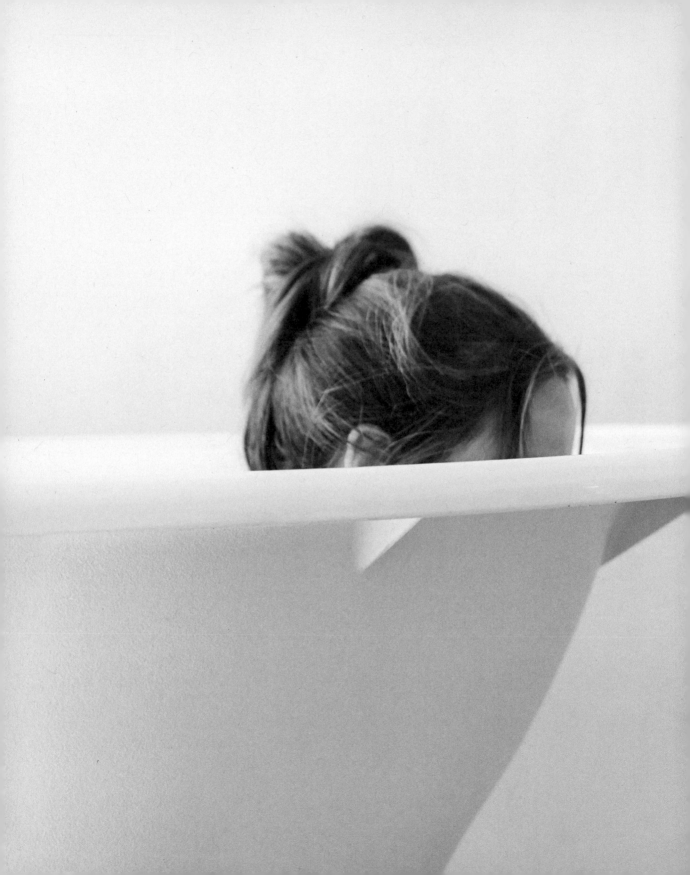

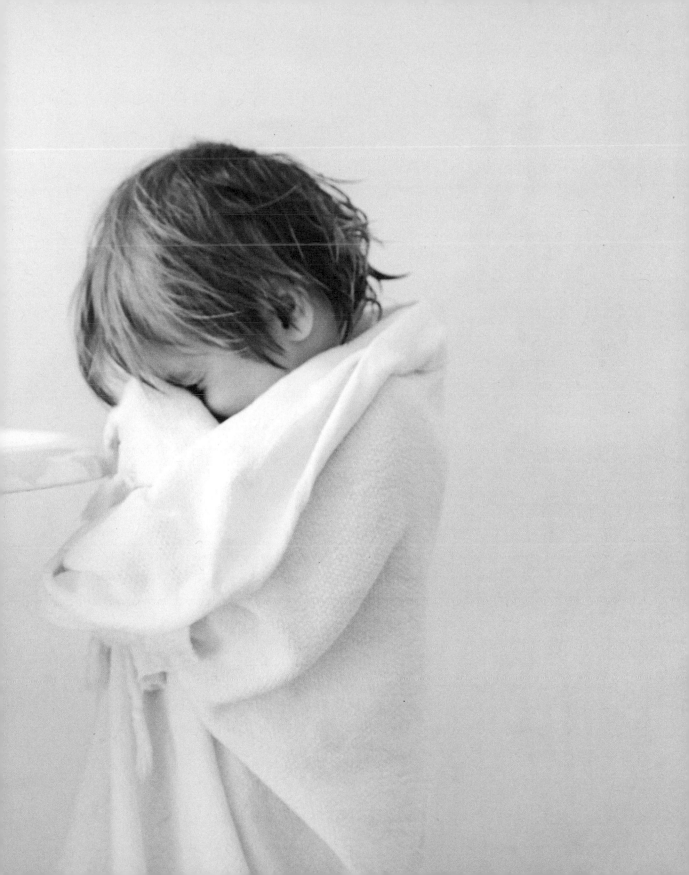

Baby's First Bath

Hold off on the splashing and fun until the remaining part of the umbilical cord falls off, which usually happens within 7 to 10 days. Until then, stick to gentle sponge baths if they are needed at all. Place a small towel or washcloth in the bottom of the tub or on the floor and softly pass a sponge or lightly wet cloth over his skin. Try not to touch the umbilical cord site, which you want to keep dry and irritation free until the cord falls off. Sometimes, though, the site can get goopy and smelly when it's close to detaching. In that case, you can dab some witch hazel at the base of the cord site.

If your baby isn't circumcised, there's no need to retract the foreskin to clean the penis. It is painful for the baby and can cause infection. Don't worry, he'll be getting busy with his penis soon enough and know innately how to move the skin the way it's supposed to move. It's another lovely reason to not have baby in a diaper all the time, because that way he can get to his penis and explore as nature intended.

Babies don't necessarily *need* a lot of baths, but they can get stinky from your super-rich milk stuck in their adorable little rolls, especially in their necks. When I first starting having bath time with Bear—at around 2 weeks old—I put just a couple inches of water in the bathtub. I would get in and have Christopher hand me the baby—that's important to remember so you don't risk slipping while getting in or out! Then I'd place Bear on his back and he'd wiggle and splash. He would laugh, make the craziest noises, and scrounge around looking for boobies, and I could lie back and have boobie time in hot water. It was sweet, relaxing, and fun. To this day, it's the only way we bathe. Usually, bath time is more for me to wash my hair and not because he's dirty, and we do it near bedtime so I can start the wind-it-down vibe.

SPECIAL BATH-TIME TREATS

Kind potions and lotions: Check out thekindlife.com for ones I love. I update the list with new favorites.

Scrumptious oatmeal bath: In addition to being incredibly kind to our insides, oatmeal has amazing skin-softening properties. Treat yourself and baby to a soothing oatmeal bath. Take a piece of cheesecloth or a cotton handkerchief, place a heaping tablespoon of oatmeal in the center, then gather up the sides and twist them once. Secure the bundle with a piece of string and drop the sachet into the water. Give it a firm squeeze to release all that good, creamy liquid, then dab it all over your skin and baby's for an extra-indulgent finishing touch.

Clean, chlorine-free water: The water we bathe our babies with should be as clean and contaminant free as the water we drink. But the same not-so-pleasant pollutants that we talked about in Chapter 5 are still floating around in our bathwater. Refer to the tips there for how to get the cleanest water for your home. Ideally, you would install a whole-house filter, but there are baby steps you can take. The Sprite Bath Ball faucet filter in chrome is one great option that is super-easy to attach to a bathtub and is handy for travel.

Baby Massage

Massage is another lovely way to calm baby and nurture his feelings of security. Studies have shown that babies who are held, massaged, and rocked grow up to have a stronger self-image and a gentler demeanor than those who aren't.[21] Massage offers amazing physical benefits like strengthened respiratory and immune systems, better circulation, and better digestion. It helps your baby grow and gain weight. And when baby is blissed out, he'll sleep more soundly and for longer periods.[22] Of course, if you're already doing a lot of skin-on-skin snuggling, your babe is reaping those same benefits, so don't stress about having something else on your to-do list.

The best time to do it is when baby is fed, happy, and relaxed but not too tired, so after a bath can be perfect. You can use any vegetable-based oil, though I like almond the best. Unscented is fine, but if your baby is over 3 months old and he can tolerate fragrance, try adding a couple of drops of lavender essential oil to your base oil for an extra-calming treat.

Sit comfortably on the floor or bed. Lay a cotton towel or blanket on your lap, then arrange baby so his feet are pointed toward you and his face is up. Rub a few drops of oil in your palms to warm them, then slowly rub it all over baby's body, starting with his shoulders. Avoid his hands, though, since they tend to end up in his mouth. Begin by gently squeezing his limbs (babies are sensitive!) starting from the tops of his arms and legs and working your way to his hands and feet. Then lightly press from the center of his body and outward, across his torso, repeating each stroke at least three times. End your session by slowly and gently stroking baby's tummy in a clockwise direction.

The 90-Minute Sleep Method

Tuning in to your baby's sleep cues is another way to make her feel heard, secure, and, most important for development, well rested! If you're listening, your baby will let you know when she needs to sleep throughout the day. Getting your baby down for good naps is key to a better night's sleep.

When a friend of mine told me about the book *The 90-Minute Baby Sleep Program* by Polly Moore, PhD, I was skeptical. I didn't like the sound of a program, but I was intrigued about what neuroscientist Dr. Moore had to say. She talks about how your baby's natural sleep cycles come in shifts of 90 minutes. (Makes sense; even we adults could use a break every 45 or 90 minutes!) That means that after your baby has been awake for an hour and a half, her internal clock will kick in and she will start to show signs of being tired—rubbing her eyes, getting fussy, yawning, pulling her ears, and so on. It's baby's way of letting you know that she's ready for a little shut-eye. If you can help her get there by offering something comforting in return—maybe some rocking or a bit of milk—then she'll drift off into the most content sleep and wake up happy and rested. You're helping baby get in tune with her body's innate rhythms.

Christopher and I decided to try out the theory. We watched the clock from the moment Bear woke up, and sure enough, 1 hour and 30 minutes later, he began rubbing his eyes and getting a little fussy. *Wow,* I thought. So I put him on the boob and he was out. It was crazy! After that, we started to see this incredible pattern emerge. Bear would wake up, he'd nurse, he'd play, then he'd get sleepy and we'd put him to bed. Repeat. So long as we caught him in that presleep sweet spot, he was never unhappy. Because, remember, a baby who feels right, acts right. All I can say is that this made the first year of his life even more amazing, and I couldn't recommend this more highly.

Soothing Baby

The womb was cozy, quiet, dark, full of mama smells and sounds, and super-safe. In fact, Harvey Karp, MD, author of *The Happiest Baby on the Block*, says the brand-new sensations of the outside world can be overwhelming for little ones, so surrounding them with the old comforts of home can bring a bit of solace when nothing else will. I highly recommend the techniques from Dr. Karp's book. They're essential for when your baby starts sending out her presleep signals (see "The 90-Minute Sleep Method" above) or when the boob, a burp, a nap, or a dry diaper just won't cut it. Try singing baby a sweet song, wrapping her in a swaddle, snuggling her in your sling, rocking and bouncing her, or making the ssshhh sound of ocean waves.

For Gentlemen Only: Welcome to the Parent Hood

This is a profound time for a man. There is nothing like sitting with your newborn and doing a little inventory on your life and where you are in your journey of manhood. It was so healing for me to give love to my son and to give him the strongest possible foundation.

—Christopher

Up until now, I've basically paraphrased some of the most essential stuff a papa needs to know. I recommend that you read this entire chapter about bonding and kind parenting. This is a journey that both you and your partner will share absolutely equally, and while you might think she has a leg up because of all that boobie goodness your baby seems to be grooving these days, there are just as many significant ways for you to be soothing and supportive and comforting to your baby.

After my baby was born, I loved knowing that my husband and I were in this together. My husband is as involved in parenting as I am. Christopher feels such a deep sense of pride and strength as a man and father when he wears our son around town or swaddles him or takes a bath with him. He's been involved since day 1, and because of that, he's really good at being a papa—and he knows it! So don't be intimidated by the special bond that every baby has with his or her mama. Babies need their papas, too. There's no replacing the very unique relationship that you and your child will always share. It will be the greatest joy in your life.

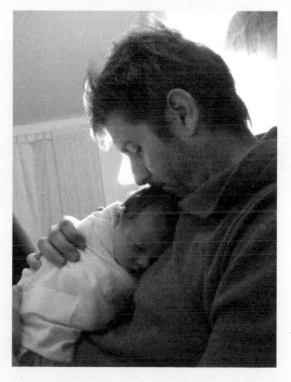

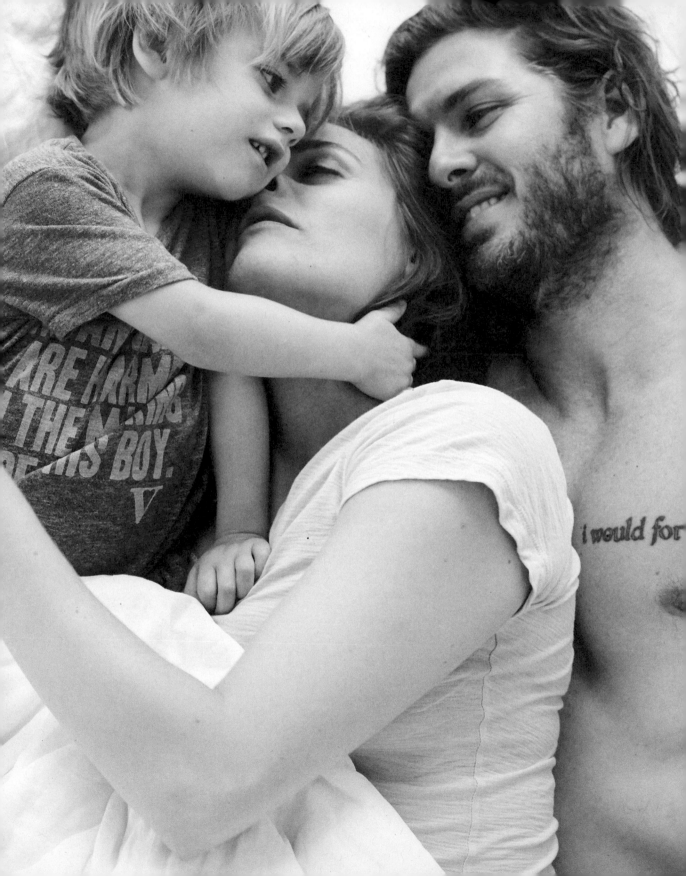

15

The Family Bed

*When I fall asleep with Bear, he feels confident, calm, and cool.
He says, "You got me, Daddy," and I say, "Yeah, I do." And then
we doze off. I can feel how good and safe he feels in my arms and
how confident it makes him. It's like meditation in a way—
you're just taking care of your baby and you're
completely present.*

—Christopher

I know the images that come to mind when people talk about "cosleeping" or "the family bed." It sounds like some kind of trippy holdover from the peace, love, and barley casserole notions of the commune-happy sixties. Okay, fine. Let's say that's the case and look at what all those crazy hippies were doing: Inviting their fresh-out-of-the-womb babies into their warm, cozy beds where they could caress and soothe and nurse whenever it was needed. Now let's consider the modern, "informed" alternative: taking a brand-new baby—a creature so small and helpless that she can't yet feed herself, communicate clearly, or even really make sense of her own tiny body—and leaving her in a barred-in box completely alone.

Parents have been sleeping with their babies for thousands of years. It was a natural, normal way to better protect their children, keep them warm, and more conveniently feed them in the wee hours.[23] But we eventually did stop doing it because as we got wealthier and wealthier and could build bigger and bigger houses, suddenly *not* giving baby her own room was terribly out of fashion. And by the time the prudish Victorians got around to making sure everyone felt guilty about their bodies and physical closeness, the family bed was officially considered a backward thing of the past.[24] By the start of the 20th century, any parents in America who were still sharing beds were encouraged to stop because it could—supposedly—spread illness, spoil their children, and cause them to suffocate.[25]

So let's go back to that first scenario: lonely crib versus warm, lovely bed. There's something innately natural about including baby in our nighttime rituals, and it shows in the research. Family-bed babies thrive, which means they not only gain weight better but they also grow to their full potential—physically, emotionally, and intellectually.[26] All that yummy skin-on-skin touching during the day benefits your baby's development; the same thing goes for nighttime. Plus, when a baby can feed on demand—and can do so in a more leisurely way because all mama has to do is roll over in bed!—the more time she'll spend nursing and the better her chances are at getting to all that scrumptious, nourishing, high-fat hind milk, which is great for physical development and helps the brain grow.[27]

Let's be clear: This is not about where the baby is physically sleeping but about accepting that parenting doesn't stop at night. Just because it's dark out doesn't mean your baby no longer has needs! She still has to be able to trust that you're going to be there for her 24 hours a day. And believe me, nothing is sweeter than your newborn sleeping on your chest.

Sharing a bed with baby means you can tune in better to her needs, which in turn builds security and trust. There's no need to worry that she'll never be able to soothe herself or that she'll grow up to be a spoiled monster of a child, because that's simply not true.[28] Think of your sleeping arrangement as an organic extension of the kind parenting you're doing during the day—the nighttime equivalent of baby wearing. It's letting your child know through your own physical closeness that you are there for her no matter what.

And babies understand that. Babies who share sleep go to sleep more happily and sleep better.[29] If she wakes in the middle of the night—which is apt to happen frequently, since babies spend most of their nights in the light part of the sleep cycle[30]—it isn't quite so scary when mama and papa are snuggled close. She can nestle into the same warmth that saw her through those blissful months in the womb, and because she's only a wiggle away from a boobie, she can nurse whenever she wants or needs. That not only makes for a happy, well-rested baby but also makes for a happier, better-rested mama. Because believe me, when you're nursing around the clock, *nothing* is sweeter—and a bigger relief—than nuzzling close to your babe, letting her nurse, then drifting back off to sleep.

YOU'RE A TOTAL FREAK AND RUINING YOUR BABY, AND OTHER SCARY MYTHS

If you ask most new moms about where their babies sleep, you'll probably hear a similar response from most of them: "Well, we bought a crib/cosleeper/bassinet, but usually we fall asleep with him in the bed." And more often than not, they feel guilty about it. Or they feel like they need to keep it a secret from their pediatricians and friends. But what all these mamas know in their hearts to be true is that bringing baby in the bed feels *good*. Maybe it's the comfort of having baby close or the deeper rest that most women and babies are able to get when they sleep together.[31] Quite likely, though, it's all the oxytocin pumping through mama's body—nature's little insurance policy that we moms will stick close by our babies.[32] At first, it's easy to honor that intuition. But soon the voices of all the sleep trainers and doctors and "experts" and naysayers might start to creep in, and the baby is banished to another room. Here are some of the reasons behind the Great Baby Bedroom Exodus:

You're a Negligent Parent/Hopeless Romantic/Naïve First-Timer

Unfortunately, this is the sentiment that many new parents walk away with after discouraging visits with their pediatricians. But consider what doctor *and* parent William Sears, MD, has to say on the matter: "Doctors do not study the answers to whether you should let your baby cry and where your baby should sleep in medical school. They are trained in diagnosis and treatment of illness, not in parenting styles."[33] And according to an article and research findings that ran in *Pediatrics*, the official journal of the American Academy of Pediatrics (!), "Many pediatricians lack sound training in developmental and behavioral pediatrics, and thus their advice is largely based on their own cultural values and beliefs in interaction with their personal and clinical experience."[34] Dr. Sears goes on to say, "If you feel that your baby, your husband, and you will all sleep better with this nighttime parenting style, then that's the right decision for you."[35]

You're Creating a Codependent Monster

Compared with much of the world, our culture puts an insane amount of pressure on parents to make "independent" babies. They're told that their infant should be sleeping through the night, equipped to soothe himself back to sleep if he wakes, and essentially able to live 12 or so hours of his life without any need for the people who provide for him. But this kind of training isn't rooted in any superior science or expertise. It started mainly after the Industrial Revolution, when people were building bigger houses, and suddenly baby wasn't welcome in the family bed anymore. This, coupled with the popular myth that women would raise needy nightmares if they held or doted too much, led to the cry-it-out fad. It was certainly easy to oblige. All mama and papa had to do was move baby's cradle a room or two away.[36]

But according to Dr. Sears and his wife, Martha Sears, RN—whose eight children qualify them as experts in this arena—you're creating *good* habits by cosleeping. The biggest reason for this is that babies have needs. It is natural, appropriate, and even beneficial for a baby to be dependent on his parents.[37] When you tend to these needs, you're letting your baby know that he can trust you, which is why family-bed children end up more independent and better adjusted later in life than those who slept without their parents.[38] "The families I see adhering to this philosophy are all happy and balanced," says pediatrician Michel Cohen, MD. "My feeling is that frequent physical contact in the first few months is essential."[39] It's most likely for these reasons that family-bed babies cry less than babies who sleep alone.[40]

When you leave a baby to cry it out, self-soothe, or otherwise independently take care of himself before he's ready, he misses out on the trust building that's crucial in infant development.[41] He's not learning how kind and giving the world is. This practice teaches a baby to devalue his own cues and his innate trust in his parents. And it teaches parents—especially mamas—to ignore their precious instincts. I hear stories about moms having to bury their heads under a pillow just to resist going to comfort their crying child. Why deny that every fiber of your truth is telling you to go to him?

It might sound convenient to have a couple of nights of fitful tears and then a lifetime of 8-hour stretches of sleep, but consider the potential long-term consequences of isolation versus the benefits of keeping him close. Studies have found that children who never slept with their parents:[42]

- Were harder to calm, less happy, had more tantrums, handled stress less well, and were more fearful than routinely cosleeping children.
- Wound up getting more professional help with emotional and behavioral problems.

But kids who *did* sleep with their parents:[43]

- Showed a feeling of general satisfaction with life.
- Had increased self-esteem and less guilt and anxiety, and were more comfortable with physical contact and affection.
- Felt they weren't as prone to peer pressure as others their age.

Besides, there's evidence that crying it out is far less effective for teaching how to self-soothe than responding immediately to baby's fussing. In a study comparing two groups of colicky babies, one group was comforted right away while the other was left to self-soothe. The babies whose cries were attended to cried 70 percent less! Those poor colicky babies left on their own, on the other hand, showed no decrease in their panicked outrage.[44]

That said, it's a reality that your baby will cry. Especially if he's tired and can't get himself to sleep. So it's important to point out that there is a vast difference between crying it out and allowing your baby to cry. While the former means letting your kid wail until he's gotten the message that nobody's coming to tend to him, the latter is far gentler. If you know your baby's needs are all met (fed, dry, warm enough, not too stimulated), then it's okay to just hold him and be present while he sorts it all out. You'll be giving him the message that it's all right to be frustrated/sad/overwhelmed and that you'll be lovingly supporting him every step of the way.

It's Not Safe

The most common concern I hear is, "Aren't you afraid you're going to smoosh him?!" I suppose in theory it's valid, but when you get into that bed with your tiny little one, it seems completely inconceivable. I mean, how on earth did the species survive? We didn't always have cribs or cosleepers or even king-size beds! As Dr. Cohen says, "Mammals have slept with their progeny since the dawn of evolution. I find it hard to imagine that something as instinctive as sleeping together could frequently lead to tragedy."[45] And according to Jay Gordon, MD, the family bed can actually help save a baby's life because you're right there to feel his every move and hear his every breath. In fact, Dr. Gordon asserts that a safely set up family bed is *safer* than solitary infant sleep.[46] Dr. Rosen agrees, saying, "As long as you don't smoke, aren't drinking alcohol or using illegal drugs, and there's no loose blankets or bedding around baby, then you can safely and successfully cosleep, which supports breastfeeding and attachment." And babies aren't entirely helpless. Even newborns have the ability to struggle, squirm, and cry to get out of what they perceive to be dangerous situations.[47]

That's a pretty all-star MD lineup supporting the family bed! The reality is that sleeping together as a family can be completely safe and completely lovely. It all comes down to our all-knowing intuition, a few precautions, and a lot of basic common sense.

Your Baby Won't Sleep through the Night

If there's one thing new mamas get asked about over and over and over again, it's "Does your baby sleep through the night?" From the time Bear was a newborn, people were constantly asking me about his sleeping habits, as though it were completely normal for a brand-new human being to enter the world and immediately understand night, day, and the merits of a full night's sleep. As any new parent can attest, babies aren't built that way. And saying good-bye to sleep as you knew it can be overwhelming. That's usually when desperate sleep-deprived couples turn to the promises of "sleep trainers" or the piles of books out there claiming that they can whip your baby into fuss-free sleep shape.

Regardless of what might be easiest for us as parents—like getting 8 hours of uninterrupted sleep—there's a *reason* why babies don't sleep through the night. It's because they need to be fed! "People don't function well if they're getting up every 2 or 3 hours, but they need to understand that if you have a newborn baby, then you're at the whim of this little creature who needs everything from you," says Dr. Rosen. "It's normal for them to eat every 1 to 2 hours, especially if you're breastfeeding." Here's what breastfeeding expert Beverly Solow has to say about it: "The breast is designed to be drained as often as the baby is designed to eat, and the feedback mechanism for how much milk to make is informed by how much milk is left in the breast. So if you sleep through the night and your milk is just sitting in your breasts, then it's telling your body to make less."

Babies who share a bed with their parents breastfeed more frequently and for longer bouts, which means giving your baby all those amazing benefits of boob food, including getting her to a healthy weight and giving her the best immunity defense against disease. Plus, when the boob is just a wiggle away, baby doesn't have to cry for it. So while they might not be getting a straight stretch of uninterrupted sleep, bed-sharing mamas can still sleep better and longer than if they had to get out of bed to nurse. And, in turn, so can baby.[48]

So why the obsession with sleep habits? According to a 2005 study published in the journal *Pediatrics*, how we interpret sleep is shaped by our culture. In Japan, for example, wakefulness during the night isn't a matter of concern, and it's definitely not something moms rush to their pediatricians to address. In contrast, because we've been told that babies *should* be able to sleep alone and *should* be able to sleep through the night without wanting attention from their parents, we see these—very natural—behaviors as a bad thing.

"The greatest anxiety and worry occur when people try to fight the natural rhythms their child has," says Dr. Rosen. "Especially before your baby is 4 months old, you're only swimming upstream if you try to fight that. But if you allow yourself to surrender, then there's a lot less stress." You can force a baby to sleep, but it comes at a price. Sleep training isn't a permanent fix—you have to do it over and over again each time there's a hiccup in the routine, like growth milestones, travel, or if your baby gets sick.

At the end of the day, no two babies will sleep alike. Just as some of us are early birds and others could stay in bed until 3:00 in the afternoon, babies have individual differences in their sleep rhythms.[49] Which is all the more reason to give a big "no thanks" to anyone who promises their special program will get your kid to sleep. Sleeping is not a behavior that seems gentle or kind to force on a baby; the best thing you can do is encourage his natural sleep rhythm and remember that this too shall pass. One day you *will* sleep again.

It's Weird

It's all relative. To many moms around the world, keeping their baby in a separate nursery is weird! Cultures in which people don't normally consult sleep experts and trainers never even consider an alternative:[50] It's natural to go from womb to breast to bed. In a survey of 186 traditional societies worldwide, mother and baby shared a bed in most of them, and none of them endorsed the Western-style nursery arrangement.[51] We're not just talking about tribes in the outback. Even technologically advanced and highly complex communities see bed sharing as the rule and not the exception. They're doing it in England, Australia, India, and Italy! An interesting distinction—as the *Pediatrics* study found—is how these cultures value dependence. In the case of the Japanese, they understand that an infant is a being who needs interdependent relationships in order to develop properly.[52]

It'll Ruin Your Sex Life

The first thing I'll say is that it'll be a little while before either of you has the energy to get frisky. But when you do want to settle back into your rhythm, most couples find that sharing a bed doesn't affect their lovemaking schedule. In fact, it's extra incentive to get a little creative. Whoever said the bed at night is the only time and place to do the deed?! You can always put the baby on blankets on the floor or something—there are many ways to be safely creative.

CREATING A SAFE FAMILY SLEEP SANCTUARY

Here are basic suggestions for keeping everybody snug and safe:

- If you're worried about your baby falling out of bed, move your mattress to the floor. That's what Christopher and I did—not only did we gain peace of mind, but it also feels like a fun kind of sleepover when we crawl into bed.

- If you're worried about the smoosh factor because you have a small bed, you can try using a sidecar or cosleeper, a little baby nook that clips on to your mattress at bed level. If you go this route, make sure it's made from safe materials: natural fabric and natural fillings and metal or solid wood. But before you buy anything, consider that my family—and a lot of families we know—has a queen-size bed, and we are perfectly comfortable.

- If your baby sinks 3 inches when you put him down because your mattress is saggy or you have an enormous, fluffy mattress topper that swallows your baby, then you don't have the best sleep conditions for him. If your bed is pushed up against the wall, make sure there's no crevice for your baby to roll into. Don't cover your baby's face with your duvet. Have I mentioned anything you wouldn't have already checked for yourself?? I honestly believe that your mama-bear protective instincts will call into question any possible hazards. But if you want to quadruple-check that you haven't overlooked anything, check out the bible on cosleeping, *Good Nights* by Jay Gordon, MD, and *Nighttime Parenting* by William Sears, MD.

You might need to play around with your arrangements before finding the most comfortable fit. At first, Christopher and I slept with Bear on our chests. Later, we put him between the two of us, up near our heads. That way we could still get cozy under our own blankets without worrying about covering his little face. For some couples, this feels like the most natural thing in the world; for others—or maybe just one partner—it can take a little getting used to. I propose giving this new setup a 30-day trial. More often than not, parents come to love having their baby so close by, all snug and secure in their bed. And when they do, it's so happy and magical.

Sudden Infant Death Syndrome

In many ways, sudden infant death syndrome (SIDS)—the unexpected and sudden death of a child under the age of 1—remains a mystery. Even though your baby's risk for it is relatively low

(6.61 in 1,000),[53] as of 2008 it was the third leading cause of infant death and the first leading cause of death among infants ages 1 to 12 months old.[54] Although we don't know what causes it, we do know how to significantly lower your baby's risk. And what's pretty great is that many of these things are inherent in being a kind parent.

The American Academy of Pediatrics acknowledges that sleeping in the same room can reduce the risk of SIDS.[55] And researchers—who recognize the many physiological benefits of cosleeping—are beginning to explore the connection between safe cosleeping and reduced risk.[56] The AAP also recommends breastfeeding as an antidote![57]

The same common sense that applied when setting up baby safely in bed goes for SIDS prevention, too: Make sure your baby sleeps on a firm mattress and in a bed that's not cluttered with suffocation hazards like cushions, stuffed animals, and synthetic fabrics. Keep your sleeping environment on the cooler side, ideally letting natural air circulate in the room and not blasting it with your central heating or air conditioner. Diet may also be a contributing factor. Since foods like simple sugars and dairy can reduce your little one's ability to absorb oxygen efficiently,[58] make sure you're not loading up on them while pregnant or breastfeeding.

HANDLING THE NAYSAYERS

Believe me, I hear you when you say how difficult it can be to make good, clear-headed decisions on weeks and weeks of no sleep. Your mind starts to wander to a place where babies magically sleep all night, and you'd do *anything* to get them there. That's when the advice of well-meaning onlookers might start to sound mighty good. It's easy to be susceptible to other people's ideas of how to parent, but their values might not be in line with yours.

Plenty of people will stick their noses in your business. But the best sleeping arrangement is, hands down, the one that works best for your family. Pay no mind to the naysayers. Instead, look around and see who has the most grounded, happy, well-adjusted, and healthy kids. Whose life inspires you? Seek out those parents—or find a forum on my Web site, thekindlife.com—and create a network so you can ask for advice about natural, intuitive parenting.

If you are considering transitioning your baby from your bed to her own space, Dr. Rosen suggests waiting until 6 months and then exploring gentler methods of helping baby sleep through the night.

BE RESOLVED

Having a baby is amazing and fulfilling and otherworldly. But when you're adjusting to your new life with baby, sleep can be hard to come by. And when sleep doesn't happen, the day suddenly doesn't look so bright and shiny. This is when it all starts to feel like *work*. It's beautiful work, but draining nonetheless. Are my husband and I often tired? Yes! Are there times when we're jealous of people who sleep train? Yes! But we know how magical our bond with our baby is, and we know it wouldn't be the same if we told him that he had to go sleep in another room.

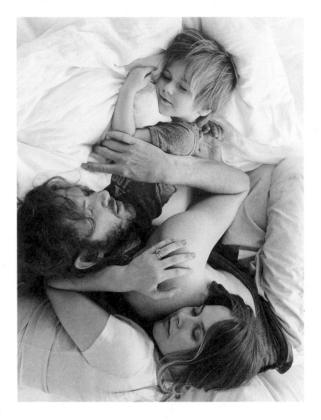

When Bear was 8 months old, I hit a rough patch with sleep. I started sending e-mails to my mama tribe at 3:45 in the morning with questions like, "Why would God make babies need their moms every 30 minutes in the night? What good does that do?" I'd start playing devil's advocate, challenging my ideas about kind parenting and wondering if maybe there was some good that could come of teaching a kid to soothe himself. Then I'd try and talk myself back in. "I don't want to be a wimp and give up on the family bed!" I'd write. I was slowly losing my mind. My friend Alanis talked me down off the ledge and reminded me why I was taking this path, with all its amazing benefits, and that I wouldn't have Bear to snuggle with forever.

And how's this for peace of mind? *Your baby will naturally learn to sleep.* According to Dr. Rosen, as babies get older, they typically learn how to stretch out their sleep cycles all on their own. At 1 to 2 months, a baby can conceivably sleep for a 4- to 6-hour stretch. On average, by 2 to 4 months, it's 6 to 8 hours, and by 4 to 6 months, it's 10 to 12. These long stretches still come with small interruptions as your baby stirs and snuggles sweetly next to you. And you'll most likely sleep with one eye open—probably until your baby's in college—which is mama's nature-given talent. Of course, this isn't written in any rule book, and timing varies from baby to baby, but I hope it reassures you that your baby will, eventually, sleep. And so will you!

Cleaner, Sweeter Dreams: Why Going Natural Makes a Difference

YOUR BED

Unfortunately, a lot of the products made for sleep—bedding, pillows, and mattresses—are doused in all kinds of chemicals that can have a serious effect on our health and our babies' health, not to mention on how well we sleep, which is a big deal given that we spend half our lives in bed!

"Wrinkle-free" and "no-iron" sheets and most conventional mattresses are made with formaldehyde, which the International Agency for Research on Cancer classifies as a known carcinogen.[59] Conventional mattresses are made using petroleum-based polyurethane foam, which off-gasses volatile organic compounds (VOCs) linked to allergies, asthma, and cancer and can be detrimental to developing nervous systems. These chemicals include fire retardants, which find their way into the air we breathe.[60]

If you've been eyeing new bedding for your family nest, think twice if it's made out of conventionally grown cotton, which represents almost a quarter of the world's consumption of insecticides and 10 percent of its pesticides.[61] While these chemicals aren't rubbing off on you while you sleep, they are being introduced into the soil where we grow our food, the water we drink, and the air we breathe.

Here's what you can do to get your nest up to kind standards.

Light Green Quick Fixes

If you're not ready to splurge on an organic mattress and new pillows, green-living expert Marilee Nelson you can still make a difference in your and your child's exposure to synthetic materials by using all-natural covers. Zip up your pillows in organic cotton protectors and wrap your mattress in a tightly woven organic cotton cover. These will reduce your exposure to contaminants that might be in your mattress by partially containing the dust particles of degrading foam and filling. (Flame retardants cling to dust particles, another reason to banish dust bunnies.) If you've already purchased nonorganic bedding, washing it will remove some of the manufacturing residues.[62] As Nelson says, "Old sheets that have been washed a million times—in fragrance-free, chemical-free laundry soaps—are fine as far as the material is concerned."

The Whole Deep Green Enchilada

Bedding: Look for sets made from unbleached, untreated organic cotton—or eco-friendly fibers like linen, hemp, and bamboo (make sure it's organic and sustainably sourced).

Pillows: Since feathers can trigger asthma and allergies—and are really bad news for the ducks and geese that are often plucked alive for years because manufacturers think it makes for better quality, despite its ripping their birds' skin to pieces[63]—look for natural fills like kapok, organic cotton, or natural latex (which, unlike its synthetic cousin, doesn't come from petroleum but from a rubber tree that can heal itself quickly). Both natural latex and kapok are naturally hypoallergenic and are inherently resistant to things like bacteria, mold, dust mites, and mildew.[64]

Mattress: Organic mattresses are free of things like flame retardants, pesticides, and toxic glues and dyes. They're made with natural materials like organic cotton, hemp, coconut husks, and natural latex, which is naturally fire resistant and deters dust mites and bacteria.[65] The only downside of buying 100 percent organic is that these mattresses are significantly more expensive. If you're on a budget, look for a version that has 65 percent natural latex mixed with 35 percent traditional foam.[66] Let it air out outdoors or in a garage for as long as you can to release any fumes and then wrap it in an organic cotton cover.

Why Wool Is Baaaad News

It's true that wool, often used in eco-friendly mattresses, is naturally flame resistant. And it's also true that it's a natural fiber. But a common misconception is that we're doing sheep a favor by shearing them. Unfortunately, these animals are often hurt in the process of collecting wool. According to PETA, there's a gruesome practice called "mulesing" that's still routinely practiced on merino sheep in Australia. Because the animals are bred to have wrinkly skin—it yields more wool—they're more susceptible not only to dying from heat exhaustion but also to an infestation of fly maggots that can eat them alive. To make the sheep less attractive to flystrike, farmers cut off (without anesthesia) chunks of skin from their lambs' backsides where maggots typically take up residence, and these wounds can become infected. Plus, when sheep have maxed out on their wool contributions, it's not like they're sent off to a nice retirement community—they're slaughtered. Even wool that's touted as kinder than kind doesn't have a happy ending.

IF YOU DO BUY A CRIB

If after reading this chapter you ultimately decide that sharing a bed with baby is not for you—or if your little one outgrows the co-sleeper really early—the next best thing is to invest in a crib that's healthy and safe. As we talked about earlier, manufactured woods—including particleboard, which is what most conventional cribs are made out of—contain formaldehyde-based carcinogenic glues that can off-gas for years.[67] Look for a naturally finished wood crib made out of sustainable wood (Forest Stewardship Council–certified products tell you the wood came from an environmentally and socially responsible source). Another option is to use a hand-me-down crib, so long as it meets current safety standards. Do a search on the US Consumer Product Safety Commission Web site (www.cpsc.gov) to make sure that model hasn't been recalled and meets the latest standards in crib safety.

As for furnishing your baby's nest with a mattress and bedding, use the same rules of thumb outlined on page 257. Pay particular attention to what's inside the mattress you purchase, because according to a report titled *The Mattress Matters: Protecting Babies from Toxic Chemicals While They Sleep,* 72 percent of mattresses on the US market contain chemicals of concern like vinyl, polyurethane, and other VOCs that have been linked to asthma attacks and suspected of even more serious health effects, including cancer.[68] Even though the worst toxic offenders in the flame retardant category have been phased out of mattress construction, the alternatives are still sometimes concerning.[69] Check out the *Mattress Matters* study's full findings for a list of mattress brands without these chemicals and other allergens: clean-healthyny .org/2011/11/mattress-matters-report.html. OMI makes a great one. You can also ask manufacturers directly to spell out what's inside their mattresses. If they don't want to tell you, it's probably not what you want to hear.

16

The First 6 Months for Mama and Baby

By the time you've made it to this point, you'll have been on the most blissful, most delicious (and very tiring) adventure of baby's first weeks. You will have birthed a beautiful baby and soaked up every minute of your lying-in, and will be ready to transition back to "normal" life. But don't worry, that doesn't mean saying good-bye to the glowing, flowing yumminess of early mamahood. It's just the next step in this incredible journey. This chapter is everything you'll need to make these next steps as smooth as possible. In the meantime, continue soaking up this adorable, milky, miraculous, sometimes exhausting, but always heavenly love affair with your baby.

YOUR BODY AFTER BABY

Within several days of birth, most new moms lose between 12 and 16 pounds. That's the weight of the baby plus the placenta, the amniotic fluid, any blood loss, and fluids that your body was retaining during pregnancy. After that, more weight seems to magically fall off. I remember not doing an ounce of exercise and dropping 25 pounds in 5 weeks. That said, the last 10 pounds are no joke. It can take another 9 months for those stubborn pounds to disappear. According to Christina Pirello, it's our body's insurance policy against running out of food. Because our system never got the memo that we can now get meals on demand, it instinctively holds on to some of the extra weight to make sure we could still produce milk if famine were to strike.

Even though your body might seem like it's returning to its original prepregnancy shape, there'll inevitably be a few small alterations. Not only will your boobs grow, but your back and hips—which widened to accommodate your growing baby—might keep their postpregnancy shape.[70] Embrace it! You are a beautiful, sexy mama. I have so much more respect for my body now after carrying my baby and delivering him into this world. So what if you're 5 or 10 pounds heavier after your baby is born?! If you're taking great care of yourself, your body will do exactly what it needs to do to support you with love. And when you're ready to get back into the world—and out of stretchy pants—it'll be ready to get moving.

Three months after Bear was born, after enough people had asked me when I was due (jerks!), I was ready for a change. Up until that point, I was happy with my new shape—I was enjoying my new big boobs—and I was so enthralled with Bear that I felt like a mommy goddess. But now I was in this weird in-between stage where my regular clothes still weren't working nor was most of my maternity gear. First, I added a few new pieces from my favorite "vintage" go-to sources, and then came to terms with the inevitable: I needed to start exercising.

Exercise and Weight Loss

The gentlest and safest way to lose baby weight is to eat as cleanly and kindly as possible, nurse your baby, and slowly—when you're ready—start moving again. But gentle exercise is an important part of the equation. Though you may not be eager to pull on your workout clothes, that postpartum movement is an amazing tonic that boosts your sanity, puts a bounce in your step, makes you more alert, calms your mind, and sharpens your focus. And what's good for you is good for baby. Because when mama can run and jump and tussle and lift and throw and cuddle all day long instead of wasting all that precious time feeling sick, fat, and tired, that's good parenting!

The important thing to gauge before doing exercise is whether your body has fully recovered from birth. Consult your caregiver, but usually 10 days is the absolute minimum amount of time you want to wait, with 6 weeks being ideal. Even then, keep your movement practice gentle, like walking with your baby in a sling. Although you'll be burning calories, moderate exercise won't negatively affect your milk production.[71] One thing to keep in mind, however, is that working out immediately after nursing is much more comfortable because your breasts won't be as full.

When starting up your movement practice again, ideally you should find something you enjoy—and something you can do with baby! I loved going for long walks with Bear, and even doing chores and tidying up with him in the Ergo helped the weight melt off. The goal is to be moderately active for at least 30 minutes a day. Or try the Baby-Love Workout (page 262).

Don't be overly hard on yourself at first. Like me, you'll get to a point where you'll think, "You know what? I'm ready." Maybe you'll get mad at your jeans, or maybe you won't love what you see in the mirror, or maybe you just want a good energy boost. But regardless, don't stress about rushing back into things. Let this part of the journey unfold at its own leisurely, natural pace.

Baby-Love Workout

A friend of mine sent me a YouTube video of someone doing these exercises, and I loved the idea of it. These simple moves make a fun—and convenient—game out of exercising. Sneak in a few sets of 15 throughout the day. It's sweet playtime for baby and getting-strong time for you.

- Lay baby faceup on the floor and do pushups directly over her, pausing at the bottom each time to give her a kiss.

- Put baby in the sling or carrier and do walking lunges around the house.

- When baby is old enough to sit up, put her on your lap as you lie back with bent knees, feet on the floor. Push your feet into the ground and lift your hips for a simple bridge pose that's also a fun ride for baby. Hold for a few seconds, then slowly lower your butt until your back is flat on the floor.

Or try these yoga poses that come from inspired yogi Desi Bartlett, who helps mamas rediscover their physical strength while bonding with baby. Baby-and-me yoga is amazing because it strengthens and tones muscles that were stretched during pregnancy, opens tight chest muscles (a side effect of breastfeeding and always curling up around baby), and tones the upper arms. Plus, there's all the time you get to spend connecting with your baby, who as Bartlett will attest, are natural yogis and gifted little teachers themselves. Just watch your baby giggle and squirm and you'll always be reminded to live freely in the present.

Flying Baby: Place your baby with his torso on your shins, draw your knees toward you, and then straighten your legs.

Boat Pose: Lift your legs to a 45-degree angle (you can bend your knees to modify) with your upper body leaning back, so that your body forms a V shape. Make sure to pull your shoulders down your back and keep your back straight. Rest your baby's back against your thighs and feel the strength in your belly as you hold your little one.

Tree Pose: Place your baby on your right hip as you lift your left foot to the inside of your standing leg, just above or below the knee. Press the foot and standing leg together to find a deep sense of inner and outer balance.

SEX AFTER BABY

I'm willing to bet that sex won't be the most appealing prospect in the world for at least the first 6 weeks—if not longer. That's okay! Don't worry if you're not feeling like a seductress, and definitely don't feel pressured to get it on—just take care of yourself. If you're not sure whether you're ready to start having sex again, do some gentle exploring. Using a light oil, tenderly massage your vaginal and perineal tissues. This will help them gain flexibility and also let you gauge whether they're—or you're—ready for someone else's touch.

And remember that it's not just about the nookie—intimacy changes after you have a baby. There isn't the luxury of lying around all afternoon and making love! I sometimes wanted nuzzle sessions with my husband after Bear was born, but I'd be *sooo* tired from the new crazy sleep schedule and from work that once we'd get in the moment, we'd end up snuggling then slipping into a delicious nap. I'd curl up on his chest and wake up in a little puddle of drool. It was intimate and nurturing in its own way.

Kinder Birth Control

While breastfeeding can be a natural contraceptive (the same prolactin hormone that stimulates milk production also prevents the release of eggs), 1 in 50 women will still get pregnant if they're relying on nursing as their primary method of birth control.[72] Not such great odds! The most natural method of birth control is to tune in to your cycle. In Chapter 5 ("Get Your Box in Check," page 58), we talked about how by listening to your body's rhythms you can chart your peak fertility. Just as you can use this method to get pregnant, it's also effective when used for birth control. Your cycle might be a little cuckoo right after you have a baby, but once you get your first period, you can start taking your daily temperature and checking your mucus. Check out Margaret Nofziger's *A Cooperative Method of Natural Birth Control* for much more info on how to do it. In the meantime, opt for condoms over methods that affect your hormones (the Pill, IUD). Condoms are the safest way to babyproof the baby house dressed up with Blossom Organics' amazing vegan lube. Check out Sir Richard's Condom Company and Glyde, two of the only brands making all-natural, vegan rubbers. You support their initiative to donate one condom to a developing country for every one that's purchased.

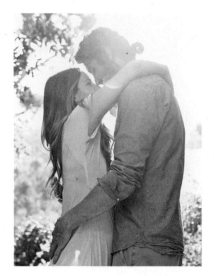

For Gentlemen Only: Bringing the Sexy Back

As your partner heals and gets some much-needed rest, know that she wants to rekindle that intimate connection just as much as you do. Embrace this time as an opportunity to woo your wife all over again. Really court her and make her feel special, and when you do finally go all the way, be gentle and slow. To be in charge of rebuilding your romance is probably the sexiest thing you could do for your woman right now.

Being kind and gentle out of the bedroom is important, too—you'll be setting a healthy example for your baby. When Christopher kisses me, Bear thinks it's cool, and then he'll kiss me, too. Sometimes, though, he doesn't want to share! The important thing is that he learns from Daddy how to be affectionate, and it's incredibly beautiful.

GETTING A LITTLE HELP

Remember when you were preparing for those blissful weeks after baby arrived, rallying your support network to lend a hand? Transitioning back to everyday life is no different. As strong and capable as we mamas are, there will come a point in every single one of our journeys when no matter how hard we push, how hard we fight, and how much we don't want to admit it, we need help. And that's okay. If we were still living in tribes, we wouldn't be having this discussion. You'd simply hand your baby over to the next mama with the understanding that you needed to bathe or visit the shaman or maybe just have 5 minutes of solitary peace in your hut. Together, you'd raise a community of babies while still preserving a distinct sense of balance in your life. You could work *and* raise a baby; maintain a sense of self *and* be a parent. Remember, it's not natural to do this all on your own.

Just as you did in the early days, make sure to call on your tribe—friends, family, neighbors—to help in any way they can. And here are other simple ways to get the support you need and protect the sacred space between you and baby:

Prioritize

Cutting back on some of the clutter in your life—including emotional and professional—might make all the difference between full-on mama meltdown and finding a little peace for yourself even without an extra set of hands. When it comes to paring down to life's essentials, there's only one tool to have in your arsenal: saying no. If an obligation/event/favor/job doesn't bring you joy, peace, happiness, necessary income, or otherwise fill your heart or change the world, then it's not worth taking the time or energy away from yourself or your baby.

A practice that's been a real lifesaver for me is setting aside big chunks of time throughout the day to do nothing but be a mom—no multitasking! We both get the gift of a scrumptious, uninterrupted love marathon. Make being a present, focused parent a priority, especially if it's only for a couple stretches of time a day. Not all of us can spend all day, every day soaking up our babies, so make the time and make it count.

Don't Underestimate the Papas

We want to be sexy, feminine partners, but we also want to make sure everything gets done right (we know best, after all!). We want to have total control over raising our babies, and yet we also want to bring home the tofu. But if we're so busy being both the woman *and* the man in our relationships, how is the man supposed to be the man? He can't!

One beautiful thing that happened in my relationship with Christopher after Bear was born was that I learned to back off (well, that's still a work in progress). I was balancing a ton of projects and deadlines and being the mama and it was so much pressure. One day, I had a toddler tantrum. I felt like I was doing everything all by myself, and that there wasn't enough of me or enough time in the day to get everything done on the ever-growing list. Christopher calmly said, "Give me your list." "You can't handle my list!" I said. He took that list and said, "Yes, I can," and I melted. I gave him the things I could delegate. And you know what? He did it! He did it faster and better than I would have. It was such a powerful and confident gesture. Your man can't reach his complete papa potential if you're trying to do it for him. Unless you let him take care of things, he can't be there to help you.

KEEPING KIND IF YOU GO BACK TO WORK

As lovely as it would be to have nothing to do but be with our babies, it's just one of our truths that one day we will likely have to return to work. Or if not work, then the demands of everyday

Hair Today, Gone Tomorrow: Hair Loss after Birth

I had been warned by a few people that this would happen, and I was feeling cocky when it hadn't occurred. But about 4 months after I had Bear, I started to notice some of my hair coming out easily into my hands when I was washing it. I wasn't concerned because I'd amassed so much while pregnant, thanks to naturally higher estrogen levels (and thanks to Mother Nature, who gave me thick hair in the first place). And, of course, thanks to my kick-ass diet, I knew it wasn't the result of some freaky vitamin deficiency. So even though I lost a few strands in the shower now and then, I was still feeling pretty cocky!

It turns out that because your estrogen levels drop after delivery, your body begins to release some of the hair it was clinging to during pregnancy. The amount you're losing should start leveling off within a year.[73] While you can't prevent it from happening, you can try to fend off too much change to your hairline by giving yourself gentle scalp massages to boost circulation, avoiding brushes that might be too rough on your hair, and maintaining your kind lifestyle. In particular, make sure you're getting plenty of biotin, omega-3s, and sulfur-rich foods, which are super-healthy for your mane. Red peppers, garlic, onions, broccoli, Brussels sprouts, nuts, brown rice, molasses, beans, cabbage, whole grains, oats, raisins, cucumbers, avocados, strawberries, alfalfa, and flaxseed oil are your new hair-care arsenal.[74] However, if your hair loss seems excessive—you're developing bald spots or losing big clumps more than 6 months after delivery—then have your caregiver check your thyroid levels, since thyroid hormone deficiency can be a factor.[75]

life. Especially if you love what you do, folding other responsibilities back into the mix is a really delicate balancing act. Believe me, I know busy. As I mentioned before, I'm not being waited on by a staff of hired help while my son is raised by a team of nannies. I am an overscheduled, under-slept working mom. I love my job and all my projects and want to help change the world. These things are my passion. But too much time away from Bear isn't an option for me. I refuse to miss moments in his life, these once-in-a-lifetime experiences. When we are together, it is so sweet and precious. I'm 1,000 percent committed to being a focused parent with him. I love everything about being his mom, from planning his meals to doing his laundry and folding his clothes.

So can you have it all? Yes. Absolutely. However, it is work—beautiful work—but hard work. You'll definitely have to get your priorities straight. And maybe you won't go shopping for a while or get to spend as much time, or any time, noodling around on the computer or socializing or watching TV. But what you can do is make time for your little one, do the best you can, and vow to get better at mastering balance as time goes on.

TAKE TIME FOR YOURSELF, TOO

If you're being a Super-Kind Mama, at some point you'll notice that your personal needs are not being met. It's amazing that you're giving so much of yourself to your baby, and your baby will thank you! But to continue being your best, most nurturing self, it's crucial that you get some of that loving, too. Don't feel guilty. Even the best mamas in the world need time for themselves! Whether it's a day, an afternoon, or a half hour; a time where you send dad and baby out of the house and have a mini-vacation; or anything else that makes your world a better place—a nap, watching your favorite show, reading a book, taking a walk—do what it takes to get back to center.

It's also important to take some time to just be with your partner. Go on a date, ride bikes to dinner, take a yoga class together—anything to maintain the special space that you two share.

LETTING BABY BE BABY: LETTING GO OF DEVELOPMENTAL MILESTONES

Mamas—and some papas—*love* to compare their babies. It's almost like getting first place in the crawling, walking, or talking department secures them early admission to Harvard. Don't be tempted to let them lure you into the baby race! There's an incredibly wide range of "normal" in terms of a baby's development, and it has absolutely no bearing on how smart and talented your child will grow up to be.[76] So why not just let go and enjoy your baby doing his own thing? It's so much more fun that way—and full of the most adorable surprises. Babies who are the product of kind parenting that includes wearing baby often show more advanced motor skills,[77] but there's no reason to go rubbing that in anyone's face.

I had no idea what to expect when it came to Bear's milestones, and I had no idea what any of the developmental "milestones" actually were. I was content letting Bear be Bear and trusted my instincts that because I was giving him everything he needed both inside and out that he would turn out fine. And not just fine—perfect and amazing. Everyone tells me how connected and focused and calm and happy and sweet and loving he is. They call him the kissing bandit! He talks up a storm and runs so fast and is strong and so smart. Not for one second do I get wrapped up in what he "should" be doing.

Here's what Dr. Lawrence Rosen has to say about it: "Child development is not a predictable linear path, and it differs from child to child. I don't like relying on strict milestones because it usually causes more anxiety."

Bottom line: Let your baby be a baby. Stop planning and looking forward, because you'll miss what's right in front of you. Savor it all while it lasts! He will learn everything he needs to learn when he's ready to learn it. And don't worry about things like tummy time or special exercises that encourage motor skill development. By simply being out and about in the world, he'll pick up all the right moves. My friend Connie once came over with her baby, who is 3 months older than Bear. When Yobi scooted up the stairs, Bear, who had never been up the stairs before, was right behind him. Yobi showed Bear how to do it. Just like that.

Dr. Rosen says that most native cultures in which babies aren't constantly barraged with developmental homework tend to have kids who move and walk at much earlier ages than in the United States. Don't overlook one precious moment of your baby's life by focusing on the next stage. We have such little time with them at each step, so drink up each moment while it lasts!

WHEN BABY GETS SICK

No matter how well you and your baby eat, it's inevitable that sooner or later he'll get sick. Christopher and I used to wonder how in the world Bear would get the sniffles, but then we'd realize, how in the world would he not get sick! He's hanging out with other babies, touching all their snot, and you never know what old, crusty food he's going to find in the corner from like 4 days ago. I'm not exactly a germ freak either, so I'm definitely not dousing him with yucky chemical hand sanitizers. Of course, he's never been sick-sick—just feeling a little off from time to time, maybe with a stuffy nose—but then it passes. Because his body is a super-clean, healthy machine, it can defend itself against and flush out all the nasty stuff much more quickly than a baby whose diet isn't as kind. He actually never had to deal with the achy ears, gooey eyes, or rashy bottom that a lot of other babies experience. And he's never had a drop of medicine. But getting a little under the weather is natural. As Dr. Rosen puts it: "Fevers and sickness are part of growing up. They help develop a healthy immune system."

A Kinder Hand Sanitizer

As I've said before, I'm no germophobe. These little critters can help us boost and acclimate our immune systems to a world where things are, well, germy. When we use conventional hand sanitizers to obliterate any and all life-forms that our kids might drag in, we're actually making our immune systems *weaker*. By not challenging our immune systems with germs, our body's defenses might lose the ability to respond effectively when confronted with a real threat. In fact, there's conjecture that our oversanitized ways (in addition to our diet!) are partially to blame for the rise in asthma and allergies.[78] Also, antibacterial products are thought to be the culprits for breeding "supergerms," or bacteria that are resistant to disinfectants and drugs. So in our effort to get as "clean" as possible, we're actually making germs stronger.[79]

Conventional hand sanitizers are super-gnarly. Triclosan, the main ingredient in most antibacterial and disinfectant products, is related to one of the deadliest pollutants out there: dioxin. (It's what's formed when triclosan mixes with water and sunlight.[80]) Studies have linked triclosan to a range of health issues like skin irritation, allergies, and endocrine disruption. Plus, it taints our water and destroys fragile aquatic ecosystems.[81]

A kinder solution: Washing your hands with good old-fashioned soap and water is just as effective for eliminating most germs.[82] Another option is to make Dr. Rosen's recipe for your own hand cleaner using essential oils that have antibacterial properties. Note that this is for mama's use only until your baby is at least 6 months old (younger babies can be sensitive to the essential oils). I've also listed some of my favorite products on my Web site, thekindlife.com.

Natural Antibacterial Spray

Add the following to a 4-ounce spray bottle:

    3 ounces filtered water
    1 teaspoon aloe vera gel
    10 drops each of cinnamon, clove, rosemary, and eucalyptus oils
    20 drops lemon oil

Just like yours, your baby's body is designed to heal. Most of the time, if nurtured with curative foods, rest, and otherwise left alone, it will mend on its own. But ironically, even though most people have been taught to believe that babies should cry it out and deal with soothing their nighttime discomfort on their own, most people will tell you that a sick baby shouldn't have to be sick. Fevers should be brought down with pain relievers, runny noses dried up with antihistamines, rashes alleviated with cortisone creams, and aches and pains remedied with anti-inflammatories. But in reality, a spike in temperature is the body's way of killing viruses, and mechanisms like a runny nose and diarrhea are its way of flushing out the bad guys. Drying up that mucus, lowering the fever, and binding loose stools only means invaders can live longer. And then there's this alarming fact: Most Western medicines are processed by the liver. The boxes, tubes, and bottles on the shelves at your local drugstore are filled with chemicals that are eventually filtered by your baby's liver, which I might remind you is very tiny and fragile. In most cases, those meds aren't necessary. Antibiotics should also be used with care. Sometimes they are truly useful and can save lives, but when we overadminister them, we challenge bacteria to grow stronger and more resistant to treatment.

"We shouldn't be so scared about childhood sickness," says Dr. Rosen. He believes that in many cases, baby's ailments can be cured by more gentle remedies. Of course, if you're ever in doubt of whether baby's illness is serious, don't hesitate to call your doctor. It's all the more reason to connect with a pediatrician you trust isn't going to pump your kid full of drugs at the first sign of discomfort. More often than not, you can make baby well with minimal medical intervention. The key is patience, love, and a few natural remedies to bring her comfort. See "Your New No-Medicine Chest" on page 328 for my favorite natural remedies gathered from healers, Dr. Rosen, and my own mama instincts.

WHEN MAMA GETS SICK

Your baby won't necessarily get sick if you happen to. Assuming you're not taking medication—ask your midwife or pediatrician about what's not safe for nursing—the best thing you can do is continue breastfeeding because those antibodies will keep baby from contracting whatever you have.[83] Your milk supply may decrease during and just after your illness, but it'll build back up again when you've recovered.[84]

Eating clean, nourishing foods and taking it easy are always going to be your life jacket in these situations. If you have a cold or deep chest cough, macrobiotic counselor Warren Kramer

The Vaccine Debate

According to Drs. Roizen and Oz, if your child gets the entire panel of recommended vaccines, that means she's getting 32 shots over 6 years and being injected with 113 vaccine antigens.[85] That's three times as many as what was recommended 20 years ago,[86] and it's a lot of chemicals going into your child's body (including aluminum and formaldehyde!). While there has not been a conclusive study of the negative effects of such a rigorous one-size-fits-all, shoot-'em-up schedule, there is increasing anecdotal evidence from doctors who have gotten distressed phone calls from parents claiming their child was "never the same" after receiving a vaccine. And I personally have friends whose babies were drastically affected in this way.

Vaccines are a very complicated issue. And it's a way too significant one just to rely on the status quo. The best thing you can do is get educated and make a decision that feels best for you. Then team up with a pediatrician who will not only help guide you but also support your choices.

For loads more information, watch Dr. Jay Gordon's vaccinations webinar on his site, drjaygordon.com; read *Vaccinations: A Thoughtful Parent's Guide* by Aviva Jill Romm and *The Vaccine Book* by Dr. Robert Sears; and visit nvic.org.

recommends you avoid baked flour products—especially "dry" foods like crackers, pretzels, bread, rice cakes, etc., because they can make your condition worse—as well as strong sweets for 3 to 4 weeks. He recommends having miso soup at least four to five times a week in addition to lots of lightly cooked vegetables, especially leafy greens, every day. He also suggests doing a daily body scrub (page 57) to help your system flush out unwanted visitors.

TEETHING

Contrary to reputation, the teething stage of your baby's life doesn't have to be not some kind of shrieking, freak-out nightmare. By continuing to keep your baby's food clean and kind, you can help her make a more gentle transition, which usually starts between 5 and 9 months until all 20 teeth emerge.[87] Teething signs include excessive drooling, swollen gums, irritability, and a slight fever.[88]

By the time Bear was teething, he'd let me know he was a bit uncomfortable every now and then, but he certainly didn't display any of the banshee howling that I'd heard about. If I ate any sugar and passed it on to him through the boob, though? Then it was on. Between keeping baby's system even-keeled with nurturing foods and some simple soothing tricks, this stage will be calmer for everyone.

Bring your diet into balance. If baby's having pain with teething, then mama might need to adjust what she's eating. Go easy on the sugar. Instead, try milder remedies like carrot juice, *amasake,* some cooked fruit, or Sweet Calming Kuzu (page 297).

Give baby the boob. Breastfeeding is the best remedy for teething discomfort. It's soothing and gives baby something to do with her mouth.

Rub baby's gums. Use your finger or a cloth to gently stimulate the offending area.

Give baby something to chew. Any household item that's not a choking hazard or made out of any of the nasty substances like soft plastic that we talked about in Chapter 10 will suffice. Bear loved gnawing on a toothbrush when he wasn't trying to (adorably) gnaw on me.

Try something cold. The cooling sensation is really pleasant. Ice in a baby sock works wonders. Or try a washcloth fresh out of the freezer.

SHOULD MY BABY BE IN THE SUN?

There are few things more delicious than soaking up warm sunshine with your little nugget—and it's good for you, too! It's emotionally healthy and physically healthy, and according to Dr. Rosen, safe for babies and kids. Indirect sunlight or short periods of direct sunlight—15 to 30 minutes a day for little ones—is great. More than that, however, can be too much for baby. So if you're at the beach, the pool, or otherwise out and about on a bright day and will be in the sun for more than 30 minutes, keep her in the shade or bring a hat. Even though these measures offer enough protection, you can also use sunscreen if it gives you peace of mind. According to Dr. Rosen, it's a myth that it's not safe to use sunblock or sunscreens for babies younger than 6 months. Just make sure it's a natural, nontoxic one—which is especially important for babies because of their extra-absorbant skin. Anything you'd use for yourself—like zinc oxide or titanium dioxide creams—is perfectly fine to share with little ones. Go to my Web site for a list of my favorite brands.

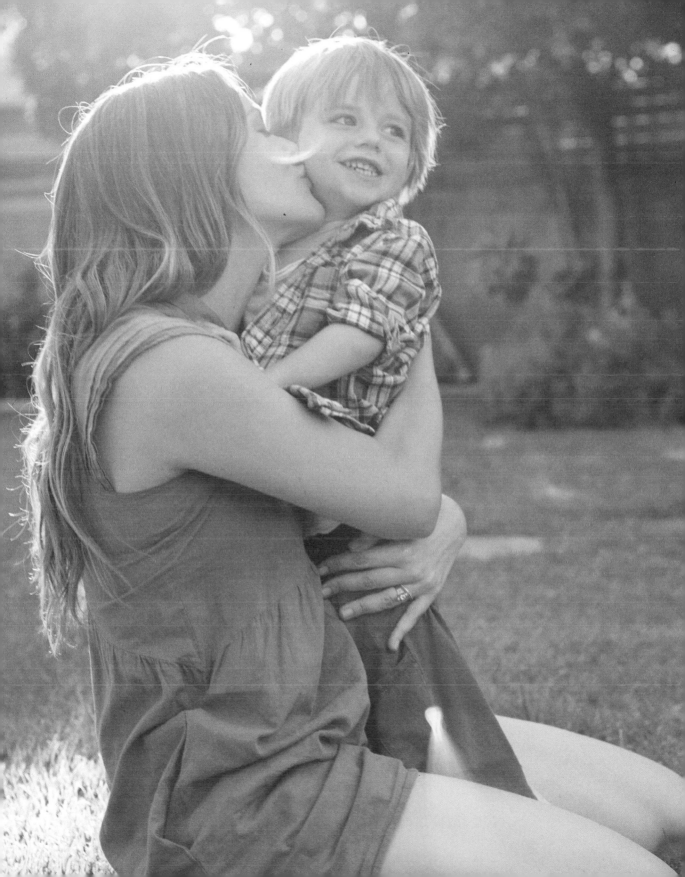

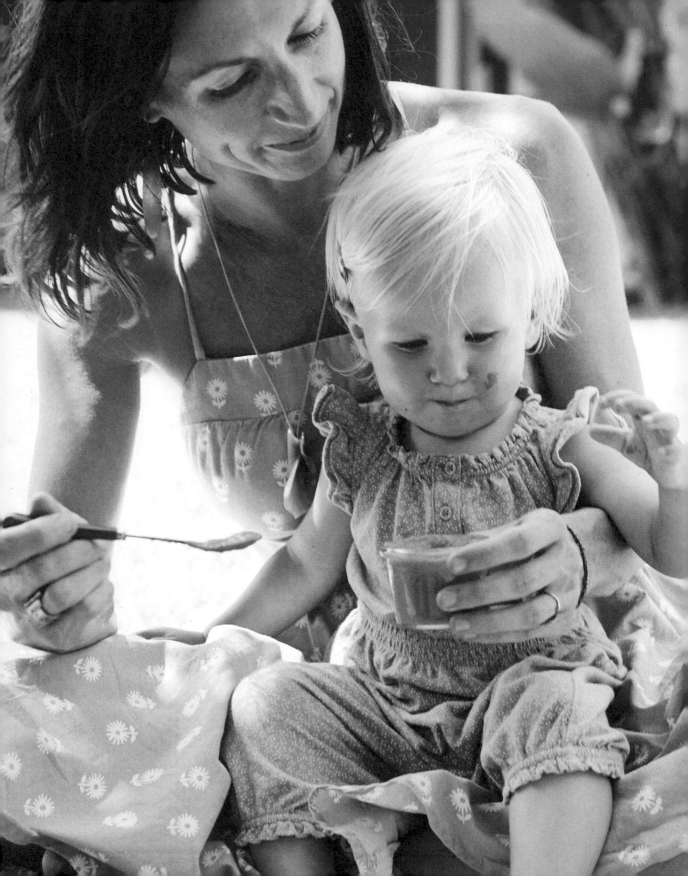

17

Baby's First Food

It's hard to believe, but one day your baby—that itsy-bitsy peanut who once couldn't so much as find her own little thumb—will want and need to start eating solids. The great news is that you already know all about the scrumptious, nurturing, superpowered foods that will give your baby the best possible head start. What's kind for you is most certainly kind for baby!

And guess what? Babies *love* food! Even better, they love planty, leafy, nourishing foods, the very same ones that you're eating. I'll tell you why certain grains and vegetables are the perfect first foods and how all the experts agree, but what's more important is that I can attest to how well Bear's done eating these things. He eats grains every day. He loves tofu and beans and veggies, and at times has been *obsessed* with cabbage. What kid on the planet is asking for cabbage for breakfast?! Before you think for 1 second that he's this sad, deprived little boy whose terrible mommy won't give him "fun" food, know that before we sit down and eat, this kid is *howling* for his cabbage or tofu or rice. That's because when you feed your baby kind foods from the start, you're not only setting up his nutrition for later, you're also setting up his taste buds. You're getting him excited to try new flavors and textures. Believe me, babies don't come out of the womb only wanting to eat Cheerios and chicken fingers! And when they grow up, if they start sneaking naughty treats when you're not looking (though many kind kids don't!), at least you know that their growing bodies were built out of the best stuff there is.

The flip side is that all the nasty foods we mention in Chapter 4 are particularly bad for little bodies. They've been linked to everything from diabetes and childhood obesity to allergies and ADHD, which is not a foundation for a happy, healthy life. So many little ones are growing up on bad food—maybe because it's the norm or maybe because their parents thought it'd be "easier." But these kids are jacked up on sugar, spazzing out and making life for Mom and Dad more difficult. And most sadly of all, they don't feel good.

The first 7 years are the most important of our lives in terms of healthy development. That's why it's so crucial that we feed our babies the most nourishing foods possible and set them up to want to eat well. Here are a few more of my favorite reasons for keeping things balanced and kind for baby:

It keeps baby healthy. Kind foods protect the body by making the immune system vibrant and strong. As your child starts eating more solids and less breast milk (though hopefully not for a while!), you'll still be giving him the best protective shield possible. Plus, these foods are good for circulation, keeping the heart strong, enhancing the quality of the blood, creating strong teeth and bones, and giving growing brains a megaboost by helping with concentration and focus.

It keeps baby happy. Kind foods are calming. They're gentle on the digestive system and keep little bodies humming along in a harmonious way, which means babies can feel more relaxed and at peace—it can be the difference between a cranky baby and a blissed-out one.

It's giving baby food that's alive. Plants are bursting with life-giving goodness. They're packed with energy and nutrients to meet your baby's growing needs. You can't say the same for animal foods or powdered concoctions.

WHEN SHOULD I START SOLIDS?

Your baby doesn't need food before she's 6 months old. And don't just take it from me—listen to the American Academy of Pediatrics, World Health Organization, UNICEF, and American Academy of Family Physicians. They all recommend that babies be exclusively breastfed for the first 6 months of life.[89] The reasons they give are:

It gives baby greater protection from illness. Even though baby will continue getting the amazing immunities from breast milk after he eats solids, the most impactful immunity happens when a baby is exclusively breastfed.[90] Plus, the early introduction of solid foods has been linked to an increased risk of diabetes, eczema, and celiac disease.[91]

It gives baby's digestive system time to mature. Introducing solids too early can cause baby a lot of discomfort, such as digestive upset, gas, and constipation.[92]

It helps protect baby from iron-deficiency anemia. Consider the alternative: Giving baby iron supplements or iron-fortified foods, especially during the first 6 months, can affect how well baby naturally absorbs iron.[93]

It keeps baby from being obese.[94] Introducing solids too early has been linked to increased body fat and weight in childhood.[95]

It helps you maintain your milk supply. Simple supply and demand—the more you're nursing, the more you're making and the longer you can give your baby this precious resource. Babies who eat solids early tend to wean prematurely.[96]

Look to your baby for cues and wait until he shows an interest in food. Otherwise, what's the point? While making food for baby is fun and rewarding, it's one more thing to do, and let's be honest, there's only so much time in the day. If he can hold his head up and sit upright, and starts stuffing his hand in his mouth, grabbing at what you're eating, or mimicking you when you're chewing, then he's probably ready to get started.

But My Pediatrician Recommended Supplementing So My Baby Will Sleep through the Night!

"Do not think that early solid food feeding will help them sleep better or make them happier babies at 4 months. Or that they'll grow better," says Lawrence Rosen, MD. "Plus, there's clear data showing that solid feeding before 4 months is an absolute no-no. There's a higher risk of allergies." He concludes that exclusively breastfeeding until 6 months is most desirable and typically recommends introducing solids before the 9-month mark.

What If My Baby Wants Food before 6 Months?

Pediatricians like Dr. Rosen agree that easing your baby into foods other than breast milk is fine just shy of the 6-month mark. So long as baby can hold his head up and sit upright, and it's not earlier than 4 months, then it's okay to honor these not-so-subtle demands.

Conversely, some babies aren't so keen to embrace something new. After all, a spoonful of mush is a far cry from mama's soft, warm boobie. Don't worry and definitely don't force it. For now, food is really just an extra treat—something to pique baby's curiosity about eating and prepare her taste buds for what's to come. If it's not happening naturally, then it wasn't meant to be yet. Feeding your baby shouldn't be a chore. It's one more fun and special thing you share.

SO WHAT SHOULD I FEED BABY?

Your Baby's New Menu

These foods are just as healing and nourishing for baby as they are for you. Here are the highlights:

Grains and vegetables: Sound familiar? Just as these foods are the foundation for your diet, they'll also help get baby off to a thriving, healthy start. We'll talk more specifics on how these foods can best be introduced—namely in grain milk and porridge—in the sections to follow.

Brown rice syrup: A naturally processed sweetener made from sprouted brown rice, it's mildly sweet and gentle on the body, which makes it perfect for adding to baby's first meals.

Barley malt: This is just like brown rice syrup only it's made from sprouted barley and has a maltlike flavor. It has protein and also helps relax digestion.

Kombu: As we talked about at the beginning of your journey, veggies from the sea are nutrient-packed gems. They are full of essential minerals and can strengthen the blood. To give your baby's grain milk a boost, add a small piece of kombu when cooking the grains. A little goes a long way, though, so you only need to do this about every other time you prepare the recipe. Another great sea veg is wakame, which is rich in protein, iron, and magnesium. You can add this when making miso soup. Even though your baby might not be able to chew these veggies, he still gets the nutrient goodness that infuses into whatever's being cooked with them.

Miso: Miso has live enzymes that are amazing for digestion, the immune system, the heart, and the blood—all while delivering protein, iron, vitamins, and minerals. What I like to do is make a batch of miso soup for myself (see recipe on page 295), then add 2 teaspoons of it to a bottle with about ½ cup of water. At the 6-month mark, your baby only needs a few teaspoons of soup a few times a week to reap all the benefits and not get overloaded on salt.

Kuzu: This root is great for digestion, supports the immune system, relaxes the muscles, and is strengthening and balancing for the whole body. You can usually find it ground into starchlike lumps. Sweet Calming Kuzu (page 297) is great to introduce to baby in addition to solid foods. It works to alkalize baby's intestines and will help baby's tummy during this transitional time when he's eating his first nonboob fare.

Sesame seeds: These are so good for baby and can be given daily. They have five times as much iron as meat, and they're a major source of calcium. Plus, they taste super-delish and add richness and texture to any dish. I toast these guys up then mash them with a mortar and pestle. You can also introduce baby to tahini, which is a sesame seed paste. Adding ½ teaspoon of this or 1 teaspoon of ground toasted sesame seeds to soft grains before sieving them into milk is a great way to add more flavor and nutrients.

Kukicha tea: This tea is made from the roasted twigs of the tea bush, so it has a nice, rich, earthy flavor. And since the caffeine is stored in the leaves, kukicha barely has any. This makes

The Powdered Food Myth

There are people out there who will tell you that, like formula, powdered cereal is the perfect food because it's made specially in a lab to suit all your child's needs. This myth took off in the 1950s, when baby food companies started loudmouthing about how easy these cereals were to digest—easier than anything you could make at home! But according to David Ludwig, MD, director of the Optimal Weight for Life program at Boston Children's Hospital, "There's no scientific basis for this recommendation. That's a myth."[97] Plus, a lot of these cereals are white rice based. That means that most of the fiber, vitamins, and other nutrients have been stripped out and then added back in artificially. This nutritionally naked rice—plus the flour that's usually added, too—turns to sugar in the body almost immediately, which raises blood sugar and insulin levels.[98] It's baby's first junk food! There are brown rice versions out there, but because even these products have been so processed, the best choice is whole grains.

it a perfect offering for babies, especially because it can calm digestion, ease colic, and relax the body. Just a few drops can be therapeutic while also alkalizing the blood, delivering calcium, and strengthening the body's systems. Add a little to Grain Milk (page 321) for a healing and tasty boost or dilute some with water in a bottle. The easiest way to make the tea is to buy the prepared bags. If you're making a cup for yourself, you can also add a little lemon or brown rice syrup every once in a while.

Grain: Why It (and Not Sweet Vegetables or Fruit) Is the Perfect First Food

According to macrobiotic wisdom, whole grains are what will lay the strongest foundation for your baby's health, with veggies coming in a close second. As Warren Kramer attests, soft grain strengthens the intestines from the very beginning while being gentle enough on your baby's still-developing system. Grains like brown rice, whole barley, whole oats, wheat berries, spelt, and whole rye are the best to start with because they break down so easily into glucose. It's the fuel we run so efficiently on, and it's the stuff that's going to help your baby's brain develop. Plus, grains are mildly sweet, which is important since baby is used to your sweet breast milk.

For those reasons, the porridge variation of Grain Milk (page 321) is the perfect first food for baby. It's both easily digestible and nourishing, and it's 100 percent better than the popular powdered cereals out there, which are mostly sugar and white rice or another refined grain. As Dr. Rosen says, "Nobody's first food should be a white powdered food!"

As for sweet veg and fruit, it's common that your mother-in-law/pediatrician/friend will recommend giving your baby foods like bananas, sweet potatoes, or avocados as a first food. The reason most often given is that babies will reject more bitter vegetables in favor of their sweeter, richer cousins. But, when you're giving your baby a wide variety of veggies from the get-go, everything is pretty easy from then on. You're not only setting up their nutrition for the rest of their lives, but you're also introducing their palate to a whole spectrum of flavors, not just sweet.

Even though fruit is a plant, the trouble is it contains fructose, a sugar. Bananas in particular, though rich in vitamins, are a naughty food for baby and should be had in moderation. They're kind of like baby's first soy ice cream: sugary and sweet, making veggies like bok choy or green beans seem less tasty. And according to macrobiotic wisdom, they can make the digestive system sluggish. Sound too New Agey? I assure you that when Bear eats bananas, he gets diarrhea. Period. His system is strong, and then he has a banana and it gets all soft. Avocados should also be a less frequent fixture on the menu. I know babies go nuts for them—Bear loved the tiny dab of guacamole I gave him when he was 5 months old and making googly eyes at a party—and they're full of good fats, but try to keep it to two to three times a week because otherwise it can steal the spotlight from the other veggies on the plate. If you feel that offering avocado even a few times is distracting baby from the main veg attraction, scale back.

Now, I'm not antifruit—and Bear *loves* him some fruit—but I don't go out of my way to give it to him. I know those apples and blueberries find their way into his little mouth one way or another. But we consider it a sweet little treat, not a way to get vegetables into his system. If you're giving your baby vegetables from day 1, then you never need to hide anything!

Bottom line: Make fruits a treat for special occasions. Considering the alternatives, how great is it that a banana can be as exciting as a cookie?! And it's relaxing for babies to have a little fruit. Bear gets 1 cup a day, which is just enough to keep him satisfied and not enough to upset his digestive system. Fruit's also a great negotiating tool for when your baby gets older. They'll forget those birthday party cupcakes even existed when you whip out fresh blueberries!

STEP 1: INTRODUCING GRAIN

Use Grain Porridge for easing baby into new foods. For his first meal, we made Bear brown rice and barley porridge and fed it to him with a spoon. It didn't all land in his mouth, but it was fun!

Keep in mind that the amount baby takes won't be more than a few teaspoons. At this point, it's really more of a fun thing to see babies eating food than it is giving them nourishment to completely sustain them. Since you're still nursing, you know your little one is getting all the nutrients she needs from your milk. For now, the boobs are the main event and everything else is just frosting on the boobie cupcake.

STEP 2: HERE COME THE VEGGIES!

After a few days of grain porridge adventures, your baby is ready to become an official member of the veggie-loving tribe. The best way to introduce this whole new world of flavors is by incorporating them into the grains. Check out my recipe for Baby's First Veggies on page 323—and find all the tools you'll need on page 284.

Great options to start with include kale, summer squash, string beans, corn, watercress, onions, leeks, parsnips, turnips, and peas. You can also introduce cauliflower, broccoli, and cabbage, but start by cooking and offering them on their own, just to make sure they aren't making baby too gassy. If they're well cooked, they're usually fine. When playing with sweeter varieties like winter squash, carrots, and sweet potatoes, make sure you're incorporating greener veggies too, like kale, watercress, or green beans. I didn't prepare these sweeter foods for Bear until he was a bit older because I wanted him to love his greens first. For a while, he was a maniac for kale and bok choy and cabbage and wouldn't touch the sweeter options, but now he loves them all.

Babies, just like adults, dislike eating the same thing every day. And they *definitely* have preferences. Introduce a wide range of new flavors and combinations. Most babies prefer sweeter-tasting vegetables like carrots, sweet potato, and squash—and these are fine to include—but make sure you're also getting in those greens. If your baby's not sure he loves a vegetable, don't try to force it. Babies change their minds all the time. Just offer the veg again in a week or so, and if they're like Bear, they'll soon be big fans of just about anything they can get their hands on.

Homemade: Healthy and from the Heart

These days, it's seemingly a cinch to feed yourself and baby. All you have to do is go to the store (or maybe shop online) and stock up on all kinds of packaged foods that come in bottles, bags, jars, and boxes. The packaging might advertise how "fresh" or "all natural" it is, it's probably pretty inexpensive, and best of all, it makes food shopping and meal prep a piece of cake. Totally ideal for the new mama, right? Well, not exactly.

Remember when we talked about processed food in Chapter 4? The same rules apply to factory-made foods that are prepared for baby. Anytime a plant has to make the transition from the soil to a package that can sit on shelves for weeks or months, most if not all of its nutritional identity is lost. A lot of these foods, particularly jarred baby foods, are made at such high heat that any vitamins once in that all-natural, organic container of butternut squash have been nearly obliterated (and then added back in artificially).[99] That's not taking into account any preservatives, additives, or stabilizers that might be tagging along for a shelf life–boosting ride. And then there's the sweeteners that are sometimes added— even the super-nasty ones we talked about in Chapter 4, like aspartame, sucralose, and saccharin.[100] (Aspartame is particularly to be avoided given the growing brains of children.[101]) Artificial sweeteners are not only terrible for your baby's health, but they can also skew your little one's taste buds. So if you start your baby on processed food, she might later turn her nose up at the actual plant version.

And if you've ever compared the consistency of a jar of food that's been industrially manufactured to the real thing, it doesn't even come close. Those peas look like sad, soupy pudding compared to the rich, creamy, and naturally lumpy goodness of hand-mashed. Plus, think about the fact that 30 percent of American's household waste is packaging— much of it food related[102]—and that in 1 year American families throw out more than two million tons of glass food containers, including baby food jars.[103] There are not enough arts and crafts projects in the world that can put that many jars to good use again!

Here's a simple solution to all of this: Make your own baby food. It's the easiest, most satisfying, and peace-of-mind-giving way of getting your baby food that's the absolute most delicious and nutritious. When you prepare baby's meals instead of scooping them out of a package, you have total control over what ingredients are going into her growing body. And you aren't littering the planet with more unnecessary waste! You can give your baby food that you're also feeding yourself, which is setting the stage for sacred and communal family mealtimes. Believe me, you aren't going to feel like a homesteading martyr, sweating over the stove, barefoot, with a baby on your hip. It's not as much work as you think it might be, yet it's a million times more rewarding than serving store-bought.

That said, if you're on the go or really in a pinch, there are some better packaged brands out there. The HappyFamily/HappyBaby brand uses organic ingredients and isn't bogged down with preservatives. Though watch out for products that contain cane sugar.

WHY ORGANIC MATTERS FOR BABY

If you thought buying organic was important for yourself—and it most certainly is!—multiply those reasons by 10. That's because the nasty chemicals used to grow conventional produce are up to 10 times more toxic to children's growing bodies than they are to adults.[104] According to the EPA's Guidelines for Carcinogen Risk Assessment, children are exposed to 50 *percent* of their lifetime cancer risks in their first 2 years of life, and research done by both the FDA and eight of the leading baby food companies has led the CDC to single out as one of the main sources, not exposure to industrial pollutants or hazardous waste, but our *food*.[105] Blood samples taken from children ages 2 to 4 showed that the concentrations of these pesticide residues are six times higher in children eating conventionally farmed fruits and veggies than in those whose parents gave them organic.[106] Yet another study tracked children who ate conventional foods over just a 3-day period, and those poor little ones had nine times more pesticide traces in theirs systems than kids who ate organically during that same period—an amount that exceeded what is considered safe by the EPA.[107]

These toxic cocktails affect how our babies grow and thrive. The first 3 years in a child's life are when his brain is undergoing significant development. Because your baby's noodle uses 60 percent of the total nutritional energy he consumes, that brain of his is literally using what he eats as building blocks.[108] If you're feeding him pesticide-ridden foods, those pesticides are poisonous to brain cells.[109] These same chemicals—namely organophosphate pesticides (OP), which account for half of the insecticides used in the United States—have been linked to behavior disorders, learning disabilities, developmental delays, and motor dysfunction.[110]

(continued)

YOUR BABY FOOD TOOL KIT

For making food: When I first started making Bear's food, I used a sieve, a food mill, and a mortar and pestle, and I still remember how precious it felt to be doing that. I could have used a blender—it wouldn't be the end of the world if it means giving my baby the best food possible. But to my mind, that takes almost as much time as using these hand tools when you factor in rounding up all the pieces, plugging it in, and cleaning it. I chose not to use a blender or food processor because of the energy these gadgets create when tearing the food apart. It's not calming. It's using something that sounds like a chain saw to pulverize some itty-bitty baby food! Working the food with my hands feels more soothing and full of intention. Plus you won't have to do it forever. Babies only need super-smooth purées for a short time.

For storage: I like to store Bear's food in glass containers in the fridge and use it right away. It might be easier for you to make a bunch in advance and freeze it, which is okay, but less ideal. It doesn't have the same vibrant energy as fresh food, but it's still a million times better than store-bought! Ice cube trays with tight-fitting lids are the perfect serving size for little mouths, so if you're going to go the freezer route, invest in a few BPA- and phthalate-free versions like those from OXO, Fresh Baby So Easy, or KidCo.

For feeding: I prefer tiny sugar spoons instead of plastic, which can contain polyvinyl chloride (PVC) or phthalates and leach into baby's food. Better yet? Use your finger! Babies love that. Or maybe your baby will surprise you one day like Bear did and come after the food you're eating—and try to eat it from your mouth! (And if you're munching on some nishime or anything not too salty or seasoned, it's completely fine to share.)

Which leads me to . . .

AM I CRAZY FOR LETTING MY BABY EAT FROM MY MOUTH?

When Bear was 7 or 8 months old, he was sitting on my lap and we were enjoying our respective meals. All of sudden, he came at my mouth and literally tried to get inside for my food! It was so hilarious and cute! I followed my motherly instinct and took his lead—and it led me to a baby who was curious and excited about the foods I was eating like greens and daikon and rice. It's not how I feed him all the time or something we were practicing; it was just something sweet and funny we did from time to time. That's what all the tribe mamas were doing back in the day. It was either that or risk your kid choking on a big piece of food! They weren't worried about whether their baby would end up perverted or socially awkward or diseased. I remember going to an audition right after I posted the video of my feeding Bear this way, and this director said to me, "Oh, aren't you the one who fed your baby out of your mouth? That's what I used to do with my kids. I'd do it with pizza." Clearly this guy wasn't some hippied-out nut, but he totally got the point. "They'd choke if I didn't do that!" he said.

But just in case you still think I'm nuts, take it from someone far smarter than I am:

"I'm totally with her on this," says Dr. Rosen. "Like a lot of kids, Bear was interested in what Alicia was eating. It's a ridiculous idea that it exposes him to bacteria. Babies are exposed to their mother's bacteria from the moment they're born! There's nothing medical, emotional, *anything* that would worry me about this. If you go to other countries and see what people are doing with bodily fluids—making soup out of placentas, sucking mucus out of a kid's stuffy nose with their mouths—that's all just normal parenting stuff. We get so freaked out about people who are close with their babies in this kind of way. But if it feels all right, and the kid's okay, then whatever." And remember that study we talked about in Chapter 12, the one saying that kids whose parents licked their pacifiers to clean them had fewer allergies, lower rates of eczema, and fewer signs of asthma? That was all thanks to "immune stimulation," or exposure to the friendly cooties that live inside our mouths.''' So there!

Helpful Hints and Tips for Feeding

- At first, introduce new foods when your baby is hungry and in a good mood and when you aren't feeling rushed. Mealtimes should be lovely and fun!

- Offer a very small spoonful at first. Don't worry if your baby is eating only a teeny-tiny amount or isn't really into food yet at 6 months. At this stage, it's more about introductions and less about well-rounded nutrition. Your boobies have him covered.

- If your baby isn't interested in a food the first time you offer it, try again in a couple of days. Babies' tastes change all the time.

- Make sure you're introducing new foods one at a time to identify or rule out anything your baby might not be tolerating well.

- Have family mealtimes! Instead of making baby eat all by himself, get everyone involved. Sure it can lead to *veeeery* long mealtimes, and it's more difficult to get food into your own mouth, but that's what made Bear so excited about food—he couldn't wait to get his hands on what we were eating. When everyone eats together, baby gets to observe and feel included. He learns about different foods and eating customs and your family's own mealtime rituals.

- It's normal for your baby's poops to change color and odor once you introduce solids, even just those tiny teaspoonfuls! If your baby gets constipated—his poops seem too firm or he doesn't go on a daily basis—make sure that the grain milk is thin enough, consider using barley or whole oats to get things moving, and include fiber-rich vegetables.

- Keep up the breastfeeding! Remember that these new foods aren't yet meant to replace your all-nourishing breast milk.

BEYOND 6 MONTHS

If it were up to me, this book would be about 1,000 pages longer and cover every single thing that you're going to experience as your little one grows. But something tells me your head would start spinning! Luckily, there's my Web site, thekindlife.com, where we can continue to share our collective wisdom. In the meantime, I'll leave you with the knowledge and support that you can absolutely raise a kind baby and child.

Some naysayers will accuse you of imposing your beliefs on your little one. To that I say: "Oh, do you mean good health and kindness?" Teaching your child the difference between nasty and kind is not the same as saying, "I hate bananas, therefore you should, too." Your values are not a whim or a thrill; they're the foundation of who you are. To me, it would seem strange *not* to share that with your child. And if you believe that things like animal and processed foods are to blame for a host of illnesses and environmental woes, then why would you give them to your precious baby? As we've talked about time and time again, your job is to protect your child's well-being, and that lies squarely with what children are putting in their bodies.

Thankfully, there's no shortage of expert opinions that support this. Babies, children, kids, teens—none of them benefit from nasty foods. Dr. Spock, the mainstream go-to for all things baby, recommended in his final revision of the classic *Baby and Child Care* that children be fed a plant-based diet. He pointed out that many health problems—heart disease, some cancers, high blood pressure, and diabetes—are largely caused by diet, and, most alarming, that many of these conditions have their roots in childhood. The beginnings of artery changes are often found *before the age of 3*, and by age 12, they are present in *70 percent* of children. By 21, they exist in almost all young adults.[112] That's a crime! Plus there's all the weight problems that are getting worse among our children and are contributing substantially to health-related difficulties later in life.

The Physicians Committee for Responsible Medicine wholeheartedly supports Dr. Spock's wisdom. They, along with the Academy of Nutrition and Dietetics (formerly the American Dietetic Association), contend that a well-planned plant-based diet can clearly meet the nutritional needs of children.[113] The academy says that plant-based eating can "satisfy the nutrient needs of infants, children, and adolescents and promote normal growth."[114] That's because plants are rich in complex carbohydrates, protein, fiber, vitamins, and minerals.[115] Children who are raised on whole grains, vegetables, fruits, and legumes have a lower risk of heart disease, stroke, diabetes, cancer, and many obesity-related illnesses compared to children who are raised on the average American diet.[116] As the PCRM so brilliantly—and tragically—puts it, "Children who acquire a taste for chicken nuggets, roast beef, and french fries today are the cancer patients, heart patients, and diabetes patients of tomorrow."[117]

Food can be just as fast/easy/fun/tasty when it's healthy as when it's not. We can raise a whole new generation of children who grow up demanding something better than "kid food" because kind food tastes better and makes them feel good. All our babies can be screaming for cabbage and mochi at mealtimes! That starts with you, one little spoonful at a time.

As for the rest? Well, that's another book!

A Little Thank You Note

In *The Kind Diet*, I told readers I believed that what we eat could lead to world peace. I know that might sound naïve, but I really meant it. By becoming a Kind Mama, you are contributing in a glowing, constructive, nurturing way. You're helping keep our planet healthy and our animals free from torment. You're setting an example that could inspire thousands of other mamas and mamas-to-be to get in touch with their truth and find a more beautiful way to carry, birth, and raise their babies. You are the new tribe leaders! And you are creating healthier, happier, more present, sensitive, compassionate little beings who know they belong, feel confident, and love themselves. Wouldn't it be nice if the world were filled with people like that? Does world peace sound so far-fetched now?

I hope we can keep in touch as you continue on this journey. Please join me on my Web site thekindlife.com. It's a place where we like-minded mamas can connect, explore, get involved, share, vent, question, and learn. I can pass along all my discoveries as my own baby gets older, and I can in turn learn from you as your little ones navigate this beautiful life. It's a heart-rich space where we can grow together in a meaningful, tuned-in way. So please continue to send me your moving stories and inspirational conquests, and in exchange I'll keep fielding your questions, passing along my breakthroughs, and cheering you on. Come and visit soon! And thank you from the bottom of my heart for making this world a better place for all of our babies.

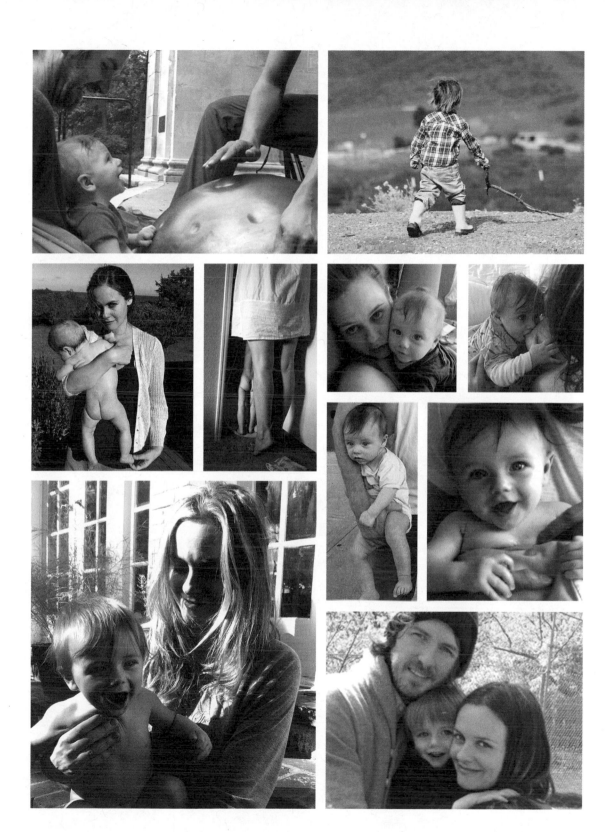

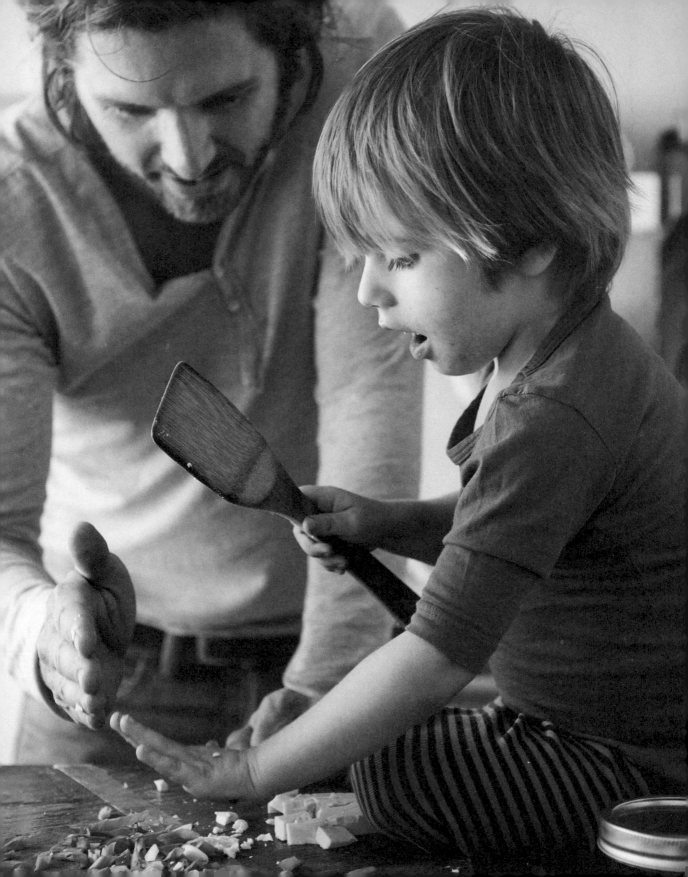

recipes

These are some of my favorite go-to dishes—not just for getting or being pregnant, but for life! From superpowered healing remedies to seriously decadent indulgences, I think you'll find a little bit of everything you're looking for. I've tested them all in my own kitchen, so I can assure you how simple and rewarding every single recipe is to make. Flip through, get inspired, and dig in!

Also, don't forget to check out thekindlife.com for additional tasty options. Or, of course, *The Kind Diet,* a great resource for food and eating in general, with even more incredible dishes to keep you nourished and satisfied.

A WORD ON INGREDIENTS

Cooking water: Yes, the water you cook your food with is an ingredient. That's because whatever's in your water is also what's ending up in your dish. Many of these recipes call for spring water, but please use tap if your water is filtered. Check out the "Clean Food Calls for Clean Water" section on page 46 for simple ways to get the cleanest water possible.

Miso: When choosing a miso, the rule of thumb is that the lighter the miso, the sweeter the taste, and the darker the miso—such as aged varieties—the more salty and savory the flavor. Aged miso is more healing than light miso because of all its concentrated, long-fermented energy. Just make sure you're buying an organic brand that says on the label that it's been naturally aged in wood using traditional techniques. And *definitely* don't buy miso that's been pasteurized. You'll miss out on all the probiotic goodness.

You'll note in the recipes that include cooking with miso that I tell you not to boil it. Doing so kills all the lovely live things that make miso so healthy. Now, if you accidentally boil your big batch of miso soup, don't throw it away! It happens. It sucks. But it's not the end of the world. Just don't make a habit of it!

Salt: Many of these recipes call for sea salt, which is the healthiest option. It contains 80 minerals needed by the human body and reflects the natural composition of our blood, unlike table salt, which has had most of those minerals removed. When shopping for ingredients, look for a salt that's unrefined.

Shoyu: This ingredient gives a dish dimension that salt can't. *Shoyu* is the Japanese word for soy sauce, which is how you'll most likely see it labeled in a health food store. It's made from soybeans, salt, and wheat—that's it. If you see anything else on the label, then keep shopping for a better alternative. A lot of cheaper brands (especially the ones that show up at the table in most

Asian restaurants) contain added sugar, alcohol, and chemical preservatives. So even though you're paying a little bit more for quality, it's worth it. My favorite is Mitoku Sakurazawa, a macrobiotic brand that you can find in some health food stores or sold online by Natural Import Company. Ohsawa and Eden also make good versions. Especially look for those that are traditionally aged for 2 to 3 years versus those that are fermented using chemical methods for only a few months. If you have a gluten intolerance, go with tamari instead, which is made without wheat.

When cooking with shoyu, remember that the really good stuff is unpasteurized, meaning it contains all kinds of friendly bacteria and enzymes. But those guys can only do their probiotic magic if they're left alive. So whenever you heat a dish with shoyu—either when cooking or reviving leftovers—make sure you do it gently, without letting it boil. But as I mentioned in the miso section, don't freak out if you accidentally let your dish boil. It's not ideal, but it's still completely worth eating the dish. Also, go easy on the salt in the recipes until you've tasted the final dish; you'd be surprised how much flavor a high-quality shoyu or tamari offers.

Ume vinegar: Shorthand for "umeboshi plum vinegar," this is the pickling brine from making umeboshi plums. I consider it a pantry must-have because it's tart and salty and crazy tasty sprinkled over steamed veggies and salads or used to add brightness to any dish (but go easy!). You can find it in most health food stores and some grocery stores in the Asian foods aisle.

Note: If you can't find any of the ingredients called for in these recipes at your local health food store, check out these online sources: Gold Mine Natural Foods, Natural Import Company, or the Kushi Store.

Buying organic. It should be assumed that all the ingredients called for in these recipes are organic. After reading the case for going au naturel on page 44, that choice should be a no-brainer, but just a friendly reminder!

Dried versus canned beans? Dried beans take longer to prepare than canned, but it's worth the wait. You don't risk nasty BPA leaching into your food, and it's cheaper! Plus, you don't need to babysit those beans once they're on the stove; you can set a timer and get on with your day while they cook. That said, if it's the difference between not making yourself something healthy to eat and using canned beans, it's okay to take a shortcut every once in a while, even if it's not ideal. But if you do use canned, go with a brand like Eden Foods, which specifically says "BPA free" on its label.

A Few Useful Techniques

Cooking veggies. It's ideal to prepare veggies fresh every day because that way they retain the most vitality-boosting nutritional value. But sometimes, you just have to say, "Screw that!" and make a big batch that'll last you 3 to 4 days. Again, it's not what would happen in the most perfect of perfect worlds, but if it's the difference between getting something healing and nutritious on the plate and ordering in, then go for it!

A note on sautéing. Whenever you sauté veggies, test to see if the oil is hot by adding a small piece of what you're cooking to the pan. It should sizzle. If the pan is too cold before you add your veg, they'll absorb way too much oil, so make sure you get that nice crackle.

Whole grain medley. Mixing grains is a great way to get variety into the rotation. You can blend any type—barley, quinoa, millet—with short or medium-grain brown rice and cook them together. Just remember to keep a basic ratio of about 80/20, so there's a majority of brown rice and 1 cup total (but no need to get super anal about it). Put the grains in a pot, cover them with water, and give them a few swirls with your hand. Drain the water, add 2 cups of fresh water, and if possible, soak the grains overnight. When ready to cook, add a pinch of salt to the pot and bring to a boil over high heat. Cover and turn the heat down as low as it will go. Simmer for 50 minutes, then turn off the heat, let it sit for a few minutes with the lid on, then remove from the pot.

Cooking grains with kombu or salt. You'll see that some of these recipes call for cooking grains with salt, while others call for kombu. Ultimately, it's up to you which you prefer, and it's nice to switch it up for variety's sake. Both carry good-for-you minerals (so long as you're using good-quality sea salt—see "A Word on Ingredients," page 292). But because both kombu and salt add sodium to the dish, make sure you're choosing one or the other.

Quick Tricks

Always make extra grain and bean dishes. I like to cook up enough for a couple of days and then use them as the base for meals, adding things like extra vegetables or other tasty toppings.

Start with a salad as your base. Fill your bowl with rice, then mound on beans, seeds, vegetables, tempeh, some flavorful lettuce like arugula or radicchio—whatever you have a taste for or is in your fridge. Throw in some raisins or pine nuts, walnuts, or almonds. Maybe drizzle the whole thing with some flaxseed or olive oil and umeboshi vinegar or lemon juice. Get creative! Sometimes the tastiest concoctions are the craziest ones.

Wrap leftovers in nori. There's almost no leftover too sad that doesn't benefit from becoming an instant burrito. This technique is great if you need to eat something on the run.

HEALING TONICS

Immune-Boosting Miso Soup   Makes 4 servings

The live enzymes from miso are so good for every inch of your body. Just one bowl can feel like a magical tonic. I recommend having at least one portion a day, four times a week. Miso soup is an incredibly nourishing breakfast! Alongside some grains and greens, it's a light and refreshing way of waking up your system after its nightly fast. And definitely treat yourself to some whenever you feel like you might be getting sick. (One bowl every day until you feel better should do the trick!) To preserve the soup's medicinal qualities, make it fresh or only store the prepared soup for one extra day and try not to boil it.

This soup is the perfect canvas for all kinds of seasonal veggies, but aim for four or five veg max per batch. Additional healing add-ins include dried shiitake mushrooms,* carrots, cabbage, leafy greens, and scallions.

This recipe calls for 6 cups of water, which makes a big batch for your tribe that lasts for a few days. If making this soup just for yourself, halve the recipe.

*When using dried shiitake, reconstitute them in warm water first. I like soaking mine overnight because they get softer and easier to slice. But if you're in a hurry, as little as 15 minutes will do. Then slice them thin.

FOR MAMA

6 cups water

1"–2" piece dried wakame

½ cup diced kabocha squash

½ cup shiitake mushrooms, stems trimmed and tops sliced

½ cup chopped red onion

1 small leek, whites only, halved and sliced into half-moons (about ½ cup) (optional)

2 tablespoons aged barley miso or white, sweet, or red miso; or a combination of the two (see page 292)

2 cups watercress, rinsed well, stems trimmed (just the bits that look a little thicker and more fibrous), and chopped for garnish

In a large saucepan, add the water and wakame. Soak the wakame for 5 minutes, then strain it out (retaining the soaking water) and chop into bite-size pieces. Set aside.

Bring the reserved soaking water to a boil over medium heat. Add the squash, mushrooms, onion, leek, and wakame and reduce the heat. Simmer for about 15 minutes, or until the vegetables have softened slightly.

Meanwhile, put the miso in a small bowl. Ladle in about ¼ cup of the hot cooking water and mix well with a spoon or fork until the miso is completely dissolved.

Add the miso to the pot. Simmer the soup for 2 minutes, then remove the pot from the heat. Garnish each serving with about ½ cup of the watercress and serve.

FOR BABY

Start by adding a couple of tablespoons of the broth mixed with double the amount of water to baby's bottle to dilute since babies and young children shouldn't be having as much salt as we do. Then, as baby grows, begin pulling out the veggies and giving them to him separately on a plate. Bear loved how they'd soaked up all the miso flavor, especially daikon.

Sweet Vegetable Drink   Makes 4 cups

This funky macrobiotic "tea" is a miracle remedy for settling both an upset tummy and a cranky sweet tooth. Drink a warm cup or two every day, if you need it.

¼ cup each: finely minced onion, cabbage, winter squash, and carrot

4 cups water

Place the veggies in a soup pot. Add the water and cover. Bring to a boil over medium heat, reduce to a gentle simmer, and cook for 20 minutes. Strain out the vegetables and store in the fridge.

Soothing Ginger Tea   Makes 1 serving

Whether you're drinking this to quiet an upset tummy, find some postpartum calm, or boost your milk supply, or you're adding it to a bath and using it as a soak for a sore bottom, this simple tea is comforting and lovely.

3″ piece fresh ginger (sliced)

1–2 cups of water

Brown rice syrup or barley malt (if drinking, optional)

Add the ginger to a saucepan with the water. Boil for 20 minutes, then serve and sip at your leisure.

If the flavor is too strong, dilute with more water. Drink the tea as is, or strain out the ginger pieces. Sweeten with a tiny bit of the brown rice syrup or barley malt, if desired.

Sweet Calming Kuzu   Makes 1 serving

If You're Craving: Sweet

Kuzu is a starch made from wild mountain kuzu root—which you can find in most natural and specialty foods stores or online—and it's incredibly strengthening and calming. This tea really does help you relax and brighten your vibe. I have this when I'm a crankypants, and Christopher and I give it to Bear whenever he seems a little off. Sip it a few times a week as a preventive remedy. Be mindful not to drink this too close to bedtime, because it might keep you up.

1 teaspoon kuzu

1 cup cool water

1–2 tablespoons brown rice syrup

In a small saucepan, add the kuzu and water. Let it sit for a moment, then stir until the kuzu is completely dissolved.

Cook over medium heat, stirring constantly so that the kuzu doesn't get lumpy. Once the liquid turns clear, add the syrup and enjoy.

Ume Sho Kuzu   Makes 1 cup

This soothing tea is a magical remedy that wards off colds and flu, strengthens digestion, and generally helps you feel well. It's a little too potent for everyday health maintenance, but any time you feel something icky coming on, drink it three days in a row or however long it takes to feel better. This tea is also nice for tummy issues, especially nausea.

1 heaping teaspoon kuzu (see above— Sweet Calming Kuzu)

½ an umeboshi plum, flesh torn or chopped small

Shoyu (see note, page 292)

Add the kuzu to a small pot with 1 cup of cool water, let it sit for a moment, then stir until the kuzu is completely dissolved.

Add the umeboshi plum to the pot and cook the mixture over medium heat, making sure to stir constantly or the kuzu will get lumpy. Once the liquid has turned clear, add 2 to 3 drops of shoyu. Bring to a simmer for 1 or 2 minutes but don't boil, and enjoy.

Watercress with Creamy Tahini Dressing and Toasted Sesame Seeds Makes 2 servings

If You're Craving: Creamy or Fresh-Flavored Yumminess

This dish is the answer to anyone who doesn't believe greens can be exciting and decadent. Peppery watercress isn't just bright and fresh, it's bursting with folate, calcium, potassium, magnesium, and vitamins A, C, E, and K! Use this veg dish as a side with any meal—even breakfast. It's delightful slathered with the rich tahini dressing, but I highly recommend you try it naked, too, when you're feeling less frisky.

Thick or thin? Try playing around with the consistency of this dressing. By adding a little water, you can take it from a thicker, creamier paste to a lighter vinaigrette.

2 teaspoons black sesame seeds	2 tablespoons sesame tahini
1 teaspoon shelled hempseed	1 teaspoon ume vinegar
½ red onion, sliced into thin rings	1 teaspoon brown rice syrup
1 bunch watercress, rinsed well and stems trimmed (just the bits that look a little thicker and more fibrous)	1½ teaspoons shoyu (see page 292)
	1 teaspoon lime zest, to finish (optional)

In a dry skillet over low heat, gently toast the sesame seeds and hempseed until just fragrant. Remove from the heat and set aside.

Fill a saucepan with water and bring it to a rolling boil. Add the onion and boil for 30 seconds, then remove with a slotted spoon or skimmer. Shake off any excess water and transfer to a bowl. Add the watercress to the boiling water and cook for about 1 minute, or until it just wilts. Scoop it out, shake off the excess water, then transfer it to a cutting board and give it a rough chop before adding it to the bowl with the onion.

Make a dressing by whisking together the tahini, vinegar, syrup, and shoyu, adding a little water if necessary to get to your desired consistency. Drizzle it over the top of the veggies. Sprinkle with the toasted seeds and lime zest (if you're in the mood—it's really nice both with and without) and serve warm.

Chunky Stewed Veggies   Makes 4 servings

Nishime (pronounced *nee-shee-may*) is a humble Japanese vegetable dish. It's calming and centering and incredibly healing for the stomach, spleen, and pancreas. It's like a little hug for your organs, which is why it's ideal to have regularly.

Feel free to mix and match with anywhere between three and five different veggies. Experiment with combinations of kabocha squash, daikon, celery, onion, sweet potato or yam, turnip, rutabaga, snow peas, green cabbage, carrot, burdock root, lotus root, and my new favorites, celery root and cauliflower. Just keep in mind that more delicate, tender veg like snow peas should be added in the last 5 minutes of cooking.

The trick is to use as little water as possible, which helps bring out the sweetness in the veg. The perfect nishime will have little to no water left at the end of cooking. That said, it's kind of a bonus if you do end up with extra liquid because you can turn it into a "gravy." But this dish is completely delicious without the gravy, too.

1 sweet potato (I prefer the white-fleshed variety over the orange, but either works), cut into 1" chunks (about 2 cups)

1 onion, cut into large chunks

2 cups chopped kabocha squash (aim for 1" chunks)

2 postage-stamp-size pieces kombu

1 generous pinch of sea salt

2 teaspoons shoyu (see page 292)

1 teaspoon kuzu

In a large, heavy-bottom pot, arrange the sweet potato and onion along one side of the pot. Add the squash to the other half of the pot, then place a piece of kombu on each side. Top with the salt.

Pour in about a cup of water, or enough to reach ¼" up the side of the pot. Bring to a boil over high heat, cover the pot, and reduce the heat to medium-low.

After 25 minutes, add 1 teaspoon of the shoyu. Cover the pot again and cook for 5 minutes.

Remove the veggies from the pan but leave any remaining liquid and small bits of veg. If you want to make a gravy, add ½ cup water and bring it to a simmer.

In a small bowl, combine the kuzu with 1 tablespoon of the simmering water and mix well before adding it to the pot. Stir the mixture constantly until it turns translucent and thick. Add the remaining 1 teaspoon shoyu, cook for 1 minute more, then pour over the veggies, if desired.

Delicate Steamed Greens with Toasted Sesame Oil Vinaigrette   Makes 2 servings (or if you're like me, 1)

I'm always surprised by how good and fresh and satisfying this simple dish can be. Perfectly steamed veg that are naturally sweet with a drizzle of tangy shoyu and brown rice vinegar. Top all that goodness with rich, nutty toasted sesame or flaxseed oil? Heaven. Below is my favorite combination, but you could try this with other varieties of greens like bok choy, radish tops, and Swiss chard.

2 cups watercress, kale, and Napa or savoy cabbage, cut into thin strips

1 large carrot, cut into matchsticks (see note, page 306)

4 radishes, halved

1 teaspoon shoyu (see page 292)

1 teaspoon brown rice vinegar

Toasted sesame or flaxseed oil, to finish (optional)

Place the watercress, kale, cabbage, carrot, and radishes in a steamer basket and cook over boiling water for 2 minutes, or until they're tender but not falling apart.

Transfer to a serving dish and sprinkle with the shoyu and vinegar, plus a drizzle of oil, if desired. Eat immediately.

AMAZING GRAINS

Sweet Rice, Amaranth, and Apricot Breakfast Porridge   Makes 2 or 3 servings

A piping-hot bowl of cooked grains is a lovely way to start the day. And by making a porridge, you're giving your body a gentler, more digestible way to soak up all that grainy goodness. Sweet rice is the real star here (it's sticky and gooey). Try swapping in other grains for amaranth, like whole barley, wheat berries, or, one of my favorites, rye. Or change up your fruits with prunes or raisins.

If you'd like a more savory porridge, top with a sprinkle of gomasio, shiso powder, or ¼ teaspoon tekka, a condiment made with root vegetables and soybean miso.

¾ cup sweet rice

¼ cup amaranth

3 cups filtered or spring water

2–3 large or 3–4 small Turkish dried apri-

cots, finely chopped

Pinch of sea salt

1–2 tablespoons toasted almonds (optional)

In a large bowl, cover the sweet rice with 2" to 3" of filtered or spring water and soak overnight. In the morning, put the amaranth in a fine-mesh sieve and rinse.

In a saucepan, add the 3 cups water, rice, amaranth, apricots, and salt. Bring to a boil, reduce to a gentle simmer, and cook for 50 minutes.

Give the mixture a stir, take it off the heat, and scoop into bowls. Garnish with the almonds or whatever sounds tasty at the moment.

Fat Fried Noodles   Makes 2 to 4 servings

If You're Craving: Meaty, Hearty, Salty, and Fried

I love these noodles—they're great and way healthier than takeout! Feel free to get creative with any veg that you have on hand or are your favorites. Bok choy, bell peppers, spinach, sprouts—they'd all work here. I like to top the whole thing with some tempeh (especially my all-time favorite teriyaki tempeh from Rhapsody Natural Foods). Practice this one often!

Udon versus soba. According to macrobiotic expert Christina Pirello, it's worth considering your "condition" as an expectant mama when choosing which of these to cook up. Soba, which are made from buckwheat, are a little more contracting in their energy than udon, which are made from wheat. If you tend to be stressed or are battling nausea, then Pirello advises sticking with udon. But if you consider yourself pretty chill and relaxed, then either would work well. When you reach the last 8 weeks of pregnancy, adding in more soba can help channel the right energy for a good labor.

- 1 package (12 ounces) Annie Chun's Japanese-style udon noodles (these send this dish over the top) or 1 package (8 ounces) whole wheat udon or soba noodles
- 1 tablespoon olive oil, toasted sesame oil, or plain sesame oil
- 1 clove garlic, minced or pressed in a garlic press (optional)
- 1 tablespoon fresh ginger, minced (optional)
- 2 tablespoons toasted sesame oil + more for finishing
- 1 onion, sliced into half-moons

- 2 pinches of sea salt
- 8 shiitake mushrooms, cleaned, stems removed, and sliced
- 2 cups carrots, cut into matchsticks (about 2 carrots) (see note, page 306)
- ½ cup red cabbage, sliced thin
- 3 teaspoons shoyu (see page 292)
- ½ cup frozen organic corn or kernels from 1 ear fresh corn
- ¼ cup spring water
- 1 scallion, chopped, for garnish
- Sesame seeds, for garnish

Cook the noodles according to package, then drain and rinse with cold water. Set aside.

Heat the olive oil in a large skillet over medium-high heat until the oil begins to shimmer. Add the garlic (if using), ginger (if using), and onion. Throw the salt into the pan to help draw out the onion's sweet juices. Keep stirring as the aromatics get soft and translucent, about 1 minute. Add the mushrooms and cook until they release their moisture and soften. Toss in the carrots and continue to stir for another few minutes before adding the cabbage. Season with 1 teaspoon of the shoyu and cook for another 2 minutes.

While the pan is still on the heat, heap the noodles on the cooked veggies, then add the corn and the remaining 2 teaspoons shoyu—but don't stir them into the vegetables. Sprinkle in a little of the water, if necessary, to make sure the vegetables on the bottom of the pan don't stick. Reduce the heat to low and cover the pot. Cook for 5 minutes, or until everything cooks together, then remove from the heat. Finish with a drizzle of toasted sesame oil and a sprinkling of scallions and sesame seeds. Serve piping hot or at room temperature.

If you're adding tempeh. If using uncooked tempeh such as Lightlife Smoky Tempeh Strips, add ½ to 1 6-ounce package to a small pan with a bit of water. Cover the pan and steam the tempeh over low heat for 15 minutes. (You could also use a steamer basket over boiling water.) Cut the tempeh into bite-size pieces and add it to the pan with your vegetables. If you're using cooked tempeh such as Rhapsody Teriyaki Tempeh, cut a ½ to 1 6-ounce package into bite-size pieces and either throw it right in with your vegetables to warm it or sear it in a small skillet with a bit of oil and serve it over the top of the dish.

Crunchy-Sweet Quinoa Couscous with Fresh Herbs   Makes 3 or 4 servings

This is one of my favorite grain salads. It's quick, full of bright, herbaceous flavor; and will easily become a staple in your rotation. Quinoa is very high in protein and fiber and also packs some iron. Pair that with protein powerhouse chickpeas, crunchy almonds, and sweet raisins, and you have a seriously rocking dish.

¼ cup dried chickpeas

1" piece kombu

¼ teaspoon sea salt

1 cup quinoa

½ cup raisins

½ cup toasted almond slices or whole almonds, chopped

¼ cup fresh parsley, chopped

½ cup fresh basil, chopped

2 tablespoons olive oil + more for finishing

½ teaspoon Herbamare seasoning, ume vinegar, or sea salt

Squeeze of fresh lemon juice, to taste (optional)

1 teaspoon orange or lemon zest, or to taste (optional)

In a large bowl, cover the chickpeas with 2" of filtered or spring water and soak overnight.

Drain the beans, add them to a medium-size soup pot, and cover with 2" to 3" of water. Bring to a rapid boil and skim any foam that rises to the surface. Add the kombu and reduce the heat to a simmer. Cook for 1 hour, checking every so often to make sure that you don't need to add more water and that the beans have cooked through. The fresher the beans, the longer they can take to cook, sometimes up to 2 hours. About 10 minutes before they're done, add the salt. Remove from the heat, drain, and set aside.

In another pot, cover the quinoa with filtered water and swirl with your hand to give the grains a nice rinse. Drain. Add 2 cups fresh water and bring to a boil. Reduce the heat to a simmer, cover, and cook for 25 minutes, or until all the water is absorbed. Transfer the quinoa to a large mixing bowl to cool.

Once the quinoa has cooled to slightly warmer than room temperature, add the raisins, almonds, parsley, basil, 2 tablespoons oil, and the Herbamare, vinegar, or salt. Finish the dish with a drizzle of oil and a splash or citrus juice or zest, if desired.

Black pepper. If you're entertaining, you can add a pinch of freshly ground black pepper at the end to taste. It's not a super-healing ingredient to have normally—and this dish tastes perfect without it—but if you want to dress it up a little for company (or you are having cravings), go for it.

Millet Mashed "Potatoes" with Mushroom Gravy

Makes 3 to 5 servings

If You're Craving: Hearty, Salty, or Creamy

Millet is such a healthy grain to have in your rotation. It's the base of this rich creamy dish (in addition to a yummy breakfast porridge in *The Kind Diet*).

Choose whichever varieties of mushrooms you like best, or try a combination. Shiitakes have a chewier texture than button mushrooms, so sometimes I'll combine them with creminis (fancy talk for regular button mushrooms), which I love.

You can make this dish pretty with something fresh and green like scallions, parsley, or chives, but it certainly doesn't lack flavor if you go without.

1 cup millet, rinsed

5½ cups water

2½ cups cauliflower (½–1 head), broken into small florets or medium-size chunks

Sea salt

1 tablespoon tahini, or to taste (optional)

1 tablespoon sesame oil

1 medium onion, diced (or ½ if you prefer a smoother gravy)

12 white button or cremini mushrooms, 8 fresh shiitake, 6 dried shiitake (reconstitute in warm water for about 10 minutes, then strain that water and use it in the gravy—instant mushroom stock!), or any combination

¼ cup shoyu (see page 292)

2 tablespoons mirin

1 drop of brown rice vinegar

2 tablespoons kuzu, diluted in ½ cup cold water

2 tablespoons scallions, chopped for garnish (optional)

2 tablespoons chopped parsley, for garnish (optional)

2 tablespoons chopped chives, for garnish (optional)

Place the millet in a heavy-bottom stockpot and toast it over medium heat for 5 to 8 minutes, or until it dries, becomes aromatic, and takes on a lightly golden color. Add 3 ½ cups of the water and the cauliflower and bring to a boil over high heat. Add 2 pinches of salt, cover, and reduce the heat to a simmer for 30 minutes. Remove from the heat.

Pass the mixture through a food mill, smooth out with a potato masher, or puree in the pot with a handheld immersion blender to your desired creaminess. If you decide to use a blender or food processor—which I don't recommend because I don't love putting hot food in a plastic container—be careful not to overblend or the mixture will get runny. Fold in the tahini, if using.

To make the gravy, heat the oil in a medium-size pan over medium heat. Add the onion and a couple pinches of salt and cook until translucent. Add the mushrooms and cook until tender, then pour in the remaining 2 cups water and bring the pan to a boil. Reduce the heat to a simmer and season with the shoyu, mirin, and vinegar. Gently cook for 5 minutes, adjust the seasoning to taste, and simmer for 5 more minutes.

Add the diluted kuzu to the mixture and bring to a boil, stirring constantly, as it thickens the gravy. Pour over the mash, garnish with the scallions, parsley, and chives, if you'd like, and serve.

PROTEIN! PROTEIN! COME AND GET YOUR PROTEIN!

Arame, Sun-Dried Tomato, and Zucchini Stir-Fry   Makes 4 to 6 servings

If You're Craving: Hearty and Salty

This is a super-yummy way to sneak sea veggies into your life. I promise if you like sun-dried tomatoes and basil and zucchini, then you will love this dish! Arame is a species of kelp that's packed with calcium, iron, vitamin A, and loads of minerals. These gems from the sea have a slightly nutty, sweet flavor and give depth and heartiness to a simple veggie stir-fry. This dish is delicious with or without tofu, so you could have it as the main event or as a great veggie side to complement another protein. It's the arame you're after, so you only need ⅓ to 1 cup on your plate to keep your meal balanced. This recipe will last you a few days.

1 pound firm tofu, drained and cut into ½" cubes

3 tablespoons tamari + more to taste

1 cup loosely packed arame

1 cup boiling water

1 tablespoon olive oil

2 large cloves garlic, minced

1 pound zucchini, sliced into ¼" half-moons (about 3 ¼ cups)

⅓ cup finely chopped sun-dried tomatoes

¼ cup fresh basil, minced

Marinate the tofu by placing it in a shallow dish or container with the 3 tablespoons tamari and letting it sit for 10 to 15 minutes. If you have a tight-fitting lid, cover the dish. Shake occasionally or simply turn the tofu.

Put the arame in a bowl and cover it with the boiling water. Let it sit for 15 minutes, then strain out the arame and reserve the soaking water. Set aside.

Meanwhile, heat the oil in a large skillet or wok over medium-high heat. Add the garlic and cook for 10 minutes, stirring constantly. Add the tofu and marinade plus the arame and cook for another minute. Stir in the zucchini and 2 tablespoons of the arame soaking water. Cover and cook for 3 to 4 minutes. Stir in the tomatoes and additional tamari to taste and cook for another minute. Take off the heat and fold in the basil. Serve hot or at room temperature.

Braised Burdock Root with Hearty Seitan
Makes 3 or 4 servings

If You're Craving: Hearty, Meaty, Salty, or Fried Goodness

Kinpira is a Japanese cooking style where veggies are sautéed, then braised in liquid. Because you're stewing the veg in their own juices, you end up with an amazingly fortifying, nutrient-dense, flavorful dish. Kinpira typically calls for burdock root, which is strengthening and good for the blood, as well as carrots, which are loaded with eye-boosting, tissue-repairing, skin-beautifying vitamin A. Seitan is an easy way to get some protein, though the dish is super-delicious without it. Know that not all seitans are created equal—some taste better than others. My favorite is Healthy Times Grilled Seitan. I suggest eating this dish at least once a month. I also recommend eating another version of this dish, Kinpira Stew, from *The Kind Diet*, at least every other week. Switch it up with this recipe for variety.

Making matchsticks. Cut your vegetables lengthwise or on a diagonal, so you have a longer slice than if you just cut them into rounds. Stack a few of the slices at a time and slice into matchstick-like pieces.

1 tablespoon toasted sesame oil + 1–2 teaspoons for finishing

1 cup burdock root, sliced into matchsticks (you don't need to peel the burdock, just gently scrub with a vegetable brush so that the skin stays intact)

½ onion, sliced into half-moons (optional)

1 cup carrots, sliced into matchsticks

1 tablespoon shoyu (see page 302)

⅓ cup water

¼–½ cup mirin (optional—but yum)

1 package (8 ounces) seitan, sliced (about 1 ½ cups)

1 teaspoon black sesame seeds, toasted

1 tablespoon cilantro, chopped (scallions and parsley would also work well)

Heat the oil in a skillet over medium heat until the oil shimmers. Add the burdock and cook for about 2 minutes. Add the onion, if using, and cook for 2 minutes. Then add the carrots and cook for 1 minute. Sprinkle in 2 dashes of the shoyu, the water, and the mirin, if using. Toss in the seitan and increase the heat until the liquid comes to a boil, then reduce the heat to a simmer and cover. Cook for 15 to 20 minutes, checking occasionally to make sure there's still liquid in the pan.

Remove the cover and taste. If your seitan is salty, you might not need to add the remaining shoyu. Otherwise, add the shoyu to taste. Cook the mixture for another minute, then take it off the heat. Finish with a drizzle of the toasted sesame oil and the sesame seeds and cilantro. Yum city!

Shoyu Broth with Wilted Arugula and Stewed Lentils   Makes 4 or 5 servings

If You're Craving: Hearty and Satisfying

This is a rich, soul-warming dish. The lentils are packed with baby-building, breast-milk-fortifying protein, and the tangy shoyu and ume vinegar give it a kick that scratches the salty itch. Plus, you can pack in all kinds of veggies to bring more depth of flavor and nutrients: cherry tomatoes, spinach, green beans, rutabagas—you can clean out your fridge into this soup! It only gets more delicious as the flavors meld together, so stew up a big pot, pack up the leftovers, and enjoy this dish for 3 to 4 days. If you reheat the soup, avoid bringing it to a boil—so you don't kill the powerful live enzymes in the shoyu.

Even though burdock root is a perfect addition because it's so strengthening and good for your blood, it is optional. This soup is still nourishing and delicious without it!

Choosing lentils. I like adding some green lentils to this dish because they give a lot of flavor to the broth, but feel free to use all French or any other color lentil here. Just note that the French kind add 15 minutes to your cooking time. So if you're not using them, you'll only need to cook the lentils for 30 minutes.

1 tablespoon olive oil

½ yellow onion, chopped

1 clove garlic, minced

½ cup diced carrots (about 1 carrot)

¼ cup chopped burdock root (you don't need to peel the burdock before chopping; just gently scrub with a vegetable brush so that the skin stays intact)

1 tablespoon dried basil (optional)

¼ cup diced celery (about 1 rib)

Kernels from ½ ear fresh corn or ¼ cup frozen

3 sun-dried tomatoes, soaked in water for about 15 minutes

¾ cup diced zucchini (about 1 zucchini)

¼ cup French lentils

¼ cup green lentils

5 cups water

1 bay leaf

1" piece kombu

2½ tablespoons shoyu (see page 292)

1 teaspoon ume vinegar

1 cup chopped arugula

In a soup pot over medium heat, gently heat the oil until it shimmers but doesn't smoke. To make sure the oil is hot enough but not too hot, throw in a piece of onion; it should sizzle.

Once the oil is ready, add the onion, garlic, carrots, burdock, and basil (if using). Cook for 2 to 3 minutes, then add the celery, corn, and tomatoes.

Cook for about 3 minutes, then add the zucchini, lentils, and water. Bring to a boil, then add the bay leaf and kombu. Reduce the heat to a simmer and cook for about 45 minutes, or until the lentils are soft. When the dish is about done cooking, add the shoyu and ume vinegar and remove from the heat.

To finish the dish, toss in the arugula so it just wilts.

Tempeh with Caramelized Onion and Braised Cabbage Makes 4 to 6 servings

If You're Craving: Hearty, Meaty, and Salty

This dish is insanely delicious. Why? Uh, caramelized onions and braised cabbage, anyone? The arame, a sea vegetable, is full of calcium and amazing for your hair, skin, nails, and bones. But the real star is the very special teriyaki tempeh made by Rhapsody Natural Foods. It's sweet and salty and so outrageously good that I order a big box of it once a year and stash it in the freezer so I can cook up some whenever the mood strikes. (I order my supply during the colder months so I don't need to worry about having it shipped overnight; and I split the order with a friend to keep costs down.)

In case you don't want to order the Rhapsody tempeh—or you just can't wait until your shipment arrives—I've included two variations for the dish: one using DIY teriyaki tempeh and another using plain tempeh.

A note on sauerkraut. Make sure you're buying the best-quality product you can find. Ideally, it would be organic, contain no sugars or funky preservatives, and be found in the refrigerated section of your grocery store. Anything that's sitting on the shelf at room temperature has been pasteurized, which means there aren't any of the live enzymes that make it so good for you.

Even though in this dish you're cooking the sauerkraut, which means some of those live enzymes are lost, it's still best to be using the cleanest, healthiest ingredients possible. Plus, you'll definitely want to top this dish with a tuft of fresh, briny 'kraut, so it's ideal to have the good stuff on hand.

⅓ cup dried arame

1 tablespoon olive oil

2 yellow or red onions, sliced into half-moons

½ head red or green cabbage, thinly sliced

½ cup high-quality sauerkraut (like Eden Foods and Gold Mine Natural Foods) + ¼–⅓ cup for garnish

1 teaspoon ume paste

1 package (6 ounces) teriyaki-flavored tempeh (I like the one by Rhapsody Natural Foods), cut into ½" cubes

¼–½ cup parsley, roughly chopped

Soak the arame in just enough filtered or spring water to cover it and set aside. It only needs to soak for about 5 minutes, but longer is fine. When done, strain out the arame, reserving the soaking liquid.

Heat the oil in a skillet over medium heat until the oil begins to shimmer, then add the onions. Cook for 3 to 5 minutes, or until soft and translucent. Adding a pinch of salt can help release the juices.

Add the cabbage plus a tablespoon or two of the reserved arame soaking liquid so the veg don't stick to the bottom of the pan. Adding a pinch of salt here, too, will help. Cook for a few minutes, then add another tablespoon of the soaking liquid and cover the pan so the veggies continue to steam, which keeps all their delicious juices in the pan. Cook for 10 minutes, then check to make sure the vegetables aren't sticking to the bottom of the pan. If necessary, drizzle in a little more soaking liquid—or water if you've run out—and replace the cover. Just be sure to not add more than ¼ cup of liquid at a time, or it will dilute the special sweetness of the dish.

After another 10 minutes, add the sauerkraut and, if necessary, more soaking liquid or water. Continue cooking for 10 minutes, or until the veggies are soft and caramelized. Reduce the heat if the veg are cooking too quickly. Add the arame, ume paste, and tempeh. Cook for 15 minutes.

Garnish with a little mound of sauerkraut and a sprinkling of fresh parsley.

IF MAKING YOUR OWN SAUCY TEMPEH

3 tablespoons olive oil or, for stronger flavor, sesame oil

¼ cup brown rice syrup

3 tablespoons shoyu (see page 292)

1 clove garlic, minced

1 package (6 ounces) unflavored tempeh (Lightlife makes a few variations of plain with things like flaxseed and wild rice), sliced

Mix the oil, syrup, shoyu, and garlic in a small bowl. Add the tempeh and stir until it's well coated. Marinate the tempeh in the bowl for 30 minutes or overnight in the fridge.

Preheat the oven to 400°F. Transfer the tempeh to a baking pan. Bake for 40 minutes, flipping the slices after 20 minutes, until most of the marinade is cooked into the tempeh. Cut into bite-size pieces.

IF USING REGULAR TEMPEH

Before adding the tempeh to the cabbage mixture, put it in a small saucepan with a little bit of water. Cover the pan and steam the tempeh over low heat for 15 minutes. (You could also heat it in a steamer basket over boiling water.) Remove, blot dry, and fry in olive oil until golden.

Black Soybean Stew Makes 5 or 6 servings

Black soybeans are packed with protein and iron, they help relieve stress on the body by healing the adrenal glands, and they are particularly good at cleansing your system if up until now you've been eating less-than-kind fare.

While black soybeans are the most antioxidant-rich of the entire legume family, you can take this up another notch and seek out the Hokkaido variety. They're even more creamy and nutritious than their regular soybean cousins, thanks to the famous volcanic soil of the Hokkaido region in Japan. Another great reason to seek them is that you can use their soaking water because it gets infused with their medicinal goodness, as opposed to regular beans, which just release their sugar, necessitating fresh water for cooking.

I recommend using a pressure cooker to get the smoothest consistency in the least amount of time. If you simmer these in a pot, and are using Hokkaido beans, just set a timer for an hour and a half, then check to see how far along things are. It could take 2 to 4 hours to cook them, but soaking them overnight will definitely help reduce that time.

This dish would be as scrumptious with any veg—diced celery, corn, sliced burdock root, a few slices of dried lotus root that you've soaked for a few minutes—clean out the fridge. And don't feel like you can't make this soup if you don't have any of the ingredients. Feel free to omit, double up, and swap.

Taking the fartiness out of beans. Beans don't have to be the musical fruit. As you'll see in the bean preparations in this book, I recommend discarding the beans' soaking water, skimming off any foam that rises to the surface as they cook, adding kombu and/or a bay leaf 15 minutes after removing the foam,* as well as tossing in a pinch of salt when the beans are about 80 percent done (doing so earlier can make the beans contract, which makes it harder for them to break down). If you're using a pressure cooker, wait until the pressure comes down before adding the salt, then cook for 10 more minutes on the stove with no pressure. (Make sure you build that additional time into how long you have the beans in the pressure cooker, or they'll get too mushy.)

These simple measures help make the beans easier to digest and reduce their hard-to-process sugars. If you're still having farty issues after taking these measures, then after you skim the foam, rinse the beans and begin the cooking process again.

*Both kombu and the bay leaf help make beans more digestible, so you can use one or both. The bay leaf will give you more flavor, while the kombu provides more minerals.

½ cup Hokkaido or organic black soybeans, soaked overnight in 5 cups spring water

5 cups spring water, if using non-Hokkaido beans, or as needed (if you're cooking the beans in a pot, you'll most likely need to add a bit more water when it's time to make the soup, since some will have evaporated)

1" piece kombu, rinsed, and/or 1 dried bay leaf

2 teaspoons sesame oil

1 cup diced onion

Sea salt

¾ cup diced carrots

1 cup diced winter squash, like kabocha or butternut

1 cup diced cabbage

1 cup fresh daikon or ½ cup dried (if dried, soak in water for 10 minutes, then cut into bite-size pieces, if desired)

5 small or 2–3 large dried shiitake mushrooms, soaked in water for 20 to 30 minutes or overnight (it's fine to soak the mushrooms and daikon together), soaking water reserved in case more is needed for soup

2 teaspoons mirin

1 tablespoon barley malt (optional)

2½ teaspoons barley miso

Scallions, whites and greens, sliced, for garnish (optional)

Arugula, for garnish (optional)

If using a pressure cooker to cook the beans: Add the black soybeans to the pot with their soaking water (if applicable) or the 5 cups spring water. Bring the beans to a boil over medium heat with the pot uncovered. Skim any foam that rises to the surface (see note on the opposite page). After 15 minutes, add the kombu and/or bay leaf.

Cover the pressure cooker, raise the heat to medium-high, and bring to pressure. Reduce the heat as low as it goes or use a flame deflector, if you have one, and cook for 45 minutes. Bring the pressure down by pouring cold water over the pot or by placing cold towels on the lid.

If not using a pressure cooker to cook the beans: Add the black soybeans to a large saucepot with their soaking water (if applicable) or the 5 cups spring water. Bring the beans to a boil over medium heat with the pot uncovered. Skim any foam that rises to the surface (see note on the opposite page). Reduce the heat to low, add ¼ cup more water, cover the pot with a lid, and simmer. After 15 minutes, add the kombu and/or bay leaf. Continue simmering until the beans are tender and creamy but not mushy. This will take about 2 hours if using regular black soybeans, closer to 4 hours if using Hokkaido.

Meanwhile, heat the oil in a large skillet over medium heat. Add the onion and cook for 2 to 3 minutes, or until translucent. Add a few pinches of salt to the pan.

Next, add the carrots and squash and cook for 3 to 4 minutes, or until they just begin to soften. Add the cabbage and cook for 3 to 4 minutes, or until it wilts. Remove from the heat and set aside until the beans are done.

Add the cooked vegetables to the beans in the pot, along with the daikon, mushrooms, mirin, and barley malt, if using, and a small pinch of salt. Cook over medium heat for 15 to 20 minutes.

In a small bowl, whisk together the miso with a few tablespoons of water until smooth.

When the bean and vegetable mixture is just about done, fold in the miso and cook gently (so you don't kill those enzymes!) for about 5 minutes.

Remove from the heat, garnish with scallions and arugula, if using, and serve.

Adzuki Bean Soup with Kabocha Squash

Makes 4 servings

Adzuki beans are very strengthening for the kidneys, and the sweet kabocha squash is packed with potassium (and insanely delicious!). This soup is soothing, restorative, and extremely nourishing.

As with black soybeans, the Hokkaido variety of adzuki beans is where it's at. Thanks to the rich volcanic farmland in the Hokkaido region of Japan, adzuki beans grown there are larger, sweeter, and more medicinal than those from anywhere else in the world. Similarly, you don't have to ditch the soaking water, since Hokkaido adzukis release extra nutrients into the water. (That said, it's not crucial that you soak them because they don't take as long as other beans to cook. So if you forget to put them in water the night before, no big deal.) If you don't want to track them down—or wait for them to arrive—it's still totally worth it to make this dish with regular adzukis, which are so good for you, too.

I like to change up this recipe with the season. That's because how you cook vegetables can alter their "energy," or how you feel after eating them. During the warmer months, we want light, bright energy that revs us up; during the colder seasons, it's all about slowing down and getting grounded. So in the spring and summer, I cut the vegetables into smaller pieces, which cook more quickly and lend a lighter energy to the dish. Fall and winter calls for large chunks of vegetables, which can simmer and stew for longer. Feel free to get creative with the veg you add. Celery would make a nice addition, as would daikon.

Try working this dish into the rotation often. Making a batch every other week or so would be great!

Do you need a pressure cooker? Even though some beans—like chickpeas and black soybeans—benefit from a pressure cooker, adzuki beans don't. They're more delicate and therefore cook more quickly, so they'll only get mushy and sad in a pressure cooker.

1 cup Hokkaido or organic adzuki beans, washed, soaked overnight, and drained (unless using Hokkaido, in which case, reserve the soaking liquid)

1" piece kombu and/or 1 dried bay leaf

½ teaspoon sea salt

1 cup diced yellow onion

½ cup washed and cubed kabocha (unpeeled) or butternut (peeled) squash

½ cup diced carrots

½ cup corn kernels, fresh or frozen and thawed

Shoyu, to taste (go easy—start with 1 teaspoon), see page 292

2 scallions, washed and finely chopped on the diagonal (a couple of tablespoons of finely chopped chives or a handful or arugula would also work well here, depending on what's in season and what you fancy)

In a large pot, add the beans and soaking liquid, if applicable. If not, add 5 to 6 cups fresh water. Bring to a boil over high heat, skimming any foam that rises to the top. After about 15 minutes, add the kombu and/or bay leaf and salt.

If making during the fall or winter: Cover the pot and reduce the heat to low, simmering the beans for 1 hour, or until they are just becoming tender but aren't completely soft. Add the onion, squash, carrots, and corn, and cook for 25 minutes. Season to taste with the shoyu and simmer for another 5 to 10 minutes.

If making during the spring or summer: Cover the pot and reduce the heat to low, simmering the beans for 30 minutes, or until they are just becoming tender but aren't completely soft. Add the onion, squash, carrots, and corn, and cook for 15 minutes. Season to taste with the shoyu and simmer for another 5 minutes.

Ladle out the soup and garnish with scallion greens (or chives or arugula).

Seitan and Veggie Mochi Melt   Makes 4 to 6 servings

If You're Craving: Hearty, Creamy, Chewy, Meaty, Salty, or Yum City!

The texture is chewy and gooey, and it's just so yum.

1 tablespoon sesame oil

1 small onion, sliced into half-moons

1 small carrot, washed and cut into matchsticks (see note, page 306)

1 cup small broccoli florets, washed

Kernels from 1 ear of corn

2 cups sliced seitan

3 teaspoons mirin

3 teaspoons shoyu (see page 292)

½ cup spring water

½ teaspoon ume vinegar (optional)

½ package mochi (about 6 ounces), diced

Heat a skillet over medium heat. Add the oil and heat until it shimmers. Add the onion and cook for 1 minute. Repeat with the carrot, broccoli, and corn.

Add the seitan, mirin, and shoyu and cook for 2 minutes. Add the water. Let simmer for another minute. If you want more salty brightness to the dish, sprinkle in the ume vinegar.

Sprinkle the mochi over the top of the vegetables and seitan and cover with a lid. Cook for 3 minutes, or until the mochi is melted. Serve straight from the skillet.

Strengthening Daikon, Carrots, and Tofu

Serves 4 to 6

This dish has all kinds of healing voodoo and is especially good to have after birth. Dried daikon is thought by experts to be even more curative than fresh because it has the ability to penetrate deep into the body and flush out any gunky toxins—and gently enough so it's safe if you're pregnant or nursing. They also believe that by layering vegetables and allowing them to cook undisturbed (as opposed to sautéing), their nutritional energy gets even more concentrated and powerful. Make this if you're just starting to clean up your act or if you've been indulging in too many naughty foods—or, of course, as nourishing maintenance to stay vibrant and well.

1 14-ounce package extra-firm or firm tofu

1 tablespoon plus 2 teaspoons shoyu (see page 292)

1 to 1½ tablespoons olive or sesame oil

2 stamp-size pieces of kombu, halved

1 onion, sliced into half-moons

1 medium carrot (about 2 cups), cut into large matchsticks (see note, page 306)

1 stalk celery, cut into ½" pieces

1 cup dried daikon, soaked in 1 cup water for 5 minutes, soaking water reserved

Drain the tofu by placing it on a plate and weight the top with another plate and a bowl. Don't completely squish it, just apply enough pressure to squeeze out any extra liquid. This will help it get nice and crispy when you fry it. Let it sit with the weight for about 10 minutes. Transfer the tofu to a cutting board and slice it into about 8 slices.

In a shallow bowl or small casserole dish, combine 1 tablespoon of the shoyu with 2 tablespoons of water and add the tofu. Flip a few times to coat.

In a large skillet, add the oil and heat over a medium-high flame. Tip the skillet away from you so the oil pools on the far side (to keep from getting splattered with oil when you add the tofu). Place a few tofu steaks in the pan—you don't want to crowd them or they'll steam and not get crispy and golden. Place the pan back down on the flame and let the tofu cook undisturbed until you can see a nice brown crust starting to climb about halfway up the tofu, about 5 minutes. Use a stainless steel spatula to turn the pieces over and repeat on the other side.

Transfer the cooked tofu to a paper towel–lined plate to blot any excess oil. Fry the remaining tofu in batches so as not to crowd the pan. Once cool enough to handle, cut each tofu steak into 8 slices, and then slice those slices into eight bite-size cubes. Set aside.

In a large saucepan, layer the ingredients in this order: kombu, onion, carrot, celery, fried tofu, dried daikon. Pour the daikon water over the top and bring to a boil over high heat. Reduce to a gentle simmer and add 1 teaspoon of shoyu. Continue cooking for another 35 minutes, then add the remaining teaspoon of shoyu. Cook for 5 minutes and remove from the heat. Serve.

IF YOU'RE FEELING NAUGHTY

Heirloom Tomato Saucy Toasts   Makes 2 to 4 servings

If you're craving creamy or cheesy, make these mini-pizzas. Nutritional yeast has a surprising cheeselike flavor, and the tahini and sesame seeds give the whole affair a decadent richness—not to mention vitamin B, calcium, and iron. If you're still feeling a little naughty, spread on a little Vegenaise.

3 tablespoons tahini

2 teaspoons organic jarred tomato sauce

4 slices sourdough bread or 2 English muffins, halved

2 to 3 tomato slices per toast

1 onion slice per toast

½–1 teaspoon nutritional yeast per toast

1 teaspoon sesame seeds per toast

Make the tahini sauce by mixing the tahini and tomato sauce. Set aside.

Warm the bread in the oven or toaster, removing it just before it's completely browned. Slather each piece with some of the tahini sauce, then load it with the tomatoes, onion, and nutritional yeast. Place under a broiler or in the oven for 3 to 4 minutes. Sprinkle it with the sesame seeds for a finishing touch, then serve.

Protein-Packed Waffles   Makes 8 large waffles

Not only are these waffles toasty and fluffy and all-around great, but they're also packed with protein because they're made with beans! Bear loves them! He calls them "fla-fels." Make a batch and keep some in the freezer to pop in the steamer or toaster on days when cooking isn't on the menu—or watch as everyone gobbles up every last one.

These are delicious plain, but feel free to dress them up with things like Earth Balance buttery spread or brown rice or maple syrup when you're feeling a little more frisky.

1 cup dried white beans (cannellini, great northern, baby lima, or navy), soaked overnight and drained

4½ cups water

3½ cups rolled oats

2 tablespoons whole flaxseed

2 tablespoons baking powder (Rumford makes an aluminum- and GMO-free version)

2 teaspoons sea salt

3 teaspoons vanilla extract or ½ teaspoon fresh vanilla bean seeds (just halve the pod and scrape the seeds out with the side of a spoon or tip of your knife)

1 teaspoon coconut oil, or more as needed

Add the soaked beans to a blender with the water (you read that right—don't cook them!) or half of each if your blender can't accommodate the volume all at once. Start on a low speed and gradually increase the speed until the beans are completely smooth, 3 to 5 minutes. Add the oats, flaxseed, baking powder, salt, and vanilla and blend until fully incorporated.

Heat the oil in your waffle iron, making sure both the top and bottom are coated. A pastry brush works well to spread the oil, as will a clean dish towel or paper towel.

When the waffle maker is fully heated, pour in just enough batter to fill the wells of the waffle mold. Cook for 8 to 10 minutes, or until the waffles are golden brown and cooked all the way through.

Variations:

- Blueberry Waffles: Fold in a handful of fresh blueberries to the batter once it's smooth.
- Apple-Cinnamon Waffles: Add 1 apple, diced small, and 2 teaspoons cinnamon (or to taste) to the batter once it's smooth.

Sausage and Sweet Potato Hash   Makes 4 servings

This dish will satisfy the urge for something meaty or salty. I like using Field Roast sausages here, which are grain based and rich and yummy, but feel free to use any other vegan sausage you fancy. This recipe also calls for sweet potatoes, which aren't to be confused with yams (I prefer white sweet potatoes).

1 tablespoon olive oil

1 small onion, chopped

2 sweet potatoes (or yams, if you must), sliced into ½" coins

½–1 bunch kale, chopped

1–2 Field Roast sausages, ideally Italian or smoked apple, sliced into nice, big, mouthful-size chunks

Shoyu, to taste (optional), see page 292

Heat the oil in a large skillet over medium-high heat until the oil just begins to shimmer. Add the onion and sweet potatoes and cook for 3 to 4 minutes. Flip the sweet potatoes over and cook for another 3 to 5 minutes, or until they are soft but not mushy and the onion is translucent.

Add the kale and sausages and cook until the kale turns bright green and the sausage is warmed through.

Add the shoyu to taste, if desired, though you most likely won't need the additional salty note if you've used the Italian variety or another saltier sausage.

Pan-Fried Tempeh with Garlic and Chiles

Makes 4 to 6 servings

When it's fried and crispy, this tempeh can be a great bacon replacement. And when you combine it with Asian flavors like garlic, hot chiles, lemongrass, and shoyu, it gives any Chinese takeout a run for its money, especially spooned over some jasmine rice with bok choy on the side.

Though this dish has a little sugar in it—making it a wee bit naughty—it is a great way to get some nourishing, protein-packed tempeh in you. So even though you should save this treat for when you have an itch for hearty, meaty, and salty, the tempeh is still giving your body lots of good energy.

1 lemongrass stalk, tough outer husk removed, cut into 2"–3" pieces

2 tablespoons sunflower oil or olive oil

2 packages (6 ounces each) unflavored tempeh, cut crosswise into ¼"–½" pieces

6 shallots, thinly sliced

4–6 cloves garlic, thinly sliced

2 red chiles, thinly sliced (wear plastic gloves when handling)

1" piece ginger, minced

½ cup water

⅔ cup brown rice syrup or maple syrup (brown rice syrup is gentler on the system)

3 tablespoons shoyu (see page 292)

First, "bruise" the lemongrass to release its flavor: Take each piece and bend it several times.

Heat the oil in a large skillet or wok over medium-high heat until the oil shimmers. A piece of tempeh should sizzle when added to the pan, just like veggies would. When it does, add the rest of the tempeh and fry until crispy, about 2 minutes a side. Remove to a paper-towel-lined plate and set aside.

Add the shallots, garlic, chiles, ginger, and lemongrass to the skillet and cook for 1 to 2 minutes, or until fragrant. Add the water, syrup, and shoyu. Cook until the liquid thickens and just coats the vegetables, mix in the tempeh, toss together, and remove from the heat.

Spoon over prepared rice, if desired, and enjoy.

Sweetly Glazed Carrots   Makes 2 servings

If You're Craving: Sweet—but aren't feeling too wild

Sometimes I just want custardy, sweet carrots. I don't know where the food memory comes from, but I've been trying to find this exact flavor for a while—and I finally got it right! Top these with a maple syrup glaze and you could serve them up for dessert just as easily as a savory side. They'd also be right at home on a holiday table.

2 medium carrots, cut diagonally into ½″ pieces

1 tablespoon Earth Balance buttery spread

2 tablespoons maple syrup

2 tablespoons water or orange juice

2 tablespoons grated ginger (optional)

Heat a medium-size skillet over medium-low heat. Add the carrots and Earth Balance. Gently cook for 1 to 2 minutes.

Add the maple syrup, water or orange juice, and ginger (if using) and cook for another minute. Cover with a lid and steam for about 2 minutes before checking on the carrots. When easily pierced with a fork, they're done.

Cheesy, Oozy Guacamole Bean Dip   Makes 8 servings

I can't think of a single craving that this dish wouldn't wallop.

1 can (16 ounces) refried beans

3 large avocados

3 tablespoons fresh lime juice

2 containers (8 ounces each) nondairy sour cream

1 packet taco seasoning (see note)

½ cup diced mild green chiles, drained

½ cup sliced black olives, or more if you like

5 tomatoes, chopped

2 cups shredded vegan Cheddar cheese

Preheat the oven to 350°F.

Spread a layer of refried beans in the bottom of a 8″ × 8″ glass baking dish. Pit and peel the avocados and place in a bowl. Mash the avocados together with the lime juice and spread on top of the refried beans. Stir together the sour cream and taco seasoning and spread over the avocado.

Sprinkle the chiles over the sour cream and top with a layer of black olives. Add the tomatoes and sprinkle with the cheese. Bake the dip for 15 to 30 minutes, or until heated through and the cheese is a bit melted.

Serve warm or at room temperature.

DIY seasoning. We use Bearitos organic taco seasoning, but it does contain a touch of cane sugar. If you're avoiding all white sugar, make your own by combining chili powder, ground cumin, onion powder, hot paprika or ground red pepper, and salt.

Variation:

- For chips, there are some pretty healthy baked organic tortilla chips on the market. But you can also make your own by cutting up Ezekiel sprouted grain tortillas and baking them in the oven until crisp or dry-roasting them in a frying pan.

SOMETHING SWEET
(NAUGHTY AND NICE)

Chocolate-Dunked Coconut Delights   Makes 12

These tasty bites are naughtier than a gentler treat, like Tangerine Kanten (below), but they beat the pants off a pint of Häagen Dazs! And they're particularly great for company—whip up a batch for a fancy tea party with girlfriends or for family coming over to rub your belly.

You'll notice that the recipe calls for whole wheat or white spelt flour. Whole wheat is the kinder option, but spelt makes for a lighter pastry.

1 cup shredded dried coconut

1 cup whole wheat pastry flour or white spelt flour

1 teaspoon baking powder

¼ cup maple syrup

1 teaspoon alcohol-free vanilla extract

¼ cup coconut oil + 1 teaspoon at room temperature

¼ cup mashed banana (optional)

1 teaspoon coconut extract (optional)

¼ cup vegan dark chocolate chips (SunSpire makes a great healthy version that's sweetened with grains. If you can't find them, ask your grocer to carry them.)

Preheat the oven to 375°F. Grease a baking sheet with coconut oil and set aside.

In a large bowl, combine the dried coconut, flour, and baking powder and mix well. In a separate bowl, whisk together the syrup, vanilla, ¼ cup coconut oil, and the banana and coconut extract, if using. Add the wet ingredients to the dry and gently stir to combine.

Using a small ice-cream scooper or large spoon, make bite-size balls of batter and place them on the prepared baking sheet. Bake for 12 minutes, or until golden brown. Remove from the oven and allow to cool.

Rest a heatproof bowl on top of a medium-size pot of water (or use a double-boiler, if you have one). Bring the water to a boil, then reduce the heat to a gentle simmer. Add the chocolate chips and the 1 teaspoon coconut oil to the bowl and stir until the chocolate melts and you get a thicky, glossy sauce.

After the cookies have cooled, dip them in the sauce and arrange them on a plate. Give them a couple of minutes so the sauce hardens, then serve. Do your best not to eat them all at once!

Tangerine Kanten   Makes 4 to 6 servings

Kanten, also known as agar-agar, is extracted from seaweed that makes liquids set like Jell-O. Unlike nasty animal-based gelatin, it's packed with calcium and minerals. My favorite brand is

Mitoku's Snow-Dried Kanten Flakes, which I buy from Gold Mine Natural Foods online. You can also find the Eden Foods version at most health food stores.

This treat is so relaxing for your system that you can indulge in every day if need be, but four times a week is optimal. Have a cup regularly to stave off urges for chocolate chip cookies, and play around with different flavors. Try making this with just apple juice and add in other fruits that you love and are in season, like strawberries or peaches. A batch of this dessert will last about a week in the fridge.

2 cups freshly squeezed tangerine or orange juice

1 cup store-bought organic apple juice

3 heaping tablespoons agar-agar (Mitoku makes a nice one)

1 tangerine or orange, peeled and divided into segments

Sprigs of fresh mint, for garnish

Pour the juices into a small saucepan and add the agar-agar. Bring the mixture to a boil over high heat, then reduce the heat to a simmer. Continue cooking until the agar-agar dissolves. To check if it's done, give the mixture a swirl and look for flakes floating around. If the mixture is clear, it's done.

Divide the fruit segments among a few pretty glasses for individual servings or one big mold or glass Pyrex dish. Pour the hot liquid over the fruit, then transfer to the fridge or leave at room temperature until set. It should be like gelatin in consistency. Add a sprig of mint to garnish and serve.

Baked Peaches with Gooey Nut Crumble

Makes 2 to 4 servings

There is nothing like peaches that have been caramelizing in their own juices, then topped with what is basically the best granola ever. I could probably eat the whole tray in one sitting.

2 peaches, cut into roughly 1" cubes (as best you can)

1½ tablespoons brown rice syrup

⅓ cup rolled oats

¼ cup almonds, chopped

¼ cup walnuts, chopped

1 tablespoon black sesame seeds

¼ cup raisins

Preheat the oven to 350°F.

Arrange the peaches in a small baking dish. Set aside.

Add the syrup to a small saucepan with ½ to ⅔ cup water and bring to a boil. Add the oats. Stir and cook for about 1 minute, or until well combined and the water is absorbed. Add the nuts, seeds, and raisins and stir to combine. Pour over the peaches and bake for 35 to 40 minutes, or until slightly browned and bubbling. Serve warm!

COOKING FOR BABY

Grain Milk   Makes 9 cups

This milk is full of nutrients and yet gentle on baby's still-developing digestive tract, and you can turn it into baby's first food by making it into a thicker porridge and adding veggies. But feel free to continue making the milk, too. It's a much healthier alternative to juices and to almond, rice, and soy milks from the container. Bear still loves drinking it sweetened with a little *amasake*—we call it his 'zake milkshake. Cook up a batch every 2 to 3 days and keep it in the fridge in a sealed glass jar. Or plan ahead for when you might be in a pinch and freeze it in serving-size portions so you can defrost just what you need.

Grain milk is also a good quick fix for dire breast milk emergencies. If you need to tide your baby over until her next boob session and you haven't pumped, or you're breastfeeding your pants off but still need a little extra milk to get baby through the day, this can be a lifesaver. Macrobiotic experts believe grain milk is nourishing enough to be a breast milk substitute for mothers who can't nurse, but only explore that option with a macrobiotic counselor.

I should note that while it's a lot easier to prepare this recipe in a blender, I prefer not to because macrobiotic wisdom considers that these appliances cause irritability and difficulty relaxing or sleeping, and the electric vibe isn't what I'm going for when I'm making food for my little one. There's something so calming and peaceful about using traditional tools like a food mill and sieve. It takes a little more time, but it allows you to infuse the process with a deep sense of intention and love—and gives your arm a little workout!

1 cup grains, such as short- or medium-grain brown rice, whole oats, whole barley, or sweet brown rice (Use them in varying combinations to make sure your baby is getting a balanced "milk," but only use up to three kinds together. You can also introduce cracked grains after baby's been eating for a month.)

1" piece kombu

Barley malt, brown rice syrup, or amasake (optional)

Place the grains in a large pot and cover with cool water. Swirl the grains with your hand to loosen any dirt or dust, pour off the water, and repeat until the water is no longer cloudy, most likely two or three more times.

Then add 10 cups water to the grains, cover with a clean dish towel or a bamboo sushi mat, and let sit for at least 3 hours to overnight.

Heat the pot over medium heat, toss in the kombu, and cover. Bring the contents to a boil and reduce the heat to as low as it will go, or use a flame deflector. Gently simmer for 1 ½ hours. If your heat is low enough, you should be able to just set a timer and go about your day.

Alternatively, you can use a pressure cooker, which is nice in the colder months when you need the warmer energy. Some macrobiotic experts believe this cooking method is more strengthening if your baby is sick or weak. Simply add the grains and water to the pressure cooker, cover, and over medium heat bring it up to pressure. Reduce the heat to low and cook for about 1 hour. Remove from the heat and let the pressure come down.

Remove the kombu from the pot and discard.

Next, pass the grains and cooking liquid through a food mill on the medium-size holes. (You can use the small holes, but it takes longer, and you're going to strain the mixture further anyway.) If it gets difficult to pass the grains through the mill, add some of the milk back into the grains. Discard any grains remaining in the mill once all the milk has been pressed out.

Now, strain the milk further through a fine-mesh sieve. The goal is to remove as much of the grain fibers as you can. This will make the milk easier to digest and help it pass through a bottle nipple. If you like, you can line the sieve with cheesecloth or use cheesecloth instead of a sieve. Just know that for some reason, the all-natural cheesecloths fall apart much more easily than the conventional kind.

Transfer the cooled strained milk to glass storage containers and stash in the fridge.

Before giving the milk to baby, take the chill off of it by warming it slightly on the stove. Add a little water or breast milk to thin it, if necessary.

Breast milk is sweet, so you can gently sweeten the grain milk and add ½ to 1 teaspoon barley malt or brown rice syrup or 2 teaspoons amasake for every cup of milk.

Pour into a bottle and watch as baby gobbles it up! The rest will last in the fridge for 3 days.

Variation:

- For a calming remedy, add a couple of teaspoons of kukicha tea for every cup of milk to baby's bottle.

BABY'S PERFECT FIRST FOOD

This is a soft, creamy porridge that you make by simply adding less water to the Grain Milk recipe. Instead of 10 cups, use 5. You can also play around with these other additions:

- For a calcium and protein boost, add either 2 drops of sesame oil and ⅛" piece of kombu, or 1 teaspoon toasted ground sesame seeds plus a postage-stamp-size piece of kombu to the grains as they cook. Remove the kombu before feeding to baby.

- Add 1 tablespoon Baby's First Veggies (below) or other soft veg to the grains before milling.
- Add ½ teaspoon tahini to the grains before milling or when heating up the porridge before giving it to baby, for a little more fat and protein.

Baby's First Veggies

The veggies below are just a suggestion—there's no end to the combinations of organic varieties you can try. See "Here Come the Veggies!" on page 281 for inspiration. Ideally you'd make this fresh daily or every other day, but if you need to make a batch and freeze it, that's okay. Whatever it takes to get your baby the best food possible!

¼ cup chopped winter squash like unpeeled kabocha or peeled butternut

1 heaping tablespoon thinly sliced string beans or carrots

1 heaping tablespoon finely chopped kale or watercress

Place the squash and string beans or carrots in a small pot. Cover the veggies with water and bring to a boil. Place the lid on the pot, reduce the heat to low, and cook for 15 minutes, or until everything is very soft. Add the kale or watercress and cook for 5 minutes. Remove from the heat. Using a sieve, *suribachi,* or baby food mill, mash the veggies well. Serve the mixture as is or add 1 tablespoon Grain Milk.

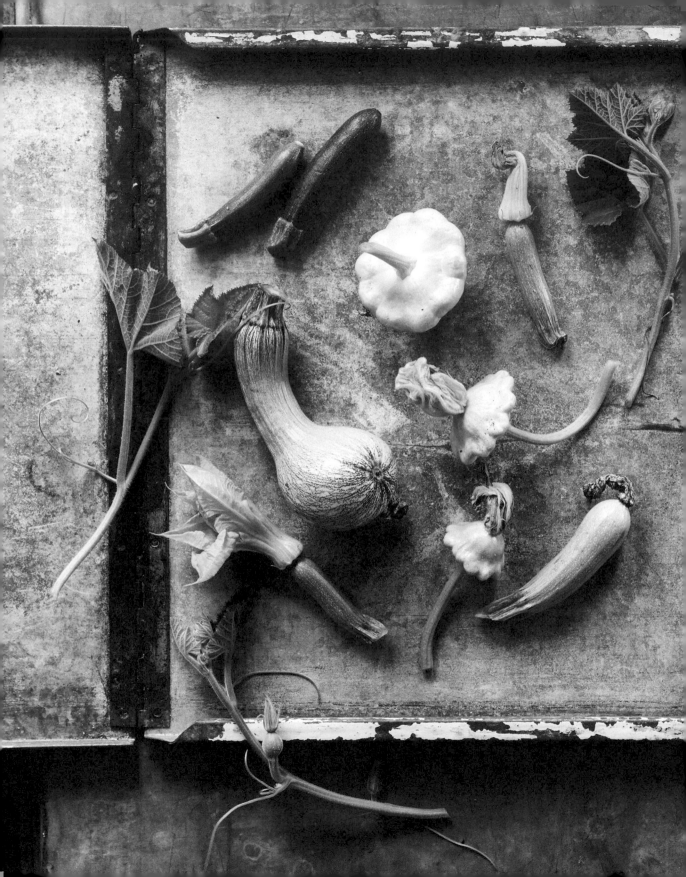

APPENDIX II

* Kind Food from A to Zinc

* Your New No-Medicine Chest

* Resources

KIND FOOD FROM A TO ZINC: Why you can absolutely get everything you need from food

THE GOOD STUFF	WHAT IT DOES	
Vitamin A	Aids in cell development and brain growth and is necessary for optimal vision. It heals body tissues, repairs the skin, and can neutralize cancer-causing radicals.	
Vitamin B₁, thiamine	Helps the body produce energy and keeps the nervous system healthy.	
Vitamin B₂, riboflavin	Helps your cells produce energy and use oxygen.	
Vitamin B₃, niacin	Helps you and your baby produce energy, stimulates circulation, prevents cramping, lowers blood pressure, and reduces cholesterol.	
Vitamin B₆, pyrodoxine	Low levels are associated with morning sickness, preeclampsia, complications during delivery, and delay in the development of baby's nervous system.	
Vitamin B₉, folate	Reduces risk of birth defects like spina bifida and cancer.	
Vitamin C	Builds connective tissue; keeps blood vessels healthy; heals wounds; boosts the immune system; fights viruses, bacteria, and fungi; and raises good cholesterol.	
Vitamin E	Prevents free radicals from developing into cancer.	
Vitamin K	Aids proper bone formation and helps blood clot.	
Calcium	Builds baby's growing bones (and fortifies yours); contributes to dental health, good circulation, and healthy body tissues.	
DHA	An omega-3 fatty acid that builds baby's growing brain.	
Iodine	Necessary for proper functioning of the thyroid gland, which regulates metabolism, produces energy, creates nerves and bones, boosts reproduction, and contributes to healthy hair, skin, nails, and teeth. Deficiency can lead to the most preventable form of brain damage in newborns.	
Iron	Carries oxygen into muscles and helps them function properly; increases your resistance to stress and disease; and staves off pregnancy symptoms like fatigue, weakness, irritability, and depression.	
Magnesium	Needed for several hundred enzyme reactions in our bodies; helps relax muscles and lower blood pressure.	
Phosphorus	Helps convert carbohydrates and fats into energy, create proteins for growth and tissue repair, contract muscles, and maintain healthy teeth and bones.	
Selenium	Can improve the body's immune response and prevent loss of tissue elasticity with aging. A deficiency can cause an increased risk for cardiovascular disease, stroke, certain cancers, and hypertension.	
Zinc	Helps build a strong immune function, the key to allergy prevention. Deficiencies are related to increased birth defects, low birth weight, miscarriage, and future behavioral problems.	

FOODS THAT DELIVER

Pumpkin, sweet potatoes, yams, squash, carrots, peaches, apricots, cherries, spinach, broccoli, seaweed

Oats, walnuts, pistachios, avocados, sesame seeds, sunflower seeds, beans, peas, citrus, soy milk, wheat germ

Whole grains, spinach, broccoli, peas, asparagus, miso

Nuts, whole grains, avocados, figs, mushrooms, legumes, prunes

Oats, bran, beans, pistachios, raw garlic, bananas, brown rice, corn, peas, yellow bell peppers, molasses, wheat germ

Oats, nuts, lentils, garbanzo and navy beans, artichokes, leafy greens, bananas, berries, pineapple, cantaloupe, oranges, Brussels sprouts, peas, asparagus, lima beans, romaine lettuce, plus bean sprouts such as soy, lentil, and mung

Whole grains, citrus, cantaloupe, kiwifruit, strawberries, green and red bell peppers, cauliflower, broccoli, tomato, cabbage, sprouted seeds

Nuts and nut butters, sunflower seeds, sweet potatoes, whole grains, avocados, soybeans, corn, wheat germ, cottonseed oils

Leafy greens, tomatoes, chickpeas, strawberries, cauliflower, asparagus, safflower oil, alfalfa, kelp, blackstrap molasses

Kale, broccoli, collard greens, sesame seeds, bok choy, and dandelion and turnip greens have a super-high calcium content. Other good sources: legumes, almonds, tofu, tempeh, corn tortillas

Walnuts, soybeans, soybean oil, hemp seed oil, flaxseed oil, chia seeds

Sea vegetables, especially kombu; sea salt

Oats; dark leafy greens like kale, collards, and dandelion greens; lentils, chickpeas, black beans, and adzuki beans; millet, buckwheat noodles, dried fruit, avocados, asparagus, beets, bok choy, lima beans, prunes, apricots, squash

Wheat germ, bran, whole grains, leafy green vegetables, okra, brazil nuts, almonds, dates, dried figs, corn

Whole grains, cashew butter, legumes, black walnuts, bran

Brown rice, firm tofu, sunflower seeds, mushrooms, molasses, Brazil nuts, brewer's yeast, wheat germ

Whole grains, nuts, legumes, popcorn

YOUR NEW NO-MEDICINE CHEST: Natural remedies for common ailments

COMMON AILMENTS	WHY IT HAPPENS	
Sniffles and Congestion	Mucus keeps germs, dirt, and bacteria from getting into our lungs. And when we get sick, our body produces even more of the gunky stuff to keep germs out.[1]	
Fever	It's the body's most effective way of combating potentially harmful invaders. This is why it's often not a good idea to use over-the-counter chemicals to artificially bring a fever down. In fact, Dr. Rosen says that fevers are rarely dangerous and usually signal that the body is fighting against infection. The major reason to treat fever, he says, is to keep your baby comfortable. And the American Academy of Pediatrics agrees![2]	
Coughing/Croup	Coughing is one of the body's genius ways of not so gently asking viruses to exit immediately.	

- **Ditch any allergen-promoting dust collectors** like fuzzy blankets, stuffed animals, and down pillows, then give your house a good airing out plus a thorough vacuuming (with a HEPA vacuum).

- To help baby breathe more easily, add a few drops of **eucalyptus oil** in a vaporizer while he sleeps or in the bottom of a bathtub with some hot water to make a DIY steam room. You can also put a few drops on his clothes or the sheets to continue opening up those little nasal passages.

- You can also just let it pass. That's what we do—**lots of boobies**, maybe some **cooled ume kuzu**, (ume sho kuzu without the shoyu) or **chamomile tea** (page 217), and **rest**, and it runs its course in no time.

For peace of mind:

- **Don't sweat it** if your baby is under 3 months and the fever is under 100.2 degrees or if your baby is over 3 months, is in good spirits, still has a good appetite, is peeing and pooping as usual, and has a temperature under 105.[3]

- **Call your pediatrician immediately** if the temperature is higher or your baby shows signs of not coping well (she's listless, not eating or pooping, or has had a febrile seizure in the past). Of course, if you have any doubts about what's going on regardless of baby's temperature, you should feel free to check in with the doc.

For relief:

- Dr. Rosen recommends **hydration** as the first and best remedy. It helps rid the body of toxins while preventing dehydration. That's great news if you're breastfeeding because your supercharged milk will automatically hydrate baby. **Cooled ume kuzu** tea (ume sho kuzu without the shoyu) in a bottle (see page 297) also works wonders.

- A neat naturopathic remedy he recommends is **soaking your baby's socks in vinegar or cold water** and putting them on/wrapping them around his feet to help bring down the fever.[4]

- **Tepid baths and cold washcloths** can help make baby feel better. Or as Christina Pirello recommends, hold a **cooled cabbage leaf** to the back of baby's head. When the leaf gets warm—usually after about 2 minutes—replace it with another cool one. Try it about five times for a total of 10 minutes, she says, and you likely won't need the doc.

For peace of mind:

- **Don't sweat it** if your baby is coughing but otherwise happy, alert, and eating well with no rattling in his chest. If your baby has croup or a "barking" cough, this will eventually go away on its own.

- **Call your pediatrician immediately** if your child is having trouble breathing.

For relief:

- Start with cooled **ume kuzu** tea (no shoyu) in a bottle (page 297) and lots of rest.

- **Elderberry drops** can reduce phlegm and relieve bronchial congestion. It's also a flu preventive and great immune booster any time of the year.

- **Try homemade drops:** Grate a teaspoon of fresh ginger and squeeze 3 or 4 drops into a teaspoon of warmed sesame oil. Use a dropper to add 3 or 4 drops per ear, 3 times a day.

- Spending time in a **steamy bathroom** is great for breaking up wet-cough phlegm.[5]

- Draw a **therapeutic bath** and add some of California Baby's delicious Eucalyptus Ease Bath Drops (or just a few drops of eucalyptus essential oil—so much gentler than the icky and often-prescribed prednisone, yet effective at thinning mucus in the lungs[6]).

(continued)

YOUR NEW NO-MEDICINE CHEST—*continued*

COMMON AILMENTS	WHY IT HAPPENS	
Earache	Babies have small tubes in their ears, which easily get clogged and cause pain.	
Tummyache/Nausea/ Vomiting	As unpleasant as they are, these reactions are the body's way of expelling toxins that are making it ill.[7]	
Sticky Eyes	Sometimes new babies will develop plugged tear ducts or "sticky eyes," which can make one or both inflamed.	
Diarrhea	This typically is a result of a virus or is sometimes caused by dietary changes, especially if baby is eating too much fruit or processed foods (more on that in Chapter 17).	
Bug Bites and Stings		
Rashes	Warm and moist (and dark) can be a breeding ground for yeast and bacteria.	
Minor Ouches		

NATURAL REMEDIES

- Squeeze a few drops of breast milk into the ear to help alleviate discomfort and clear the tubes.

- Make sure your baby is getting plenty of fluids via the amazing healing tincture that is your breast milk.

- A cold compress to the head can quell nausea.

- Try any of the tummy-soothing remedies recommended in the colic section on page 217.

If your child is vomiting for more than several hours or if it's accompanied by dehydration, diarrhea, or a high fever, consult your pediatrician.

- Having ruled out pink eye, you can administer a few drops of breast milk into the eyes—or put the drops on your finger and let them roll into baby's eyes—up to six times a day, and it'll clear right up.[8]

- You can also try gently wiping the eye with a warm compress.

- Dr. Rosen suggests using a probiotic like Klaire Labs Ther-Biotic Infant Formula, but you should consult your pediatrician for dosage on children under 2 years old.[9]

- Macrobiotic counselor Warren Kramer recommends kukicha tea or a tiny bit of diluted miso soup.

- Paring down on fruit—even if baby is only eating ½ cup of apple a day—is where I'd start, followed by some Sweet Calming Kuzu (page 297).

If the symptoms last longer than a few days, dehydration is a concern, so call your doctor.[10]

- Breast milk, in addition to tea tree and lavender oils, have anti-inflammatory properties that offer some comfort.

- Air and sunlight—nature's own antibiotics—are better than any topical remedy.

- Breast milk can also do the trick.

- In the case of cradle cap—or thick, scaly dandruff on baby's head—apply a dab of olive oil. Leave the oil on the affected area for a couple of hours to soften the skin, rub firmly with a dry towel, then wash and dry his hair.

- Coconut oil has natural antiyeast properties. Slather a little on affected areas.

- Lots of hugs and kisses can sometimes do the trick, as does an ice pack (they love these for just about everything), especially for bruising, and "magic cream" (which is really just any natural cream).

- For split skin, skip the triple antibiotic ointment (which contains an alphabet soup of active ingredients and can cause mild side effects like minor burning and redness or less common but serious side effects like allergic reactions and severe irritation and burning).[11] Instead use a soothing, nonmedicinal cream like calendula. Dr. Rosen recommends applying it to the affected area three to four times a day.[12]

Resources

For even more information and inspiration about the topics discussed here, check out some of my favorite books, documentaries, and organizations:

Natural Birth

Books

Birthing from Within: An Extra-Ordinary Guide to Childbirth Preparation by Pam England and Rob Horowitz
Ina May's Guide to Childbirth by Ina May Gaskin
Orgasmic Birth: Your Guide to a Safe, Satisfying, and Pleasurable Birth Experience by Elizabeth Davis and Debra Pascali-Bonaro
Your Best Birth by Ricki Lake and Abby Epstein

Documentaries

Birth Story by Sara Lamm and Mary Wigmore
The Business of Being Born by Ricki Lake and Abby Epstein
Orgasmic Birth by Debra Pascali-Bonaro

Organizations

American College of Nurse-Midwives: midwife.org
DONA International: www.dona.org

Breastfeeding

Book

The Womanly Art of Breastfeeding by Diane Wiessinger, Diane West, and Teresa Pitman

Organizations

Holistic Moms Network: holisticmoms.org
Kelly Mom: kellymom.com
La Leche League International: llli.org

Kind Parenting

Books

The Attachment Parenting Book by William Sears, MD, and Martha Sears, RN
The Continuum Concept by Jean Liedloff
Diaper Free: The Gentle Wisdom of Natural Infant Hygiene by Ingrid Bauer
Good Nights: The Happy Parents' Guide to the Family Bed (and a Peaceful Night's Sleep!) by Jay Gordon, MD, and Maria Goodavage
The Happiest Baby on the Block by Harvey Karp, MD
The 90-Minute Baby Sleep Program by Polly Moore, PhD
Treatment Alternatives for Children by Lawrence Rosen, MD, and Jeff Cohen

Organizations

Attachment Parenting International: attachmentparenting.org
Babywearing International: babywearinginternational.org
DiaperFreeBaby: diaperfreebaby.org

To Find Out More from Our Experts

Suzanne Gilberg-Lenz, MD: thedrsuzanne.com
Jay Gordon, MD: drjaygordon.com
Margo Kennedy, CNM, MSN: margokennedycnm.wordpress.com
Lawrence Rosen, MD: wholechildcenter.org
Beverly Solow, IBCLC: bevsolow.com
Katherine Thurer, MD, ACOG: rabyintegrativemedicine.com

Notes

Part 1

1 Deborah Kotz, "Fighting Infertility May Be Easier Than You Think," *US News and World Report,* April 29, 2007, http://health.usnews.com/usnews/health/articles/070429/7infertility1/43.htm.

2 "Reproductive Health: Infertility FAQs," 2011, CDC, http://www.cdc.gov/reproductivehealth/infertility/.

3 Michio Kushi and Aveline Kushi, *Macrobiotic Pregnancy and Care of the Newborn* (New York: Harper & Row, 1984), 32. "Causes of Irregular Periods," Fibroids & Endometriosis Help, http://www.fibroids-and-endometriosis-help.com/causes-of-irregular-periods.html.

4 T. Colin Campbell, PhD, and Thomas M. Campbell II, MD, *The China Study* (Dallas: BenBella Books, 2006), 160.

5 P. H. Gann et al., "The Effects of a Low-Fat/High-Fiber Diet on Sex Hormone Levels and Menstrual Cycling in Premenopausal Women: A 12-Month Randomized Trial (the Diet and Hormone Study)," *Cancer* 98, no. 9 (November 1, 2003): 1870–79.

6 M. Muñoz-de-Toro et al., "Organochlorine Levels in Adipose Tissue of Women from a Littoral Region of Argentina," Environmental Research 102, no. 1 (September 2006): 107–12.

7 Jorge E. Chavarro, MD, ScD, Walter C. Willett, MD, DrPH, and Patrick Skerrett, *The Fertility Diet* (New York: McGraw-Hill, 2008), 94.

8 D. W. Cramer, H. Xu, and T. Sahi, "Adult Hypolactasia, Milk Consumption and Age-Specific Fertility," *American Journal of Epidemiology* 139, no. 3 (February 1, 1994): 282–89, http://aje.oxfordjournals.org/content/139/3/282.short.

9 "Reproductive Health: Infertility FAQs."

10 Ibid.

11 "Public Data," Google, www.google.com/publicdata.

12 Pauline W. Chen, MD, "Teaching Doctors about Nutrition and Diet," *New York Times,* September 16, 2010, http://www.nytimes.com/2010/09/16/health/16chen.html?1/4r=0.

13 "Fertility Treatment: Artificial Insemination (IUI)," BabyCenter, http://www.babycenter.com/01/4fertility-treatment-artificial-insemination-iui1/44092.bc?page=1.

14 Stephanie Saul, "21st Century Babies: Grievous Choice on Risky Path to Parenthood," *New York Times,* October 12, 2009, http://query.nytimes.com/gst/fullpage.html?res=9F0DE1D8163BF931A25753C1A96F9C8B63&ref=assistedreproductivetechnology.

15 Stephanie Saul, "The Gift of Life, and Its Price," *New York Times,* October 11, 2009, http://www.nytimes.com/2009/10/11/health/11fertility.html?pagewanted=all.

16 Ibid.

17 "In Vitro Fertilization," FertilityFactor.com, http://www.fertilityfactor.com/infertility1/4in1/4vitro1/4fertilization.html.

18 Saul, "Gift of Life."

19 Chavarro, Willett, and Skerrett, *Fertility Diet,* 208.

20 Campbell and Campbell, *China Study,* 230.

21 Chavarro, Willett, and Skerrett, *Fertility Diet,* 208.

22 "Treating for Two: Safer Medication Use in Pregnancy," National Center on Birth Defects and Developmental Disabilities, http://www.cdc.gov/ncbddd/birthdefects/documents/ncbddd1/4birth-defects1/4eiationuseonepager1/4cdcrole.pdf/. Jane E. Brody, "Too Many Pills in Pregnancy," *New York Times,* February 25, 2013, http://well.blogs.nytimes.com/2013/02/25/too-many-pills-in-pregnancy/.

23 Campbell and Campbell, *China Study,* 184.

24 Gann et al., "Effects of a Low-Fat/High-Fiber Diet."

25 Campbell and Campbell, *China Study,* 7.

26 D. A. Ehrmann, "Polycystic Ovary Syndrome," *New England Journal of Medicine* 352, no. 12 (March 24, 2005): 1223–36.

27 "Soy and Your Health," Physicians Committee for Responsible Medicine, http://pcrm.org/search/?cid=145.

28 F. Parazzini et al., "Selected Food Intake and Risk of Endometriosis," *Human Reproduction* 19, no. 8 (August 2004): 1755–59.

29 Campbell and Campbell, *China Study,* 89.

30 Chavarro, Willett, and Skerrett, *Fertility Diet,* 44.

31 Campbell and Campbell, *China Study,* 93.

32 Michael F. Roizen, MD, and Mehmet C. Oz, MD, *You: Having a Baby* (New York: Free Press, 2009), 36.

33 Ibid., 79.

34 Ibid., 2.

35 Ibid., 66.

36 Jorge E. Chavarro, MD, Walter C. Willett, MD, and Patrick Skerrett, "Fat, Carbs, and the Science of Fertility," *Newsweek,* December 10, 2007, 58.

37 N. Maconochie et al., "Risk Factors for First Trimester Miscarriage—Results from a UK-Population-Based Case-Control Study," *BJOG* 114, no. 2 (February 2007): 170–86, http://www.ncbi.nlm.nih.gov/pubmed/17305901.

38 "Position of the American Dietetic Association: Vegetarian Diets," *Journal of the American Dietetic Association* 109, no. 7 (July 2009): 1266–82.

39 "Doctors Endorse Vegan and Vegetarian Diets for Healthy Pregnancies," Physicians Committee for Responsible Medicine, http://www.pcrm.org/media/news/doctors-endorse-vegan-and-vegetarian-diets-for.

40   Kushi and Kushi, *Macrobiotic Pregnancy*, 6.
41   "Position of the American Dietetic Association: Vegetarian Diets."
42   Campbell and Campbell, *China Study*, 205.
43   Roizen and Oz, *You: Having a Baby*, 50
44   Ibid.
45   Susan Levin, MS, RD, CSSD, Physicians Committee for Responsible Medicine, e-mail interview, May 6, 2013.
46   Milton R. Mills, MD, "The Comparative Anatomy of Eating," VegSource.com, http://www.vegsource.com/news/2009/11/the-comparative-anatomy-of-eating.html.
47   Holly Roberts, DO, *Your Vegetarian Pregnancy* (New York: Simon & Schuster, 2003), 148.
48   Karl Weber, ed., *Food, Inc.* (New York: Public Affairs, 2009), 23. Robert W. Sears, MD, FAAP, and Amy Marlow, MPH, RD, CDN, *HappyBaby: The Organic Guide to Baby's First 24 Months* (New York: William Morrow Paperbacks, 2009), 24.
49   M. Hansen et al., "Potential Public Health Impacts of the Use of Recombinant Bovine Somatotropin in Dairy Production," Prepared for a Scientific Review by the Joint Expert Committee on Food Additives, Consumers Union, September 1997, http://www.consumersunion.org/news/potential-public-health-impacts-of-the-use-of-recombinant-bovine-somatrotropin-in-dairy-production-part-1/.
50   E. F. Orlando et al., "Endocrine-Disrupting Effects of Cattle Feedlot Effluent on an Aquatic Sentinel Species, the Fathead Minnow," *Environmental Health Perspectives* 112, no. 3 (March 2004): 353–58.
51   "Meat-Eating Moms Have Less Fertile Sons," Physicians Committee for Responsible Medicine, April 3, 2007, http://www.pcrm.org/health/medNews/meat-eating-moms-have-less-fertile-sons.
52   R. Sears and Marlow, *HappyBaby*, 25.
53   "Meat-Eating Moms Have Less Fertile Sons."
54   "Meat on Drugs," Consumer Reports, June 2012, http://www.consumerreports.org/content/dam/cro/news1/4articles/health/CR%20Meat%20On%20Drugs%20Report%2006-12.pdf.
55   Weber, *Food, Inc.*, 20.
56   R. Sears and Marlow, *HappyBaby*, 27.
57   "Abuse of Antibiotics at Factory Farms Threatens the Effectiveness of Drugs Used to Treat Disease in Humans," Sierra Club, http://www.sierraclub.org/factoryfarms/factsheets/antibiotics.asp.
57   Roberts, *Your Vegetarian Pregnancy*, 148.
58   "A Cesspool of Pollutants. Now Is the Time to Clean Up Your Body," *McDougall Newsletter*, August 17, 2004, http://www.nealhendrickson.com/PDF/PDFMc040800NL.pdf.
59   "Dioxin & Furans: The Most Toxic Chemicals Known to Science," Energy Justice Network, http://www.ejnet.org/dioxin.
60   Arnold Schecter et al., "Intake of Dioxins and Related Compounds from Food in the US Population," *Journal of Toxicology and Environmental Health* 63, no. 1 (May 11, 2001): 1–18, http://www.ejnet.org/dioxin/dioxininfood.pdf.
61   "Dioxin & Furans."
62   "The Natural Human Diet," PETA, http://www.peta.org/living/vegetarian-living/the-natural-human-diet.aspx.
63   Weber, *Food, Inc.*, 22.
64   "Consumer Reports Investigation: Talking Turkey," Consumer Reports, http://www.consumerreports.org/turkey0613.
65   Neal Barnard, MD, "Meat Too Tough to Eat," *Hartford Courant*, August 28, 2006, http://www.pcrm.org/media/commentary/meat-too-tough-to-eat.
66   "Natural Human Diet."
67   Ibid.
68   "Natural Human Diet."
69   Colin Beavan, *No Impact Man* (New York: Picador, 2010), 55.
70   Muñoz-de-Toro et al., "Organochlorine Levels in Adipose Tissue." G. M. Louis et al., "Environmental PCB Exposure and Risk of Endometriosis," *Human Reproduction* 20, no. 1 (January 2005): 279–85.
71   Hope Ferdowsian, MD, and Susan Levin, RD, "Fish Still Not a Healthy Choice," *Providence Journal*, October 24, 2006, http://www.pcrm.org/media/commentary/fish-still-not-a-healthy-choice.
72   Levin interview.
73   "Lard," EatThisMuch.com, http://www.eatthismuch.com/food/view/lard,272/.
74   "Lead Contamination of Chicken Eggs and Tissues from a Small Farm Flock," *Journal of Veterinary Diagnostic Investigation* 15, no. 5 (September 2003): 418–22, http://vdi.sagepub.com/content/15/5/418.full.pdf.
75   Weber, *Food, Inc.*, 23.
76   Michael Pollan, *The Omnivore's Dilemma: A Natural History of Four Meals* (New York: Penguin, 2006), 139.
77   Campbell and Campbell, *China Study*, 186.
78   Mark Bittman, "Got Milk? You Don't Need It," *New York Times*, July 7, 2012, http://opinionator.blogs.nytimes.com/2012/07/07/got-milk-you-dont-need-it/.
79   Mark Hyman, MD, "Dairy: 6 Reasons You Should Avoid It at All Costs or Why Following the USDA Food Pyramid Guidelines is Bad for Your Health," HuffPost Healthy Living, http://www.huffingtonpost.com/dr-mark-hyman/dairy-free-dairy-6-reason1/4b1/4558876.html.
80   Bittman, "Got Milk?"
81   Ibid.
82   Mayim Bialik, PhD, CLEC, *Beyond the Sling* (New York: Simon & Schuster, 2012), 24.
83   Weber, *Food, Inc.*, 25.
84   Weber, *Food, Inc.*, 121.
85   Beavan, *No Impact Man*, 126.
86   Mayim Bialik, PhD, CLEC, *Beyond the Sling* (New York: Simon & Schuster, 2012), 24.
87   Chavarro, Willett, and Skerrett, *Fertility Diet*, 44.
88   Kate Johnson, "High Sugar, Fat Intake During Early Pregnancy Increases Preeclampsia Risk," *OB GYN News*, May 15, 2000, http://findarticles.com/p/articles/mi1/4m0CYD/is1/4101/435/ai1/462827604/.
89   Jessica Porter, *The Hip Chick's Guide to Macrobiotics* (New York: Avery, 2004), 126–27.
90   Ibid.
91   Ibid.
92   "Ask Dr. Sears: Artificial Sweeteners for Kids?," Parenting, http://www.parenting.com/article/ask-dr-sears-artificial-sweeteners-for-kids.

93   "Trans Fats," American Heart Association, http://www.heart.org/HEARTORG/GettingHealthy/FatsAndOils/Fats101/Trans-4UCM1/43011201/4Article.jsp.

94   "Trans Fat Is Double Trouble for Your Heart Health," Mayo Clinic, http://www.mayoclinic.com/health/trans-fat/CL00032.

95   Ibid.

96   Chavarro, Willett, and Skerrett, "Fat, Carbs, and the Science of Fertility."

97   R. L. Blaylock, "A Possible Central Mechanism in Autism Spectrum Disorders, Part 3," *Alternative Therapies in Health and Medicine* 15, no. 2 (March–April 2009): 56–60, http://www.ncbi.nlm.nih.gov/pubmed/19284184.

98   Marilee Nelson, interview, November 19, 2012.

99   Ibid.

100 Ibid.

101 Ibid.

102 Ibid.

103 "Organic Authority.com: 5 Food Labels That Mean Nothing," HuffPost Food, January 12, 2012, http://www.huffingtonpost.com/organic-authoritycom/5-food-labels-that-mean-n1/4b1/41202681.html.

104 Andrea C. Gore, PhD, *Endocrine-Disrupting Chemicals: From Basic Research to Clinical Practice* (New York: Humana Press, 2007).

105 National Toxicology Program, *CERHR Expert Panel Report for Bisphenol A*, US Department of Health and Human Services, November 26, 2007. Breast Cancer Fund, *Disrupted Development: The Dangers of Prenatal BPA Exposure*, September 2013, http://www.breastcancerfund.org/assets/pdfs/publications/disrupted-development-the-dangers-of-prenatal-bpa-exposure.pdf.

106 Nicholas Bakalar, "BPA Levels Tied to Obesity in Youths," *New York Times*, September 24, 2012, http://well.blogs.nytimes.com/2012/09/24/bpa-levels-tied-to-obesity-in-youths/?ref=health.

107 "Bisphenol A (BPA): Use in Food Contact Application," FDA, http://www.fda.gov/%20newsevents/publichealthfocus/ucm064437.htm.

108 Jon Hamilton, "FDA Bans Chemical BPA from Sippy Cups and Baby Bottles," NPR, July 17, 2012, http://www.

npr.org/blogs/alt/2012/07/17/156916616/fda-bans-chemical-bpa-in-sippy-cups-and-baby-bottles.

109 Breast Cancer Fund, *Disrupted Development.*

110 Ibid.

111 Roizen and Oz, *You: Having a Baby*, 38.

112 Nelson interview.

113 X. Weng, R. Odouli, and D. K. Li, "Maternal Caffeine Consumption during Pregnancy and the Risk of Miscarriage: A Prospective Cohort Study," *American Journal of Obstetrics and Gynecology* 190, no. 3 (March 2008): 279.e1–8.

114 Physicians Committee for Responsible Medicine, "Endometriosis," T. Colin Campbell Foundation, http://www.tcolincampbell.org/courses-resources/article/endometriosis-1/category/gynecology-and-obstetrics-1/.

115 M. M. Perper et al., "MAST Scores, Alcohol Consumption, and Gynecological Symptoms in Endometriosis Patients," *Alcoholism, Clinical and Experimental Research* 17, no. 2 (April 1993): 272–28.

116 F. Grodstein, M. B. Goldman, and D. W. Cramer, "Infertility in Women and Moderate Alcohol Use," *American Journal of Public Health* 84, no. 9 (September 1994):1429–32.

117 Michael Pollan, *Food Rules* (New York: Penguin, 2009), 67–68.

118 E. M. Bell, I. Hertz-Picciotto, and J. Beaumont, "A Case-Control Study of Pesticides and Fetal Death Due to Congenital Anomalies," *Epidemiology* 12, no. 2 (March 2001): 148–56.

119 Ibid.

120 Pollan, *Omnivore's Dilemma*, 181.

121 Ibid., 182.

122 "EWG's 2012 Shopper's Guide to Pesticides in Produce," Environmental Working Group, http://www.ewg.org/foodnews/.

123 Rebecca Wood, *The New Whole Foods Encyclopedia* (New York: Penguin Books, 2010), 129.

124 Ibid.

125 Christopher Gavigan, *Healthy Child Healthy World* (New York: Plume, 2009), 173.

126 Gavigan, *Healthy Child Healthy World*, 176.

127 Ibid.

128 Ibid.

129 Ibid.

130 Roberts, *Your Vegetarian Pregnancy*, 84.

131 Alicia Silverstone, "Kind Classics: Vegan Pregnancy Q&A (Part 1)," The Kind Life, http://thekindlife.com/blog/2012/01/kind-classics-vegan-pregnancy-q/.

132 Alicia Silverstone, *The Kind Diet* (Emmaus, PA; New York: Rodale, 2009), 61.

133 "Soy and Your Health," Physicians Committee for Responsible Medicine, http://pcrm.org/search/?id 145.

134 Roberts, *Your Vegetarian Pregnancy*, 53.

135 Silverstone, "Kind Classics."

136 Mike Adams, "Vitamin B-12 Warning: Avoid Cyanocobalamin, Take Only Methylcobalamin," NaturalNews.com, http://www.naturalnews.com/0327661/4cyanocobalamin1/4vitamin1/4B-12.html.

137 "Seven Revolutionary Tips to Improve Brain Health," Physicians Committee for Responsible Medicine, August 2013, http://pcrm.org/media/online/aug2013/seven-revolutionary-tips-to-improve-brain-health.

138 Roizen and Oz, *You: Having a Baby*, 141.

139 Pirello interview.

140 Roberts, *Your Vegetarian Pregnancy*, 52.

141 Ibid., 78.

142 Ibid., 78.

143 Ibid., 79.

144 Mark Hyman, MD, "Nutrition Tips: Folic Acid: Killer or Cure-All?," HuffPost Healthy Living, http://www.huffingtonpost.com/dr-mark-hyman/nutrition-tips-folic-acid1/4b1/4601126.html.

145 Ibid.

146 Katherine Thurer, MD, interview, November 8, 2012.

147 Pirello interview.

148 "Position of the American Dietetic Association: Vegetarian Diets."

149 Pirello interview.

150 Siverstone "Kind Classics" interview

151 Neal Barnard, MD, "Going Vegan FAQs," Oprah.com, http://www.oprah.com/health/Frequently-Asked-Questions-About-Going-Vegan#ixzz2QCAim6fp.

152 Suzanne Gilberg-Lenz, MD, "Why I Love When My Patients Meditate," MindBodyGreen, May 2, 2013, http://www.mindbodygreen.com /0-9302/why-i-love-when-my-patients-meditate-an-md-explains.html.
153 Thurer interview.
154 Gilberg-Lenz, "Why I Love When My Patients Meditate."
155 Chavarro, Willett, and Skerrett, *Fertility Diet*, 201.
156 Kushi and Kushi, *Macrobiotic Pregnancy*, 25.
157 Margaret Nofziger, *A Cooperative Method of Natural Birth Control* (Summertown, TN: Book Publishing Company, 1992), 84.
158 Susan Dudley, Salwa Nassar, and Emily Hartman, "Tampon Safety," National Research Center for Women & Families, http://center4research.org /i-saw-it-on-the-internet/tampon-safety/.
159 "Cumulative Exposure and Feminine Care Products," Campaign for Safe Cosmetics, http://safecosmetics.org /article.php?id=777.
160 "Ladies only!," Daily Kos, http://www.dailykos.com/story/ 2008/06/06/530793/-Ladies-only.
161 Ibid.
162 "Pre-Conception Health For Men," American Pregnancy Association, http://www.americanpregnancy.org/ gettingpregnant/menpreconception.htm.
163 Roizen and Oz, *You: Having a Baby*, 381.
164 "New Ad Links Meat-Eating and Impotence," Physicians Committee for Responsible Medicine, February 9, 2004, http://pcrm.org/media/news/new-ad-links-meat-eating-and-impotence. "A Vegetarian Diet Can Help with Impotence," PETA, http://www.peta.org /living/vegetarian-living/Impotence.aspx.
165 Chavarro, Willett, and Skerrett, *Fertility Diet*, 153.

Part 2

1 Roizen and Oz, *You: Having a Baby*, 76.
2 Ibid.
3 Meredith F. Small, "The Biology of...Morning Sickness," *Discover*, September 2000, http:// discovermagazine.com/2000/sep /featbiology.

4 Roberts, *Your Vegetarian Pregnancy*, 143.
5 Roizen and Oz, *You: Having a Baby*, 75.
6 Roberts, *Your Vegetarian Pregnancy*, 144.
7 Roizen and Oz, *You: Having a Baby*, 86.
8 Roberts, *Your Vegetarian Pregnancy*, 169.
9 "Miscarriage," American Pregnancy Association, http://americanpregnancy. org/pregnancycomplications/miscarriage. html. Margo Kennedy, interview, December 7, 2012.
10 Julia Moskin, "The Weighty Responsibility of Drinking for Two," *New York Times*, November 29, 2006, http://www.nytimes.com/2006/11/29 /dining/29preg.html?1/4r=0.
11 "Alcohol During Pregnancy: How Dangerous Is It Really?" Huffington Post, April 6, 2011, http://www .huffingtonpost.com/2011/04/06 /alcohol-during-pregnancy1/4n1 /4845103.html.
12 " 'Moderate' Drinking During Pregnancy Has No Effect on Young Children: Study," *US News and World Report*, June 20, 2012, http://health. usnews.com/health-news/news/articles/ 2012/06/20/moderate-drinking-during-pregnancy-has-no-effect-on-young-children-study.
13 Alexandra Spunt, *No More Dirty Looks* (New York: Da Capo, 2010), 4.
14 Ibid.
15 "PABA," Cosmeticdatabase.com
16 Ruth Winter, MS, A *Consumer's Dictionary of Cosmetics Ingredients* (New York: Three Rivers Press, 2009), 32.
17 "Pthalates," Human Toxome Project at Environmental Working Group, http://www.ewg.org/sites /humantoxome/chemicals/ chemical1/4classes.php?class=Phthalate.s
18 "Common Chemical Increases Risk of Boys Genital Deformity," Environmental Health News, http://www.environmentalhealthnews .org/ehs/newscience/phthalates-increase-hypospadias-risk.
19 C. Testa et al., "Di-(2-ethylhexyl) Phthalate and Autism Spectrum Disorder," *ASN Neuro* 4, no. 4 (May 30, 2012): 223–29, http://www.ncbi.nlm .nih.gov/pubmed/22537663.

20 S. M. Duty et al., "Phthalate Exposure and Human Semen Parameters," *Epidemiology* 14, no. 3 (May 2003): 269–77, http://www.ncbi .nlm.nih.gov/pubmed/12859026. Shawn Dell Joyce, "Hidden Dangers of Phthalates," *Paramus Post*, March 8, 2010, http://www.paramuspost.com /article.php/201003080729337.
21 E. E. McCall, A. F. Olshan, and J. L. Daniels, "Maternal hair Dye Use and Risk of Neuroblastoma in Offspring," *Cancer Causes and Controls* 16, no. 6 (August 2005): 743–48, http://www .ncbi.nlm.nih.gov/pubmed/16049813.
22 Gavigan, *Healthy Child Healthy World*, 23.
23 "Laser Hair Removal and Pregnancy," American Pregnancy Association, http://americanpregnancy .org/pregnancyhealth/hairremoval.htm.
24 *Teratology Society Position Paper: Recommendations for Vitamin A Use during Pregnancy*, Teratology Society, 1987, http://teratology.org/pubs/vitamina.htm.
25 Roizen and Oz, *You: Having a Baby*, 187.
26 "Cell Phones/Radiation," Environmental Health Trust, http://ehtrust .org/cell-phones-radiation-3/.
27 Michael Segell, "Is Dirty Electricity Making You Sick?," *Prevention*, November 2011, http://www.prevention .com/health/healthy-living/ electromagnetic-fields-and-your-health.
28 "IARC Classifies Radiofrequency Electromagnetic Fields as Possibly Carcinogenic to Humans" (press release), International Agency for Research on Cancer, May 31, 2011, http://www.iarc .fr/en/media-centre/pr/2011/pdfs/ pr2081/4E.pdf.
29 "Protect Your Family: Cell Phone Radiation," Environmental Health Trust, http://ehtrust.org/protect-your-family-cell-phone-radiation/.
30 G. Chevalier et al., "Earthing (Grounding) the Human Body Reduces Blood Viscosity—A Major Factor in Cardiovascular Disease," *Journal of Alternative and Complementary Medicine* 19, no. 2 (February 2013): 102–10, http://online.liebertpub.com/doi /pdf/10.1089/acm.2011.0820. G. Chevalier and S. Sinatra, "Emotional Stress, Heart Rate Variability, Grounding, and Improved Autonomic

Tone: Clinical Applications," *Integrative Medicine* 10, no. 3 (June–July 2011): 16–21, http://imjournal.com/pdfarticles /IMCJ101/431/4p161/424chevalier.pdf.

31   "UCLA Psychology Study Finds Resonance with Buddhist Teachings," UCLA International Institute, http://www .international.ucla.edu/buddhist/article .asp?parentid=72539.

32   Committee of Obstetric Practice, "ACOG Commitee Opinion: Exercise During Pregnancy and the Postpartum Period," *International Journal of Gynaecology and Obstetrics* 77, no. 1 (April 2002): 79–81, http://www.acog .org/Resources1/4And1/4Publications /Committee1/4Opinions/Committee1 /4on1/4Obstetric1/4Practice/Exercise1 /4During1/4Pregnancy1/4and1/4the1 /4Postpartum1/4Period.

33   Roizen and Oz, *You: Having a Baby*, 108–9.

34   Gabrielle Birkner, "Home Births on the Rise for New York Families," *Wall Street Journal*, August 25, 2013, http:// online.wsj.com/article/SB100014241278 8732363970457901690283439742.

35   Ricki Lake and Abby Epstein, *Your Best Birth* (New York: Wellness Central/ Grand Central Publishing, 2010), 11.

36   Mother's Index 2013, Save the Children, http://www.savethechildren.org /site/c.8rKLIXMGIpI4E/b.8585863 /k.9F31/State1/4of1/4the1/4Worlds1 /4Mothers.htm.

37   Ibid.

38   Ibid.

39   Ina May Gaskin, *Ina May's Guide to Childbirth* (New York: Bantam Dell, 2003), 276.

40   Ibid.

41   American College of Obstetricians and Gynecologists Task Force on Cesarean Delivery Rates, *Evaluation of Cesarean Delivery*, 2001, 25–26.

42   Ellen Chuse, inteview, January 9, 2013.

43   *Orgasmic Birth*, 35

44   "Study Finds Adverse Effects of Pitocin in Newborns" (press release), ACOG, May 7, 2013, http://www.acog. org/About1/4ACOG/News1/4Room /News1/4Releases/2013/Study1/4Finds1 /4Adverse1/4Effects1/4of1/4Pitocin1 /4in1/4Newborns.

45   Lake and Epstein, *Your Best Birth*, 120.

46   E. R. Declercq et al., *Listening to Mothers III: Pregnancy and Birth* (New York: Childbirth Connection, 2013).

47   Mary Kroeger, *Impact of Birthing Practices on Breastfeeding: Protecting the Mother and Baby Continuum* (Sudbury, MA: Jones and Bartlett, 2004).

48   "Using Narcotics for Pain Relief during Childbirth," American Pregnancy Association, http://americanpregnancy .org/labornbirth/narcotics.html.

49   Ibid.

50   http://www.medsmilk.com

51   Lake and Epstein, *Your Best Birth*, 123.

52   Ibid.

53   K. Johnson and B.-A. Daviss, "Outcomes of Planned Home Births with Certified Professional Midwives: Large Prospective Study in North American" *British Medical Journal* 330, no. 7505 (June 18, 2005): 1416.

54   E. D. Hodnett et al., "Continuous Support for Women During Childbirth," *Cochrane Review* 3 (2003).

55   Patricia A. Janssen et al., "Outcomes of Planned Home Birth with Registered Midwife versus Planned Hospital Birth with Midwife or Physician," *Canadian Medical Association Journal* 181, no. 6–7 (September 15, 2009). doi: 10.1503/cmaj.081869

56   Bialik, *Beyond the Sling*, 38.

57   Eugene Declercq, "Birth By the Numbers," Orgasmic Birth, http://www .orgasmicbirth.com/birth-by-the- numbers.

58   "Infant and Neonatal Mortality for Primary Cesarean and Vaginal Births to Women with 'No Indicated Risk,' " *Birth* 33, no. 3 (September 2006): 175–82, http://onlinelibrary.wiley.com/ doi/10.1111/j.1523- 536X.2006.00102.x/abstract;jsessionid= B9196B0659B0ACDDDDEAFF350CF. d01t03.

59   E. Kuklina et al., "Severe Obstetric Morbidity in the United States: 1998– 2005," *Obstetrics and Gynecology* 113, no. 2 (Feb. 2009): 293–99.

60   Cara Birnbaum, "What Doctors Don't Tell You about C-Sections," Health, Octoer 2009, http://www.health. com/health/article/0,,20412033,00.html.

61   Ibid.

62   Gaskin, *Ina May's Guide to Childbirth*, 289.

63   Ibid., 289–90.

64   Roizen and Oz, *You: Having a Baby*, 241.

65   "OB Gyns Issue Less Restrictive VBAC Guidelines" (press release), ACOG, July 21, 2010, http://www.acog. org/About1/4ACOG/News1/4Room /News1/4Releases/2010/Ob1/4Gyns1 /4Issue1/4Less1/4Restrictive1/4VBAC1 /4Guidelines.

66   Davis and Pascali-Bonaro, *Orgasmic Birth*, 42.

67. *American Family Physician*. "ACOG Issues: Guidelines on Fetal Macrosomia." July 1, 2001, 64 (1): 169–70.

68   Gaskin, *Ina May's Guide to Childbirth*, 170.

69   Lake and Epstein, *Your Best Birth*, 112.

70   Ibid., 111.

71   "Anesthesia and Queen Victoria," UCLA Department of Epidemiology and School of Public Health, http://www.ph .ucla.edu/epi/snow/victoria.html.

72   Gaskin, *Ina May's Guide to Childbirth*, 230.

73   Ibid., 229.

74   "The High Cost of Medical Procedures in the US," *Washington Post*, http://www.washingtonpost.com/wp-srv /special/business/high-cost-of-medical- procedures-in-the-us/.

75   Lake and Epstein, *Your Best Birth*, 35–36.

76   Lake and Epstein, *Your Best Birth*, 40.

77   Talk by Sheila Kitzinger paraphrased by Ellen Chuse, in Chuse interview.

78   William Sears, MD, and Martha Sears, RN, with Robert Sears, MD, and James Sears, MD, *The Baby Book* (New York: Little, Brown and Company, 2003), 22.

79   Ibid., 79.

80   Gaskin, *Ina May's Guide to Childbirth*, 307.

81   Kushi and Kushi, *Macrobiotic Pregnancy*, 109–10.

82   Gaskin, *Ina May's Guide to Childbirth*, 306.

83   Lake and Epstein, *Your Best Birth*, 86.

84   Ibid., 80.

85   Lake and Epstein, *Your Best Birth*, 14–15.

86   Ibid.

87　Roizen and Oz, *You: Having a Baby*, 196.

88　Roberts, *Your Vegetarian Pregnancy*, 162.

89　Ibid., 164.

90　R. Sears and Marlow, *HappyBaby*, 45.

91　Pam England, CNM, and Rob Horowitz, PhD, *Birthing from Within* (Albuquerque, NM: Partera Press, 1998), 271.

92　E. Bergroth et al., "Respiratory Tract Illnesses during the First Year of Life: Effect of Dog and Cat Contacts," *Pediatrics* 130, no. 2 (August 2012): 211–20. doi: 10.1542/peds.2011-2825

93　"Body Burden—the Pollution in Newborns," Environmental Working Group, July 14, 2005, http://archive .ewg.org/reports/bodyburden2/ execsumm.php.

94　"Pregnant Women," CDC, http://www.cdc.gov/nceh/lead/tips /pregnant.htm.

95　Mary Cordaro, "The Parent Trap: Avoid Mistakes in Nursery Projects by Following Three Basic Principles," Green Home Guide, October 3, 2012, http://greenhomeguide.com/know-how /article/the-parent-trap-avoid-mistakes- in-nursery-projects-by-following-three- basic-principles.

96　Gavigan, *Healthy Child Healthy World*, 179.

97　Ibid., 52.

98　Kim Barnouin, *Skinny Bitch: Home, Beauty, and Style* (New York: Running Press, 2011), 71.

99　"Toxic Chemicals in Our Couches," NRDC, http://www.nrdc.org/health /flame-retardants/toxic-couch.asp.

100　Gavigan, *Healthy Child Healthy World*, 226.

101　Ibid., 2.

102　Nicholas D. Kristof, "New Alarm Bells about Chemicals and Cancer," *New York Times,* May 6, 2010, http://www .nytimes.com/2010/05/06/ opinion/06kristof.html.

103　"The Inside Story: A Guide to Indoor Air Quality," EPA, www.epa.gov /iaq/pubs/insidestory.html.

104　*EWG Cleaners Database Hall of Shame,* Environmental Working Group, 2012, http://static.ewg.org/reports/2012 /cleaners1/4hallofshame /cleaners1/4hallofshame.pdf.

105　Roizen and Oz, *You: Having a Baby*, 141.

106　Ibid.

107　Ibid., 142.

108　Afsha Bawany, "Steamed, Dehydrated, or Raw: Placentas May Help Moms' Post-Partum Health," UNLV News Center, February 27, 2013, http://news.unlv.edu/article/steamed- dehydrated-or-raw-placentas-may-help- moms'-post-partum-health.

109　Nicholas Bakalar, "US Circumcision Rates Are Declining," *New York Times,* August 22, 2013, http://well .blogs.nytimes. com/2013/08/22/u-s-circumcision-rates- are-declining/?1/4r=0.

110　William Sears, MD, "Dr. Sears Statement on Circumcision," Peaceful Parenting, October 27, 2009, http:// www.drmomma.org/2009/10/dr-sears- statement-on-circumcision.html.

111　Ibid.

112　England and Horowitz, *Birthing from Within*, 188.

113　"Incisive Arguments," *Economist*, July 7, 2012, 51.

114　Jill Tucker, "Pre-Birth Maternity Leave Aids Babies, Moms," SFGate, January 8, 2009, http://www.sfgate.com /bayarea/article/Pre-birth-maternity- leave-aids-babies-moms-3177455.php.

115　England and Horowitz, *Birthing from Within*, 182.

116　Jenny McCarthy and Jerry Kartzinel, MD, *Healing and Preventing Autism* (New York: Plume, 2010), 279.

117　A. Stevens Wrightson, MD, "Universal Newborn Hearing Screening," *American Family Physician* 75, no. 9 (May 1, 2007): 1349–52, http://www. aafp.org/afp/2007/0501/p1349.html.

118　William Sears, MD, and Martha Sears, RN, *The Attachment Parenting Book* (New York: Little, Brown and Company, 2001), 38.

119　Roizen and Oz, *You: Having a Baby*, 132.

120　W. Sears and M. Sears, *Attachment Parenting Book*, 39.

121　Ibid.

122　Ibid.

123　Davis and Pascali-Bonaro, *Orgasmic Birth*, 43.

124　Marie F. Mongan, MEd, MHy, *HypnoBirthing* (Deerfield Beach, FL: Health Communications, Inc., 2005), 200.

125　"2011 Childrens Car Seat Findings," HealthyStuff.org, http://www .healthystuff.org/findings.080311 .carseats.php.

126　"PVC Policies across the World: PVC Factsheet," CHEJ, http://www.chej .org/pvcfactsheets/PVC1/4Policies1 /4Around1/4The1/4World.html.

127　Roizen and Oz, *You: Raising Your Child*, 257..

128　Bialik, *Beyond the Sling*, 168. Roizen and Oz, *You: Raising Your Child*, 62.

129　Bialik, *Beyond the Sling*, 168.

130　Tina Rosenberg, "The Power of Talking to Your Baby," *New York Times,* April 10, 2013, http://opinionator.blogs .nytimes.com/2013/04/10/the-power-of- talking-to-your-baby/.

131　National Toxicology Program, *CERHR Expert Panel Report for Bisphenol A.*

132　"Introduction: Chemicals of Concern," HealthyStuff.org, http://www. healthystuff.org/chemicals.introduction. php.

133　Gavigan, *Healthy Child Healthy World*, 127.

134　R. Sears and Marlow, *HappyBaby*, 15.

135　Daniel Steinway, "Trashing Superfund: The Role of Municipal Solid Waste in CERCLA Cases," *CCM,* November 1999, http://library.findlaw. com/1999/Nov/1/130490.html.

136　R. Sears and Marlow, *HappyBaby*, 15.

Part 3

1　Tucker, "Pre-birth Maternity Leave Aids Babies, Moms."

2　Melanie Waxman, *Bless the Baby* (London: Carroll and Brown, Ltd., 2001), 68–70.

3　Ibid.

4　Ibid.

5　Kushi and Kushi, *Macrobiotic Pregnancy*, 137.

6　Waxman, *Bless the Baby*, 71.

7　Kushi and Kushi, *Macrobiotic Pregnancy*, 137.

8　Ibid.

9　Ibid.

10　Pirello interview.

11　"AAP Breastfeeding Recommendation: Statement Reaffirms Babies Should be Breastfed for 6

Months," HuffPost Parents, February 28, 2012, http://www.huffingtonpost .com/2012/02/28/aap-breastfeeding-recommendation1/4n1/41307866.html.

12   Jill Lepore, "Baby Food," *New Yorker,* January 19, 2009, http://www. newyorker.com/reporting/2009/01/19/0 90119fa1/4fact1/4lepore#ixzz26C6L 8MR9

13   Ibid.

14   Alissa Quart, "The Milk Wars," *New York Times,* July 15, 2012, http:// www.nytimes.com/2012/07/15/opinion /sunday/the-breast-feeding-wars.html.

15   "Up to What Age Can a Baby Stay Well Nourished by Just Being Breastfed?," World Health Organization, July 2013, http://www.who.int/features /qa/21/en/index.html.

16   Quart, "The Milk Wars."

17   World Health Organization, *International Code of Marketing of Breast-Milk Substitutes,* 1981, http://www.who .int/nutrition/publications/ code1/4english.pdf.

18   Bialik, *Beyond the Sling* 70.

19   England and Horowitz, *Birthing from Within,* 272–74.

20   Bialik, *Beyond the Sling,* 69–70.

21   England and Horowitz, *Birthing from Within,* 272–74.

22   Solomon, "Controversy over Infant Formula."

23   L. A. Hanson et al., "The Mammary Gland–Infant Intestine Immunologic Dyad," *Advances in Experimental Medicine and Biology* 478 (2000): 65–76.

24   S. Schwartz et al., "A Metagenomic Study of Diet-Dependent Interaction between Gut Microbiota and Host in Infants Reveals Differences in Immune Response," *Genome Biology* 13, no. 4 (April 30, 2012): r32, http:// genomebiology.com/2012/13/4/r32.

25   W. A. Walker, "Host Defense Mechanisms in the Gastrointestinal Tract," *Pediatrics* 57, no. 6 (Jun. 1976): 901–16; W. A. Walker, "Absorption of Protein and Protein Fragments in the Developing Intestine," *Pediatrics* 75 (January 1985): 167–71. A. Rigas et al., "Breast-Feeding and Maternal Smoking in the Etiology of Crohn's Disease and Ulcerative Colitis in Childhood," *Annals of Epidemiology* 3, no. 4 (July 1993): 387–92. S. Koletzko et al., "Role of

Infant Feeding Practices in Development of Crohn's Disease in Childhood," *BMJ* 298, no. 6688 (June 1989): 1617–18.

26   "Why Breastfeeding is Important," WomensHealth.gov, http://www .womenshealth.gov/breastfeeding/why-breastfeeding-is-important/.

27   F. R. Greer et al., "Effects of Early Nutritional Interventions on the Development of Atopic Disease in Infants and Children," *Pediatrics* 121, no. 1 (January 1, 2008): 183–91, http:// pediatrics.aappublications.org/ content/121/1/183.short. Silverstone, "Kind Classics."

28   R. Sears and Marlow, *HappyBaby,* 59.

29   M. P. Degano and R. A. Degano, "Breastfeeding and Oral Health. A Primer for the Dental Practitioner," *New York State Dental Journal* 59, no. 2 (Feb. 1993): 30–32. Danielle Rigg, "Get Inspired by Your Mom-Made Wonder Food," Best for Babes, http://www. bestforbabes.org/your-mom-made-wonder-food.

30   J. Freudenheim et al., "Exposure to Breastmilk in Infancy and the Risk of Breast Cancer," *Epidemiology* 5, no. 3 (May 1994): 324–31.

31   B. B. Osinaike et al., "Effect of Breastfeeding during Venepuncture in Neonates," *Annals of Tropical Paediatrics* 27, no. 3 (September 2007): 201–5.

32   J. Cubero et al., "The Circadian Rhythm of Tryptophan in Breast Milk Affects the Rhythms of 6-Sulfatoxymelatonin and Sleep in Newborn," *Neuro Endocrinology Letters* 26, no. 6 (December 2005): 657–61.

33   E. S. Mezzacappa, "Breastfeeding and Maternal Stress Response and Health," *Nutrition Reviews* 62, no. 7, pt. 1 (July 2004): 261–68.

34   W. Sears et al., *Baby Book,* 7.

35   England and Horowitz, *Birthing from Within,* 272–74.

36   T. Doan T et al., "Breast-Feeding Increases Sleep Duration of New Parents," *Journal of Perinatal & Neonatal Nursing* 21, no. 3 (July–September 2007): 200–6.

37   Roizen and Oz, *You: Having a Baby,* 252.

38   R. Sears and Marlow, *HappyBaby,* 60.

39   Bialik, *Beyond the Sling,* 59.

40   R. Sears and Marlow, *HappyBaby,* 61.

41   R. Sears and Marlow, *HappyBaby,* 69.

42   Ibid., 64–66.

43   Solow interview.

44   Roizen and Oz, *You: Having a Baby,* 252.

45   R. Sears and Marlow, *HappyBaby,* 60.

46   Kushi and Kushi, *Macrobiotic Pregnancy,* 157.

47   Ibid.

48   Ibid.

49   Bialik, *Beyond the Sling,* 63.

50   Kushi and Kushi, *Macrobiotic Pregnancy,* 157.

51   R. Sears and Marlow, *HappyBaby,* 65.

52   Silverstone, "Kind Classics."

53   Roberts, *Your Vegetarian Pregnancy,* 313.

54   Silverstone, "Kind Classics."

55   Kushi and Kushi, *Macrobiotic Pregnancy,* 156.

56   Ibid.

57   Ibid.

58   Ibid.

59   Ibid.

60   Ibid.

61   Ibid.

62   Warren Kramer, interview.

63   R. Sears and Marlow, *HappyBaby,* 137.

64   R. Sears and Marlow, *HappyBaby,* 84.

65   Emily Sohn, "Even BPA-Free Plastic Not Always Safe," Discovery News, July 15, 2011, http://news. discovery.com/human/health/bpa-plastic-food-hormones-chemicals-110715.htm.

66   R. Sears and Marlow, *HappyBaby,* 83.

67   C. R. Howard et al., "Randomized Clinical Trial of Pacifier Use and Bottle-Feeding or Cupfeeding and their Effect on Breastfeeding," *Pediatrics* 111, no. 3 (Mar. 2003): 511–18. C. G. Victora et al., "Pacifier Use and Short Breastfeeding Duration: Cause, Consequence, or Coincidence?," *Pediatrics* 99, no. 3 (March 1997): 445–53.

68   R. Sears and Marlow, *HappyBaby,* 76.

69   Ibid., 82.

70   "Storing and Transporting Breast Milk," AskDrSears, http://www.askdrsears.com/topics/breastfeeding/while-working/storing-transporting-breast-milk.

71   Solomon, "Controversy over Infant Formula."

72   Ibid.

73   Ibid.

74   Campbell and Campbell, *China Study*, 205.

75   England and Horowitz, *Birthing from Within*, 272–74.

76   Solomon, "Controversy over Infant Formula."

77   R. Sears and Marlow, *HappyBaby*, 67.

78   Roizen and Oz, *You: Having a Baby*, 123.

79   Thomas W. Hale, *Medications and Mothers' Milk 2012* (Amarillo, TX: Hale Publishing, 2012), 417–19. Nicki Heskin, "Drinking While Breastfeeding—Pumping and Dumping," BellaOnline, http://www.bellaonline.com/articles/art174499.asp.

80   "What About Drinking Alcohol and Breastfeeding?" La Leche League International, http://www.lalecheleague.org/faq/alcohol.html.

81   Ibid.

82   Kelly Bonyata, IBCLC, "Plugged Ducts and Mastitis," KellyMom, July 27, 2011, http://kellymom.com/bf/concerns/mother/mastitis/.

83   Solow interview.

84   Bonyata, "Plugged Ducts and Mastitis."

85   Solow interview.

86   "Vegetarian Diets for Children: Right from the Start," Physicians Committee for Responsible Medicine, http://pcrm.org/search/?cid=263.

87   Lisa Marasco, "Common Breastfeeding Myths," *Leaven* 34, no. 2 (April–May 1998): 21–24, http://www.llli.org/nb/lvaprmay98p21nb.html.

88   "AAP Breastfeeding Recommendation."

89   Quart, "The Milk Wars."

90   A. S. Goldman et al., "Immunologic Components in Human Milk during Weaning," *Acta Paediatrica Scandinavica* 72, no. 1 (Jan. 1983): 133–34.

91   Katherine A. Dettwyler, PhD, "A Time to Wean," *Breastfeeding Abstracts* 14, no. 1 (August 1994): 3–4, http://www.llli.org/ba/aug94.html.

92   Ibid.

93   "Would Weaning Make My Life Easier?" La Leche League International, http://www.llli.org/faq/wean.html.

94   W. Sears et al., *Baby Book*, 195.

95   Roberts, *Your Vegetarian Pregnancy*, 324.

96   Kushi and Kushi, *Macrobiotic Pregnancy*, 175.

97   Lawrence Rosen, MD, and Jeff Cohen, *Treatment Alternatives for Children* (New York: Alpha Books), 3.

98   B. Hesselmar et al., "Pacifier Cleaning Practices and Risk of Allergy Development," *Pediatrics* 131, no. 6 (June 2013): e1829–37, http://pediatrics.aappublications.org/content/early/2013/04/30/peds.2012-3345.abstract.

99   T. Berry Brazelton, "A Child-Oriented Approach to Toilet Training," *Pediatrics* 29, no. 1 (January 1, 1962): 121–28, http://pediatrics.aappublications.org/content/29/1/121.

100   R. Sears and Marlow, *HappyBaby*, 277.

101   "Municipal Solid Waste in the United States, 2007," Environmental Protection Agency, http://www.epa.gov/osw/nonhaz/municipal/pubs/msw07-rpt.pdf.

102   R. Sears and Marlow, *HappyBaby*, 277.

103   C, Lehrburger, J. Mullen, and C. V. Jones, *Diapers, Environmental Impacts and Lifecycle Analysis* (Philadelphia: Report to the National Association of Diaper Services, 1991).

104   R. Sears and Marlow, *HappyBaby*, 277.

105   Gavigan, *Healthy Child Healthy World*, 134.

106   "Glossary of Volatile Organic Compounds," CDC, http://www.cdc.gov/nceh/clusters/fallon/glossary-voc.pdf.

107   Gavigan, *Healthy Child Healthy World*, 134.

108   "Choose Chlorine-Free Diapers," Healthy Child Healthy World, January 7, 2013, http://healthychild.org/easy-steps/choose-unscented-chlorine-free-diapers/.

109   C. J. Partsch, M. Aukamp, and W. G. Sippell, "Scrotal Temperature Is Increased in Disposable Plastic Lined Nappies," *Archives of Disease in Childhood* 83, no. 4 (Oct. 2000): 364–68.

110   R. Sears and Marlow, *HappyBaby*, 283.

111   Kimberly Delaney, *Knack Clean Home Green Home* (Guilford, CT: Globe Pequot, 2008), 98.

112   Gavigan. *Healthy Child Healthy World*, 134.

113   Jean Liedloff, *The Continuum Concept* (New York: De Capo Press, 1986).

114   R. Sears and Marlow, *HappyBaby*, 16.

115   Gavigan, *Healthy Child Healthy World*, 113.

116   Ibid.

Part 4

1   W. Sears et al., *Baby Book*, 318.

2   Ibid., 12.

3   Bialik, *Beyond the Sling*, 221

4   R. Sears and Marlow, *HappyBaby*, 51.

5   W. Sears et al., *Baby Book*, 17.

6   Ibid., 14.

7   R. Sears and Marlow, *HappyBaby*, 51.

8   W. Sears et al., *Baby Book*, 14.

9   Ibid., 12.

10   Bialik, *Beyond the Sling*, 20.

11   Mongan, *HypnoBirthing*, 275.

12   Sindya N. Bhanoo, "In Parents' Embrace Infants' Heart Rates Drop," *New York Times*, April 23, 2013, http://www.nytimes.com/2013/04/23/science/picking-up-infants-calms-by-slowing-heart-rates.html?_r=0.

13   Ibid.

14   Roizen and Oz, You: Having a Baby, 122.

15   W. Sears and M. Sears, *Attachment Parenting Book*, 71.

16   W. Sears et al., *Baby Book*, 318.

17   W. Sears and M. Sears, *Attachment Parenting Book*, 71–72.

18   Bialik, *Beyond the Sling*, 84.

19   Ibid., 88.

20   Roizen and Oz, *You: Having a Baby*, 132.

21   Waxman, *Bless the Baby*, 80–85.

22   Ibid.

23   Harvey Karp, MD, *The Happiest Baby on the Block* (New York: Bantam Books, 2002), 222.

24   Bialik, *Beyond the Sling*, 92.

25   Karp, *Happiest Baby on the Block*, 222.

26   W. Sears and M. Sears, *Attachment Parenting Book*, 94.

27   Ibid.

28   Bialik, *Beyond the Sling*, 96.

29   W. Sears and M. Sears, *Attachment Parenting Book*, 92.

30   Ibid.

31   Ibid., 331.

32   Gordon and Goodavage, *Good Nights*, 11.

33   W. Sears et al., *Baby Book*, 337.

34   "Children's Sleep: An Interplay between Culture and Biology," *Pediatrics* 15, no. 1 (January 2005): 204–16, http://pediatrics.aappublications.org/content/115/Supplement_1/204.full.

35   W. Sears et al., *Baby Book*, 337.

36   Aletha Jauch Solter, *The Aware Baby* (Goleta, GA: Shining Star Press, 2001).

37   W. Sears and M. Sears, *Attachment Parenting Book*, 335.

38   Gordon and Goodavage, *Good Nights*, xiv.

39   "The New Basics: Family Bed," Tribeca Pediatrics, https://www.tribecapediatrics.com/TPeds/book-excerpt/family-bed/.

40   Gordon and Goodavage, *Good Nights*, xiv.

41   W. Sears and M. Sears, *Attachment Parenting Book*, 335.

42   Gordon and Goodavage, *Good Nights*, 23.

43   Ibid.

44   W. Sears et al., *Baby Book*, 406–7.

45   "The New Basics: Co-Sleeping," Tribeca Pediatrics, https://www.tribecapediatrics.com/TPeds/book-excerpt/cosleeping/.

46   Gordon and Goodavage, *Good Nights*, xiv.

47   Ibid., 58.

48   Ibid., 13–16.

49   W. Sears et al., *Baby Book*, 335.

50   Ibid.

51   Ibid., 336.

52   "Children's Sleep: An Interplay Between Culture and Biology."

53   SIDS Resource Center Statistics, www.sidscenter.org/statistics.html.

54   Ibid.

55   J. Laughlin et al., "Prevention and Management of Positional Skull Deformities in Infants," *Pediatrics* 128,

no. 6 (December 1, 2011): 1236–20, www.pediatrics.org/cgi/doi/10.1542/peds.2011-2220.

56   J. J. McKenna, "An Anthropological Perspective on the Sudden Infant Death Syndrome (SIDS): The Role of Parental Breathing Cues and Speech Breathing Adaptations," *Medical Anthropology* 10, no. 1 (winter 1986): 9–53.

57   "Prevention and Management of Positional Skull Deformities in Infants."

58   Kushi and Kushi, Macrobiotic Pregnancy, 200.

59   "IARC Classifies Formaldehyde as Carcinogenic to Humans" (press release), International Agency for Research on Cancer, June 15, 2004, http://www.iarc.fr/en/media-centre/pr/2004/pr153.html.

60   Mindy Pennybacker, "Green Sleep: Mattress Matters," HuffPost Green, April 18, 2013, http://www.huffingtonpost.com/mindy-pennybacker/green-sleep-mattress-matters_b_3107096.html.

61   Gavigan, *Healthy Child Healthy World*, 132.

62   Gavigan, *Healthy Child Healthy World*, 216.

63   "Down and Silk: Birds and Insects Exploited for Feathers and Fabric," PETA, http://www.peta.org/issues/Animals-Used-for-Clothing/down-and-silk-birds-and-insects-exploited-for-fabric.aspx.

64   Barnouin, *Skinny Bitch*, 40.

65   Ibid., 42. Gavigan, *Healthy Child Healthy World*, 215.

66   Barnouin, *Skinny Bitch*, 43.

67   Ibid.

68   Ibid.

69   Ibid.

70   Roizen and Oz, *You: Having a Baby*, 195.

71   R. Sears and Marlow, *HappyBaby*, 37.

72   Ibid., 260.

73   Roizen and Oz, *You: Having a Baby*, 281.

74   Roberts, *Your Vegetarian Pregnancy*, 337.

75   Roizen and Oz, *You: Having a Baby*, 281.

76   W. Sears et al., *Baby Book*, 522.

77   Ibid.

78   Gavigan, *Healthy Child Healthy World*, 47.

79   Ibid.

80   Ibid., 49.

81   "Triclosan," Beyond Pesticides, http://www.beyondpesticides.org/antibacterial/triclosan.php.

82   Gavigan, *Healthy Child Healthy World*, 48.

83   "When a Nursing Mother Gets Sick," BreastfeedingBasics, http://www.breastfeedingbasics.com/articles/when-a-nursing-mother-gets-sick.

84   Ibid.

85   Roizen and Oz, *You: Having a Baby*, 393.

86   Ibid.

87   Rosen and Cohen, *Treatment Alternatives for Children*, 12.

88   Ibid.

89   "Why Delay Solids?" KellyMom, August 2, 2011, http://kellymom.com/nutrition/starting-solids/delay-solids/.

90   Ibid.

91   Douglas Quenqua, "Infants Are Fed Solid Food Too Soon, CDC Finds," *New York Times*, March 25, 2013, http://www.nytimes.com/2013/03/25/health/many-babies-fed-solid-food-too-soon-cdc-finds.html?_r=3&.

92   "Why Delay Solids?"

93   Ibid.

94   Quenqua, "Infants Are Fed Solid Food Too Soon."

95   "Why Delay Solids?"

96   Ibid.

97   Pirello interview.

98   Ibid.

99   R. Sears and Marlow, *HappyBaby*, 170.

100   "Artificial Sweeteners and Other Food Substitutes: Dangerous to Your Health?" October 15, 2010, http://www.doctoroz.com/videos/artificial-sweeteners-and-other-food-substitutes-dangerous-your-health.

101   "Ask Dr. Sears: Artificial Sweeteners for Kids?"

102   "Municipal Solid Waste Generation, Recycling and Disposal in the United States," Environmental Protection Agency, http://www.epa.gov/epawaste/nonhaz/municipal/pubs/msw07-fs.pdf.

103   R. Sears and Marlow, *HappyBaby*, 171.

104   Weber, *Food, Inc.*, 104.

105   Ibid.

106   C. L. Curl, R. A. Fenske, and K. Elgethun, "Organophosphorus Pesticide Exposure of Urban and Suburban

Preschool Children with Organic and Conventional Diets," *Environmental Health Perspectives* 111, no. 3 (March 2003): 377–82.

107   Ibid.

108   W. Sears et al., *Baby Book*, 465.

109   R. Sears and Marlow, *HappyBaby*, 147.

110   Weber, *Food, Inc.,* 104.

111   Hesselmar, "Pacifier Cleaning Practices."

112   Benjamin Spock, MD, "Good Nutrition for Kids," *Good Medicine* 7, no. 2 (spring–summer 1998), http://pcrm.org /search/?cid=1509.

113   "Vegetarian Diets: Advantages for Children," Physicians Committee for Responsible Medicine, http://pcrm.org /search/?cid=264.

114   Ibid.

115   Ibid.

116   Ibid.

117   Ibid.

Appendix

1   Rosen and Cohen, *Treatment Alternatives for Children*, 48.

2   Ibid., 88–89.

3   Roizen and Oz, *You: Having a Baby*, 173.

4   Rosen and Cohen, *Treatment Alternatives for Children*, 88–89.

5   Ibid., 72, 74.

6   Ibid.

7   Ibid., 100.

8   Ibid., 98.

9   Ibid.

10   Ibid., 9.

11   Ibid., 190.

12   Ibid.

Index

Underscored page references indicate boxed text and tables. **Boldface** references indicate photographs.

Acknowledgments

This book would not have been possible without the support and inspiration of many people. I'd like to offer my deepest gratitude to:

Laura Dern, Deborah Frank, Lesa Carlson, Roxanne Klein, Mina Dobic, Rhonda Fehr, and Ricki Lake for planting the seed that there's a healthier and more natural way to have babies.

OG Kind Mamas Laura Louie and Lalanya Bridges for being my greatest inspiration and sharing your wisdom.

My Tribe Mamas Fatime Kramer, Alanis Morissette, Heather Mancini, and our family's trusted community: Alexandra Keeling Thompson; Heather David; Suzanne Lutz; Claire Weiss; Calvin and the Lapidus family; Marty, Alleza, Jazz, and Tess Callner; Marina Black; Renee Loux; and Anna Avelar.

My birth team, Margot Kennedy and Kelly Dietzen, for being so loving and wise. Dr. Ronald Wu for being such a great doctor—and the nurses at Glendale Hospital.

Carrie Gordon and Amanda Nesbitt and all the ladies at 42 West. Plus Andrea McNicol, Jennifer Rudolph Walsh, Bianca Levin, Jason Weinberg, Guy Oseary, Donovan Daughtry, and Ruthanne Secunda for helping me put all the pieces together.

My collaborator, Rachel Holtzman, for being so smart, warm, passionate, organized, and all-around great to work with. And, of course, for birthing this book with me—even when you were birthing your own baby!

My editor, Alex Postman, for taking the greatest care with every detail and being so kind through it all; Kara Plikaitis and Yelena Nesbit for their dedication and creativity; and Nancy Bailey, Paula Brisco, Brent Gallenberger, Mary Ann Naples, and the rest of the Rodale team—I so appreciate working with a company that takes its mission of health so seriously.

Amy Neunsinger, for your amazing photos, good vibes, sweet spirit, and generosity. Jeanne Kelly for your careful kind food prep; Kate Martindale for your beautiful treasures; and Lisa Thompson, Lydia Burkhalter, Andrew Mitchell and Marc Levy, for helping our shoot go so smoothly.

Jill Lincoln, Alyssa Sutter, Alex Elian, Alana Cain, Marco Berardini, Heather Currie, and Soleil Moon Frye—plus Jude, Wyler, Blue, and Calhoun.

Dr. Neal Barnard, Marilee Nelson, Dr. Lawrence Rosen, Bonnie Solow, Dr. Katherine Thurer, Dr. Suzanne Gilberg-Lenz, Susan Levin, Ellen Chuse, Dr. Randine Lewis, and Melanie Waxman for lending your invaluable expertise. Warren Kramer for being my sage guide in wellness, and Diane Avoli, for sharing your gifts before leaving this world.

Christina Pirello, for being my big sister in health and answering my endless questions.

Dr. Jay Gordon, for your brilliance, and Lorri Horn, for making sure all my questions get answered.

Karen Bryson, for helping me create many of the delicious recipes in this book and keeping us so well fed. And Ty Nasief for feeding me so well post-birth! And Rebecca Benenati for teaching the most yummy prenatal yoga classes.

Brian Ray and the Garden of Life team, for helping me share even more love and health with the world.

The Kind Life Community for their motivation and fire; and all the mamas for so bravely telling their stories in the book and who move me to keep seeking.

Nora Smithson, Helen O'Connell, and Garnet Batinovich for being my loving aunties when I was a little girl.

My Spina family for being such a loving bunch—to each other, and to me.

Mom, for breastfeeding me, doing bedoos together, and tickling my back before bed.

Dad, for being such a good "doctor" when I was sick or hurt, for taking me traveling, and for passing down your drive and encouraging my career choice.

Christopher, for surprising me in Detroit. And for being the best dad in the world to Bear.

Bear, for being the most precious, scrumdiliumptious being ever. You ground me, focus me, and make my heart explode with joy. I'm in love with you forever; thank you for coming into my life.